Handbook
of Informatics
for Nurses and Health
Care Professionals

Handbook
of Informatics
for Nurses and Health
Care Professionals

Second Edition

Toni Hebda, RN, MSIS, PhD
Systems Analyst
Allegheny General Hospital
and
Associate Professor
Duquesne University, PA

Patricia Czar, RN
Manager of Clinical Systems, Information Services
St. Francis Medical Center, Pittsburgh, PA

Cynthia Mascara, RN, MSN, MBA
Senior Implementation Consultant
Siemens Medical Solutions (SMS)

Prentice
Hall

Upper Saddle River, NJ 07458

Library of Congress Cataloging-in-Publication Data

Hebda, Toni.
　Handbook of informatics for nurses and health care professionals / Toni Lee Hebda,
Patricia Czar, Cynthia M. Mascara.—2nd ed.
　　p. ; cm.
　Includes bibliographical references and index.
　ISBN 0-13-031102-2 (alk. paper)
　　1. Nursing informatics—Handbooks, manuals, etc. 2. Medical informatics—
Handbooks, manuals, etc. I. Czar, Patricia. II. Mascara, Cynthia. III. Title.
　[DNLM: 1. Medical Informatics. 2. Nursing. WY 26.5 H443h 2001]
　RT50.5.H43 2001
　610.73′0285—dc21

　　　　　　　　　　　　　　　　　　　　　　　　　　　　　　　　　　　　　00-052408

Publisher: *Julie Alexander*
Executive Editor: *Maura Connor*
Director of Production and Manufacturing: *Bruce Johnson*
Managing Production Editor: *Patrick Walsh*
Manufacturing Manager: *Ilene Sanford*
Production Liaison: *Julie Boddorf*
Production Editor: *Karen Fortgang, bookworks*
Creative Director: *Marianne Frasco*
Cover Design Coordinator: *Maria Guglielmo*
Cover Designer: *LaFortezza Design Group*
Director of Marketing: *Leslie Cavaliere*
Marketing Coordinator: *Cindy Frederick*
Editorial Assistant: *Beth Romph*
Composition: *Rainbow Graphics*
Printing and Binding: *R. R. Donnelley & Sons*

Prentice-Hall International (UK) Limited, *London*
Prentice-Hall of Australia Pty. Limited, *Sydney*
Prentice-Hall Canada, Inc., *Toronto*
Prentice-Hall Hispanoamericana, S.A., *Mexico*
Prentice-Hall of India Private Limited, *New Delhi*
Prentice-Hall of Japan, Inc., *Tokyo*
Prentice-Hall Singapore Pte. Ltd., *Singapore*
Editora Prentice-Hall do Brasil, Ltda., *Rio de Janeiro*

10 9 8 7 6 5 4 3 2

ISBN 0-13-031102-2

Contents

PREFACE xvii

ACKNOWLEDGMENTS xxi

ABOUT THE AUTHORS xxiii

SECTION ONE
General Computer Information 1

CHAPTER 1
Informatics in the Health Care Professions 2

Applications of Nursing Informatics 4
  *Nursing Practice 4 • Nursing Administration 4 • Nursing Education 5
  • Nursing Research 5*
The Current Status of Health Care Delivery 6
Benefits of Nursing Informatics for Other Health Care
Professionals 6
The Role of the Nurse in Information Handling 8
The Role of the Nursing Informatics Specialist 10
Case Study Exercise 11
Summary 11
References 11

CHAPTER 2
**Hardware, Software, and the Roles of Support
Personnel   13**

Hardware   14
   *Input Devices 14 • Central Processing Unit (CPU) 15 • Secondary
   Storage 15 • Output Devices 16*

Computer Categories   16

Table 2-1 Types of Computers   17

Peripheral Hardware Items   18

Networks   20

How Computers Work   22

Box 2-1 Binary Representation of an Arabic Number   22

Selection Criteria   23
   User Needs 24 • Physical Constraints 25

Box 2-2 Measures to Reduce Computer-Related Discomfort   25

Software   25

Table 2-2 Examples of Ergonomic Devices   26

Operating Systems   26

Application Software   27
   Utility Programs 27

Box 2-3 Common Types of PC Software Applications   28

Roles of Support Personnel   28
   *Superuser 29 • Help Desk Technician 29 • Microcomputer or PC
   Specialist 29 • Analyst 29 • Clinical Liaison 29 • Programmer 30
   • Network Administrator 30 • Trainer 30 • Security Officer 30
   • Chief Information Officer (CIO) 30
   • Webmaster 31*

Case Study Exercises   31

Summary   31

References   31

CHAPTER 3
Ensuring the Quality of Information   33

Table 3-1 Example of Coded Data: Employment Status Codes   35

Table 3-2 Examples of Data and Information   35

Data Integrity   35
   Ensuring Correct Data Collection and Entry 36

Data Management   38
   Data Storage 38 • Outsourcing Data Management and Storage 39

Table 3-3 Storage Media   40
   Data Retrieval 41 • Data Exchange 42

Characteristics of Quality Information   43

Box 3-1 Threats to Information Quality, Availability, and Confidentiality   44

Case Study Exercises   45

Summary   46

References   47

CHAPTER 4
Electronic Communication and the Internet   48

The Internet   50
  E-mail 51

Box 4-1 E-Mail: Advantages and Disadvantages   52
  File Transfer 53

Box 4-2 Informal Rules for E-Mail Use   54
  The World Wide Web 54

Box 4-3 The World Wide Web: Advantages and Disadvantages   55

Box 4-4 Steps in Creating, Posting, and Maintaining a Home Page   58
  *Browsers 59 • Search Tools 60 • Listservs 60 • News Groups 61
  • Bulletin Board Systems 62 • Access to Health Care Information 62
  • On-Line Publication and Journals 65 • Marketing Services 66
  • E-health 67*
  Concerns Related to the Use of the Internet   69
  *Firewalls 69 • Web Security 70 • Organizational Policy 71
  • Overload 72 • Viral Contamination 72*

The Development of Intranets   72
  Purpose 73

Box 4-5 Advantages of Intranets   73
  Problems 74

Extranets   74

Case Study Exercises   74

Summary   75

References   76

SECTION TWO
Health Care Information Systems   81

CHAPTER 5
Health Care Information Systems   82

Clinical Information Systems   83
  Nursing Information Systems 85

Box 5-1 Advantages of a Nursing Information System   86

Box 5-2 Automation of Traditional Nursing Documentation Methods   87

Clinician Information Systems 88 • Monitoring Systems 88 • Order Entry Systems 89

Box 5-3 Features of Monitoring Systems 89
Laboratory Systems 89 • Radiology Systems 90 • Pharmacy Systems 92 • Other Clinical Systems 93

Box 5-4 Using Information Systems to Reduce Medication Errors 93

Administrative Systems 94

Box 5-5 Other Common Clinical Systems 94

Box 5-6 Administration Information Systems Used in the Hospital Setting 94

Decision Support and Expert Systems 95
Registration Systems 95 • Scheduling Systems 95

Decision Support and Expert Systems 95

Case Study Exercises 97

Summary 97

References 97

CHAPTER 6
Strategic Planning 99

The Mission 100

Box 6-1 Mission Statement of St. Francis Medical Center, Pittsburgh, PA 101

Goals and Objectives 101

Developing Strategies 102

Table 6-1 Areas of Potential Strategic Planning 102

Strategic Planning for Information Systems 103

Steps of the Strategic Planning Process 104
Identification of Goals and Scope 105 • Scanning the External and Internal Environments 105 • Data Analysis 106 • Identification of Potential Solutions 107 • Selecting a Course of Action 107

Box 6-2 Information Technology Considerations for Strategic Planning 108

Box 6-3 Pros and Cons Associated with the Outsourcing of Services 109
Implementation 109 • Ongoing Evaluation and Feedback 110

Box 6-4 Measures to Ensure a Positive Outsourcing Experience 111

Case Study Exercises 111

Summary 112

References 112

CHAPTER 7
Selecting a Health Care Information System 114

Needs Assessment 115
The Steering Committee 117 • Consultants 118 • Developing a Common Vision 118

Box 7-1 Qualities of an Effective Consultant 119
Understanding the Current System 119 • Determining System Requirements 119

Table 7-1 Sample of Criteria Defining "Musts" and "Wants" 120

System Selection 124
Additional Sources of Information 125 • Request for Information 125

Box 7-2 System Selection Criteria 125
Request for Proposal 126 • Evaluation of RFP Responses 128

Box 7-3 Questions to Ask During a Site Visit 129
Contract Negotiations 130

Case Study Exercises 130

Summary 130

References 131

CHAPTER 8
System Implementation and Maintenance 132

System Implementation 133
Develop an Implementation Committee 133 • Install the System 133

Box 8-1 Characteristics of a Successful Implementation Committee 134
Analyze Hardware Requirements 136 • Develop Procedures and Documentation 136 • Testing 137 • Provide Training 137 • Go-Live Planning 138 • Common Implementation Pitfalls 139

Maintenance 140
User Feedback and Support 140 • System Maintenance 141 • Technical Maintenance 141 • The Information System's Life Cycle 142

Case Study Exercises 142

Summary 143

References 144

CHAPTER 9
Information Systems Training 145

Identification of Training Needs 147
User Needs 147

Box 9-1 Who Might Need Training? 148
Training Class Content 149 • Class Schedules 151

Table 9-1 Sample Screen Options for Reviewing Lab Results 151
Hardware and Software Requirements 152 • Training Costs 152 • A Training Center 152 • Training Approaches 153

Box 9-2 Selecting a Training Site: Factors to Consider 153

Box 9-3 Selecting a Training Method: Factors to Consider 154

Table 9-2 Training Approaches: Advantages, Disadvantages, and Tips 155

Proficiency Testing 157

Box 9-4 Selecting a Trainer: Factors to Consider 158

Additional Training Considerations 158

Training Students 159

Case Study Exercises 160

Summary 160

References 161

CHAPTER 10
Information Security and Confidentiality 163

Privacy, Confidentiality, and Security 164

Information System Security 165

Security Risks 165

Table 10-1 Characteristics of Malicious Programs 168

Security Mechanisms 168

Box 10-1 Tips for How to Avoid Malicious Programs 169

*Physical Security 169 • Passwords and Other Means
of Authentication 169*

Box 10-2 Recommendations for Password Selection and Use 170

Firewalls 171 • Application Security 171 • Antivirus Software 172

Administrative and Personnel Issues 172

*Level of Access 173 • User Authentication 174 • Personnel Issues 174
• System Security Management 176 • Audit Trails 177*

Handling and Disposal of Confidential Information 177

*Computer Printouts 178 • Faxes 178 • E-mail and the Internet 180
• Web-Based Applications for Health Care 180 • Electronic
Storage 180*

Case Study Exercises 180

Summary 181

References 182

CHAPTER 11
Network Integration 185

Interface Engines 187

Box 11-1 The Benefits of Integration 187

Box 11-2 Interface Engine Benefits 188

Integration Issues 189

Box 11-3 Factors That Slow Integration 189

The Need for Integration Standards 190
Data Dictionary 190 • Master Patient Index 190 • Uniform Language 191 • Data Exchange Standards 191

Benefits of Integration 192

Integration Implications for Nursing 193

Emerging Integration Solutions 194

Case Study Exercises 194

Summary 194

References 196

CHAPTER 12
The Computer-Based Patient Record 197

Definitions 198

Characteristics of the CPR 199

Benefits of the CPR 203

Current Status of the CPR 204

Box 12-1 Qualities of a Successful CPR 205
Impediments to CPR Development 205

Concerns Associated with the CPR 206
Data Integrity 207 • Ownership of the Patient Record 207 • Privacy and Confidentiality 207 • Electronic Signature 208

Smart Cards 208

Considerations for the Future 208

Case Study Exercises 209

Summary 209

References 210

CHAPTER 13
Regulatory and Accreditation Issues 211

Privacy and Confidentiality Issues 212

Table 13-1 Previous Attempts at Legislation to Protect the Privacy of Medical Records 213

Box 13-1 ACLU Principles for Formulating a Health Information Privacy Policy 214

The Health Insurance Portability and Accountability Act 215
HIPAA Standards 215 • HIPAA Compliance 216 • Accreditation and Reimbursement Issues 216

Box 13-2 Evaluation of Current Security Measures for HIPAA Compliance 217
JCAHO 217 • CARF 219 • Reimbursement Issues 219

Box 13-3 Minimum Data Set for Nursing Home Resident Assessment and Care 220

Special Facility Issues   221
   Geriatric and Long-Term Facilities 222 • *Psychiatric Facilities 223*
Case Study Exercises   223
Summary   224
References   224

CHAPTER 14
Community Health Information Networks   226

Components of a CHIN   227
Box 14-1 Information Available in a CHIN Data Repository   229
Box 14-2 Services Provided by CHINs   229
Development of a CHIN   229
   Connectivity 229 • *Data Elements 229* • *Centralized Data
   Repository 229* • *CHIN Developers 229*
Benefits Associated with CHINs   231
   Access to Client Information 231 • *Cost Reduction 231*
Limiting Factors   232
   Client Confidentiality Issues 232 • *Ownership of the CHIN 232*
   • *Initial Development Costs 232*
Current Status of CHINs   233
Case Study Exercises   233
Summary   233
References   234

CHAPTER 15
Disaster Planning and Recovery   235

What Is Disaster Planning?   236
Advantages of Disaster Planning   237
Environmental Disaster versus System Failure   238
Table 15-1 Threats to Normal System Operation   239
Box 15-1 Suggested Areas for Yearly Review to Avert System Disasters   240
Steps of the Disaster Planning Process   240
   Identification of Essential Information 240 • *IS Policy and Procedure
   Development 241* • *Backup and Storage 243*
Manual versus Automated Alternatives   244
Box 15-2 Recommended PC Maintenance   245
Box 15-3 Ways to Increase Disaster Awareness and Successful Recovery   246
Recovery   247
   Salvaging Damaged Records 248

Box 15-4 General Salvage Rules   248
Recovery Costs 249

Box 15-5 Recommended Storage Media Recovery Techniques   249
Restarting the System 250

Table 15-2 Recommended Insurance Coverage   250

Using Postdisaster Feedback to Improve Planning   252

Case Study Exercises   252

Summary   252

References   254

SECTION THREE
Specialty Applications   257

CHAPTER 16
Using the Computer to Support Health Care Education   258

Box 16-1 Applications of Computers in Health Care Education   260

Potential Audiences for Educational Computer Uses   262
Formal Nursing Education 262

Box 16-2 Evaluation Criteria for Instructional Software   263

Box 16-3 Features to Look for in Computerized NCLEX-RN Preparation Programs   264
Continuing Education 265 • Client Education 265

Instructional Applications of Computer Technology   266
*Computer-Assisted Instruction (CAI) 266 • Multimedia 267
• Teleconferencing 268*

Box 16-4 Strategies to Maximize the Benefits of Multimedia Instruction   268
Distance Learning 269 • Web-Based Instruction (WBI) 269

Box 16-5 Key Points for Students Involved in Distance Learning   270
Computer Labs 271

Box 16-6 Do's and Don'ts for Developing a Web-Based Course   272

Box 16-7 Evaluation Criteria for a Computer Lab   273

Educational Opportunities in Nursing Informatics   274

Case Study Exercises   274

Summary   275

References   276

CHAPTER 17
Telehealth   279

Terms Related to Telehealth   280

Box 17-1 Some Common Telehealth Terms 281
*Teleconferencing 281 • Videoconferencing 282 • Desktop
Videoconferencing (DTV) 282*

Historical Background 282

Driving Forces 283

Applications 284

Box 17-2 Telemedicine Benefits 284
On-Line Databases and Tools 284

Box 17-3 Current and Proposed Telehealth Applications 285
Education 286 • Continuing Education 287 • Home Health Care 287

Legal and Privacy Issues 287
Referral and Payment 287 • Support Personnel 288 • Liability 289

Box 17-4 Barriers to the Use of Telehealth Applications 290
Licensure Issues 290 • Confidentiality/Privacy 290

Establishing a Telehealth Link 291
*Formulating a Telehealth Plan 291 • Building the Supporting
Framework 292*

Box 17-5 Strategies to Ensure Successful Teleconferences 292
*Human Factors 293 • Equipment 294 • Telehealth Costs 294
• Technology Issues 294*

Box 17-6 Basic DTV Components for Telehealth Applications 294

Telenursing 295
Future Development 296

Case Study Exercises 297

Summary 297

References 298

CHAPTER 18
Research 302

Using Computers to Support Research 303
Identification of Research Topics 303

Box 18-1 Computer Applications That Support Nursing Research 304
Literature Searches 305

Box 18-2 Suggested Health Care Informatics Research Topics 305

Box 18-3 Pros and Cons of On-Line Literature Searches 306
Data Collection Tools 306

**Box 18-4 Tips for Design and Administration of Web-Based Data Collection
Tools 309**
*Data Analysis 309 • Data Presentation: Graphics 311
• Computer-Aided Research in Nursing (CARIN) 312 • On-Line Access
to Databases 313*

Impediments to Health Care Research 313
Box 18-5 Possible Funding Sources for Nursing Research 314
   Unified Language Efforts 314 • *Multi-Institutional Research 315*
Box 18-6 Some Databases That Support Nursing 316
   Research in Real Time 316 • *Collaborative Research 317*
Students Using Computers for Research 317
Case Study Exercises 318
Summary 318
References 319

APPENDIX A: INTERNET PRIMER 322

APPENDIX B: CAREER RESOURCES ON THE INTERNET 331

APPENDIX C: INTERNET RESOURCES FOR NURSES AND HEALTH CARE
   PROFESSIONALS 335

APPENDIX D: CASE STUDY EXERCISES—SUGGESTED RESPONSES
349

GLOSSARY 367

INDEX 379

Preface

The original idea for this book came from the realization that there were few comprehensive sources available with practical information about computer applications and information systems in health care. From its inception this book was envisioned as a guide for nurses and other health care professionals who needed to learn how to adapt and use computer applications in the workplace. As the outline developed it became apparent that this book could also serve as an informatics text for students in the health care professions. This second edition contains updates and revisions to reflect changes that have occurred in the rapidly evolving technology and health care field since the book was first written.

Each of the authors has a long-standing interest and involvement in nursing informatics. In fact, the same idea that inspired this book also led a group of nurses that included the authors to form the Tri-State Nursing Computer Network user group in 1988. This organization remains active, and has recently changed its name to Tri-State Healthcare Informatics Professionals, with an expanded focus to include other informatics professionals in addition to nurses.

This book is divided into three sections. The first section, General Computer Information, reviews information common to all information systems. It assumes no prior knowledge of or experience with computers. Chapter 1 introduces the reader to the role of informatics in contemporary health care. Chapter 2 reviews basic information and terminology related to computer hardware and software. The section on the roles of various support personnel has been expanded. Chapter 3 emphasizes the importance of maintaining data integrity and suggests some practical steps to ensure current, accurate data in health care information systems. The fourth chapter addresses basic Internet use to support health care. The discussion on search tools and intranets has been expanded and content has been added on portals, e-health, and e-care. Additional information on Internet use and resources are found in the appendices at the end of the book.

The second section, Health Care Information Systems, covers information and issues related to the use of computers and information systems in health care. This section bridges the gap between the theory and practice of nursing informatics. Chapter 5 covers basic information on health care information systems, including decision support and expert systems. Chapters 6 through 15 discuss all aspects of selecting, implementing, and operating these systems. Chapters 6 through 9 discuss the processes of overall and system strategic planning, system selection, implementation, and training. Chapter 8 now contains additional information on testing, system evaluation, and strategies to implement system changes after system installation. Other pertinent topics are addressed in the remaining chapters. Chapter 10 discusses information security and confidentiality; Chapter 11, system integration; and Chapter 12, the computerized patient record. Chapter 13, Regulatory and Accreditation Issues, has been updated to include a review of the Health Insurance Portability and Accountability Act (HIPAA) and its implications for nursing informatics and health care professionals. Chapter 14 covers community health information networks and Chapter 15 covers disaster planning and recovery.

Section III covers three specialty applications of computers in health care. Chapter 16 discusses ways that computers can support health care education. It now contains content on Web-based education. The title of Chapter 17 has been changed since the first edition from Telemedicine to Telehealth to reflect the growing acceptance of telehealth as a broader term. This chapter explores the growing field of telehealth, which uses computer and teleconferencing technology to provide top-quality health care to clients all over the world. Chapter 18 looks at ways that computers are increasingly being used in nursing and other health care research.

Four appendices are included at the end of the book. The first three provide detailed information on getting up and running on the Internet, using the Internet to perform a job search, and Internet resources of special interest to health care professionals. The fourth appendix provides suggested answers to the case studies that are found at the end of every chapter.

Each chapter contains pedagogical aids that help the readers learn and apply the information discussed. Learning objectives let the readers know what they can expect to learn from the chapter. Case studies at the end of each chapter discuss common, real-life applications, which review and reinforce the concepts presented in the chapter. Each chapter also includes a summary and list of references. The Glossary at the back of the book serves to familiarize readers with the vocabulary used in this book and in health care informatics.

We recognize that health care professionals have varying degrees of computer and informatics knowledge. One of the features of this book is that it does not assume that the reader has prior knowledge of computers. All computer terms are defined in the text and in the Glossary. This book may be used the following different ways:

- It may be read from cover to cover for a comprehensive view of nursing informatics.
- Specific chapters may be read according to reader interest or need.
- It may serve as a reference for nurses and other clinicians involved in system design, selection, and implementation.
- It may be useful for the educator or researcher who wants to make better use of information technology.
- It can serve as a review for the American Nurses Association's Informatics Credentialing examination.

Toni Hebda
Patricia Czar
Cynthia Mascara

Acknowledgments

We acknowledge our gratitude first and foremost to our families for their support as we wrote and revised this book. We are grateful to our co-workers and professional colleagues who provided encouragement and support throughout the process of conceiving and writing this book. Finally, we thank the staff at Prentice Hall for their encouragement, suggestions, and support as we developed this second edition.

When this project began, the three of us knew each other only on a professional basis. As we worked together to write this book, we found that our varied professional backgrounds, experiences, and personalities complemented each other well and added to the quality of the final product. The best part of this project, however, has been the close friendship that we have developed as we have worked together.

About the Authors

Toni Hebda has been a nurse educator for most of her career. Toni did a descriptive study on the use of computers in nursing education for her dissertation in the mid 1980s and later served as a founding member of Tri-State Nursing Computer Network. She subsequently returned to graduate school to earn a master's degree in information science and is certified as an Informatics Nurse by the American Nurses Credentialing Center. She has used information systems for data collection, order entry, and documentation in the clinical setting. She presently works in the information services department of West Penn Allegheny Health System and teaches in the postgraduate informatics certificate program at Duquesne University School of Nursing in Pittsburgh.

Patricia Czar established a solid reputation in clinical practice and nursing administration prior to her move into informatics. She was a Nurse Manager of a medical/surgical unit for 12 years, and also was the Project Director for Policies and Procedures for 2 years. She has maintained an active role with computers in health care since 1980. Patricia first served as a Nurse Analyst during the implementation of an order entry system. She was responsible for planning, design, implementation, and ongoing support. Patricia also earned a Microcomputer Specialist certificate. In subsequent years she has increased her level of knowledge and responsibility and is now Manager of Clinical Systems at St. Francis Health System in Pittsburgh. She has been an active member and leader in local and international computer user groups. Patricia has served as guest lecturer and mentor for students in several local colleges and universities.

Cynthia Mascara also had a significant history of clinical and administrative nursing practice prior to entering nursing informatics in 1989. She was a staff nurse for 6 years, and a nursing supervisor/administrator for 4 years at the University of Pittsburgh Medical Center. Cynthia then moved into the role of Nursing Informatics Specialist. Her responsibilities included the planning, design and implementation of an order entry system, as well as end-user training and support. She also served as a liaison between nursing staff and information services department. Cynthia is now employed as a senior consultant for the health care information solutions vendor Shared Medical Systems (SMS). She has experience with project management as well as the design and implementation of clinical information systems. Cynthia holds a Master of Nursing Science degree with a focus in nursing administration, as well as a Master of Business Administration degree from Duquesne University. She has also presented at local, national, and international nursing informatics conferences.

Handbook
of Informatics
for Nurses and Health
Care Professionals

One

General Computer Information

Informatics
in the Health Care
Professions

After completing this chapter, you should be able to:

- Define *nursing informatics*.

- List several examples of how nursing informatics affects practice, administration, education, and research.

- Understand the implications of the current status of the health care delivery system for informatics.

- Discuss the relevance of nursing informatics for other health care providers.

- Identify the role of the nurse in handling information.

- Recognize nursing informatics as a core nursing competency and an area of nursing specialization.

Nursing informatics may be broadly defined as the use of computer technology to support nursing, including clinical practice, administration, education, and research. This reflects one of the earliest definitions of nursing informatics, Scholes and Barber's 1980 statement that nursing informatics is the "application of computer technology to all fields of nursing." In subsequent years, the definition of nursing informatics has come to include specific tools and functions that support nursing. For example, Hannah (1985) states that nursing informatics includes the information that nurses use to make client care decisions. Graves and Corcoran (1989, p. 227) further refined the definition to include "a combination of computer science, information science and nursing science designed to assist in the management and processing of nursing data, information and knowledge to support the practice of nursing and the delivery of nursing care." More recently, the American Nurses Association (ANA) (1994) defined nursing informatics as "the development and evaluation of applications, tools, processes, and structures which assist nurses with the management of data in taking care of patients or supporting the practice of nursing." According to Turley (1996), nursing informatics borrows theory from cognitive science, computer science, and information science and places it on a base of nursing science. Figure 1–1 displays the nursing informatics model as presented by Turley. More recently, the Nursing Informatics Special Interest Group of the International Medical Informatics Association (1998) amended their definition of Nursing Informatics. This definition states that nursing informatics is the integration of nursing, its information, and information management with information processing and communication technology, to support the health of people worldwide.

The definitions listed above demonstrate that the concept of nursing informatics continues to evolve to reflect advances in nursing practice and technology. A recent example of this is seen in the effort of the Na-

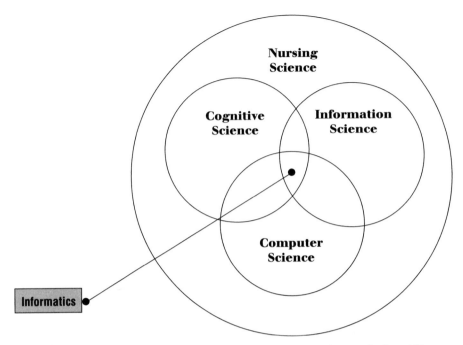

FIGURE 1–1 • Nursing Informatics Model (Turley 1996; reprinted by permission of Sigma Theta Tau International)

tional Nursing Informatics Project of Canada to develop a current definition of nursing informatics (Hebert 1999). The goals of this group include defining nursing informatics and recommending informatics competencies for nurses in all areas of practice.

APPLICATIONS OF NURSING INFORMATICS

Automation offers many solutions for nursing issues that allow the nurse to work more efficiently, allocate resources more effectively, and improve client care. Nursing informatics is applied to all areas of nursing, including practice, administration, education, and research. Some examples of how nursing informatics and computers are used to support the various areas of nursing follow.

Nursing Practice

- Worklists to remind staff of planned nursing interventions
- Computer-generated client documentation
- Monitoring devices that record vital signs and other measurements directly into the client record
- Computer-generated nursing care plans and critical pathways

- Automatic billing for supplies or procedures with nursing documentation
- Reminders and prompts that appear during documentation to ensure comprehensive charting
- Quick accessibility to computer-archived patient data from previous encounters.

Nursing Administration

- Automated staff scheduling
- Electronic mail for improved communication
- Cost analysis and finding trends for budget purposes
- Quality assurance and outcomes analysis

Nursing Education

- Computerized record-keeping
- Computer-assisted instruction
- Distance learning in the form of teleconferencing
- Internet resources and Web-based education
- Presentation software for preparing slides and handouts

Nursing Research

- Computerized literature searching
- The adoption of standardized language related to nursing terms
- The ability to find trends in **aggregate** data, which is data derived from large population groups
- Use of the Internet for obtaining data collection tools and conducting research

These examples demonstrate the importance of information sharing. Nursing informatics, through the use of computers, can facilitate and speed information sharing in all practice areas. For this to be most effective, nurses must have a basic understanding of informatics. An assessment conducted in 1995 by Arnold (1996) to determine the informatics educational needs of professional nurses found that identified needs varied by practice area. In the area of nursing practice, nurse managers identified the following as their top needs for informatics education:

- *Presentation graphics.* Managers can use computer graphics to give stronger presentations to other hospital administrators and nursing colleagues.
- *Clinical data analysis.* This includes compiling and analyzing patterns of data to improve client care.

- *Electronic communication*. Innovations like electronic mail can make communications between health care professionals more efficient.

Arnold's survey also addressed the informatics needs of nurse educators. The following areas were identified as their top needs:

- *Presentation graphics*. Like administrators, educators identified their need to learn to use presentation graphics **software,** or computer programs, to prepare visual aids to supplement lecture material.
- *Computer-assisted instruction (CAI) critique*. Educators are in a position to select CAI as a teaching tool. They need parameters for selecting effective, well-designed CAI to meet the learning objectives of students.
- *Decision support*. Analysis of data can support educators and students in making the best clinical decisions.

THE CURRENT STATUS OF HEALTH CARE DELIVERY

Managed care and consumer demands for quality are the driving forces in health care delivery. Limits to what providers can charge and capitated reimbursement plans that provide coverage for a particular diagnosis at a set rate force institutions to increase efficiency in order to maintain profitability. Downsizing, acquisitions, and mergers represent attempts to increase efficiency. Other methods include automation and cross-training personnel. Simply put, downsizing means that fewer people do more work. Unfortunately, the clinician also faces higher client acuity levels in many managed care scenarios. Acquisitions and mergers also allow providers to extend their reach by offering a more comprehensive set of services and encouraging clients to stay within the health care network. Smaller providers form alliances for the same purposes.

Alliances such as these encourage the sharing of information. The advantages of acquisitions and mergers may be minimized by the problem of having different computer systems from different organizations begin to work together. In an attempt to operate more efficiently, administrators are turning to information technology as a tool. The following represent current and emerging technological tools: client server computing; thin client technology; wireless systems; document imaging for the storage of records on optical disks; optical scanning; digital picture archiving of diagnostic images; bar coding for demographic, insurance, and prescription information; handheld computers for material management; and telemedicine, voice recognition, and the use of Internet technologies.

BENEFITS OF NURSING INFORMATICS FOR OTHER HEALTH CARE PROFESSIONALS

Nursing informatics may also benefit other health care providers. For example, other providers can use data collected and documented by nurses using automated systems. In addition, multidisciplinary critical pathways are used by nurses and providers to plan and document care for a client. The aggregate critical pathway data may be analyzed for trends related to overall effectiveness of client care.

Other health care disciplines may have information systems that use data collected by nursing systems. For example, pharmacy information systems make use of data collected by nursing information systems such as current medications, allergies, client demographic information, and diagnosis. This feature eliminates redundant data collection by different professionals, saving them time. Laboratory information systems may also connect to nursing systems. When a laboratory test is ordered and entered into the computer on the patient unit, the information is transferred to the laboratory computer system. This replaces handwritten paper requisitions, saving time and improving communication. Similarly, other hospital departments may receive requests for consults.

Other uses of automation within health care may also improve communication and increase profitability. One example is inventory control. Health care product suppliers use technology to decrease administrative costs and to attract customers with improved inventory control. Specifically, suppliers can more quickly fill orders, check hospital inventory, and allow customers to receive prices, place orders, and confirm orders through information systems. Some suppliers provide the inventory system for customer use. Customers get a more accurate inventory, automatic replacement of supplies as they are used, and the ability to maintain a smaller inventory to reduce costs (Dellecave 1995, DePompa 1996, Gambon 1995). Thus, patient care and consumer demands drive the health care delivery system toward working smarter, which is often best accomplished through automation.

Many of the benefits of automation in health care are seen with the development of the **electronic medical record,** which is an electronic version of the client data found in the traditional paper record (Mancilla 1995). Some specific benefits of electronic medical records include the following (DePompa 1996; Dexter 1995; and Pabst, Scherubel, and Minnick 1996):

- *Improved access to the medical record.* The electronic medical record can be accessed from several different locations simultaneously, as well as by different levels of providers.
- *Decreased redundancy of data entry.* For example, allergies and vital signs need be entered only once.
- *Decreased time spent in documentation.* Automation allows direct entry from monitoring equipment, as well as point-of-care data entry.
- *Increased time for client care.* More time is available for client care because less time is required for documentation and transcription of physician orders.
- *Facilitation of data collection for research.* Electronically stored client

records provide quick access to clinical data for a large number of clients.

- *Improved communication and decreased potential for error.* Improved legibility of clinician documentation and orders is seen with automated information systems.
- *Creation of a lifetime clinical record facilitated by information systems.*

Other benefits of automation are related to **decision-support software,** computer programs that organize information to aid in decision making for client care or administrative issues. Some of the benefits that can be realized with these systems include the following (Dexter 1995):

- Decision-support tools as well as alerts and reminders notify the clinician of possible concerns or omissions. For example, the client states an allergy to penicillin, and this is documented in the computer system. The physician orders an antibiotic that is a variation of penicillin, and this order is entered into the computer system. An alert informs the clinician that a potential allergic reaction may result and asks for verification of the order.
- Effective data management and trend-finding include the ability to provide historical or current data reports.
- Extensive financial information can be collected and analyzed for trends. Information related to costing by diagnosis and treatment can be more easily tracked using computer systems. For example, one can determine the least expensive drug that is effective for a particular diagnosis.
- Data related to treatment such as inpatient length of stay and the lowest level of care provider required can be used to decrease costs.

THE ROLE OF THE NURSE
IN INFORMATION HANDLING

The traditional role of the nurse as a handler of information has been to collect and document client data. This is accomplished as the nurse completes the following aspects of care and documentation:

- Initial patient history and allergies
- Initial and ongoing physical assessment
- Vital signs such as blood pressure and temperature
- Response to treatment
- Client's understanding of education

Until recently, this information has been recorded in a structured format on paper and placed in the client record. Market forces and technological innovations provide the ability to automate this process, moving from paper-based to computer-based records. With paper records, nurses could independently design or revise the documentation format. Automated documentation, however, requires collaboration with technical personnel and more extensive planning regarding what information to include, the source of the information, and how it will be used. As a result, nurses may feel they have less control over the format for nursing documentation. This need not be the case, however. Nurses must be active participants in the design of automated documentation. This will ensure that information obtained by nurses is recorded appropriately and in a format that can be accessed and useful to all health care providers.

Harsanyi, Lehmkuhl, Hott, Myers, and McGeehan (1994) argue that understanding current and evolving technology for the management and processing of nursing information helps the nursing profession assume a leadership position in health reform. If nurses understand the power of technology they can play an active role in evaluating and improving the quality of care, cost containment, and other consumer benefits. For example, nurses who are able to understand and use an information system that analyzes trends in client outcomes and cost can initiate appropriate changes in care. Nurses empowered by information technology may also design computer applications that enhance client education, such as individualized discharge instructions, medication instructions and information, and information about diagnostic procedures. In these and other ways, nurses can integrate information technology into nursing practice and administration as a means to manage client care, document observations, and monitor client outcomes for ongoing improvement of quality.

Nurses also handle information in the roles of educator and researcher. For example, educators must track information about students' classroom and clinical performance. Computers facilitate this process and allow educators to compare individuals to group norms. Nursing education must also prepare students to handle data. This is accomplished in several steps: teaching basic computer literacy, using nursing information systems, realizing the significance of automated data collection for quality assurance purposes, and recognizing the benefits of using computers to manage clinical data for research.

Researchers use computers to expedite the collection and analysis of data. One possible project, for example, uses data obtained from nursing documentation systems to study the relationship between frequent turning and positioning and the client's skin integrity. Nursing information systems are rich in data to support this type of research, and the growing prevalence of information systems increases research opportunities. As a result, nurses are able to expand the scientific base of their profession.

THE ROLE OF THE NURSING INFORMATICS SPECIALIST

Nursing informatics affects all nurses in some way because all nurses deal with data. Informatics offers advantages to nurses in project management, consultation, and marketing, as well as clinical practice, administration, education, and research. For these reasons, all nurses need to establish at least a minimal level of awareness and competence in informatics (Canavan 1996). Because of the increased importance of informatics as a tool, a new role has emerged, the **nursing informatics specialist.** This specialist is a nurse with formal education and practical experience in using computers, who supports the automation needs of all facets of nursing practice. According to the American Nurses Association (1994), some of the basic functions of the nursing informatics specialist may include the following:

- *Theory development.* The nursing informatics specialist contributes to the evolving knowledge base related to nursing informatics.
- *Analysis of information needs.* This involves the identification of the information that nurses need to do their work, encompassing client care, education, administration, and research.
- *Selection of computer systems.* The nursing informatics specialist guides the user in making informed decisions related to the purchase of computer systems.
- *Design of computer systems and customizations.* The nursing informatics specialist collaborates with users and programmers to make decisions about how data will be displayed and accessed.
- *Testing of computer systems.* Systems must be checked for proper functioning before they are made available for use. For example, nursing documentation of vital signs must be tested to ensure that the nurse can enter and retrieve the values in the system.
- *Training users of computer systems.* Users must be taught how the system works, the importance of accurate data entry, and how the system may benefit them.
- *Evaluation of the effectiveness of computer systems.* The nursing informatics specialist is in a unique position to conduct this process. The combined knowledge of computers and nursing provides the informatics nurse with specialized ability to evaluate systems.
- *Ongoing maintenance and enhancements.* This involves ensuring that the system continues to work properly. In addition, the nursing informatics specialist explores possible enhancements to the system that may better serve the needs of the users.
- *Identification of computer technologies that can benefit nursing.* The nursing informatics specialist must keep abreast of technology changes, including new hardware and software applications that may benefit nurses.

Presently, there is little agreement regarding what constitutes core nursing informatics competencies. Few graduate informatics programs exist. Undergraduate and graduate computer and informatics classes vary greatly in content. As a result, most nurses practicing informatics today are self-schooled. Now that the American Nurses Association recognizes nursing informatics as a specialty, it is expected that content-specific knowledge and practice requirements will shape the objectives for formal course offerings (Romano 1996). The ANA now offers certification as an informatics nurse through the American Nurses Credentialing Center. This action will help to define the role of nurses in terms of how technology can serve them.

CASE STUDY EXERCISE

A client arrives in the emergency department short of breath and complaining of chest pain. Describe how informatics can help nurses and other health care providers to more efficiently and effectively care for this client.

SUMMARY

- Nursing informatics is the use of computer technology to support nursing.
- Nursing informatics supports all areas of nursing, including practice, education, administration, and research.
- Nursing informatics is a necessity, not a luxury, in today's rapidly changing health care delivery system.
- Computer technology facilitates the collection of data for analysis, which can be used to justify the efficacy of particular interventions and improve the quality of care.
- Other health care providers also benefit from nursing informatics.
- Nursing informatics allows nurses to have better control over data management.
- The nursing informatics specialist supports nurses in the design, development, use, and evaluation of computer technologies.

REFERENCES

American Nurses Association. (1994). *The scope of practice for nursing informatics*. Washington, DC: American Nurses Association.

Arnold, J. M. (1996). Nursing informatics educational needs. *Computers in Nursing, 14*(6), 333–339.

Canavan, K. (November/December 1996). New technologies propel nursing profession forward. *The American Nurse*, 1–2.

Dellecave, T. Jr. (18 September 1995). Technology: The best remedy. *InformationWeek*, 126–130.

DePompa, B. (9 September 1996). Sharing the cost of recovery. *InformationWeek*, 146, 148, 150.

Dexter, I. (1995). Worth the hassle. *Nursing Times*, *91*(35), 44, 46.

Gambon, J. (18 September 1995). *InformationWeek*, 164, 166, 168.

Graves, J. R., and Corcoran, S. (1989). The study of nursing informatics. *Image: Journal of Nursing Scholarship*, *21*, 227–231.

Hannah, K. (1985). Current trends in nursing informatics: Implications for curriculum planning. In K. Hannah, E. Guillemin, and D. Conklin (Eds.), *Nursing uses of computer and information science. Proceedings of the IFIP-IMIA International Symposium on Nursing Uses of Computers and Information Science*. Amsterdam: Elsevier Science.

Harsanyi, B. E., Lehmkuhl, D., Hott, R., Myers, S., and McGeehan, L. (1994). Nursing informatics: The key to managing and evaluating quality. In S. J. Grobe and E. S. P. Puyter-Wenting (Eds.), *Nursing informatics: An international overview for nursing in a technological era. Proceedings of the Fifth IMIA International Conference on Nursing Use of Computers and Information Science*, San Antonio, TX, 655–659.

Hebert, M. (1999). *National Nursing Informatics Project Discussion Paper*. On the Internet at: *http://www.coachorg.com/nisig/nationat-nursing-informatics-project/*.

Mancilla, D. (1995). The electronic patient record maze: Where is the beginning—and is there an end? *Journal of AHIMA*, *66*(3), 48–50.

Nursing Informatics: Special Interest Group of International Medical Informatics Association (IMIA-NI) (1998). *Proceedings of the General Assembly Meeting*, Seoul, Korea.

Pabst, M. K., Scherubel, J. C., and Minnick, A. F. (1996). The impact of computerized documentation on nurses' use of time. *Computers in Nursing*, *14*(1), 25–30.

Romano, C. (October 1996). *Nursing informatics*. Paper presented at MISA/MISPA International Conference, Nashville, TN.

Scholes, M., and Barber, B. (1980). Towards nursing informatics. In D. A. Lindberg and S. Kaihari (Eds.), *Medinfo, 80* (pp. 70–73). London: North-Holland.

Turley, J. P. (1996). Toward a model of nursing informatics. *Image: Journal of Nursing Scholarship*, *28*(1), 309–313. Reprinted by permission of Sigma Theta Tau International.

2

Hardware, Software, and the Roles of Support Personnel

After completing this chapter, you should be able to:

- Explain what computers are and how they work.

- Describe the major hardware components of computers.

- Understand what networks are, and list the major types of network configurations.

- List the advantages and disadvantages of mainframe, client/server and thin client technology.

- Explain some considerations for choosing and using a computer system.

- Understand the major types of software commonly used with computer systems.

- Discuss the roles and responsibilities of various computer support personnel.

A **computer** is an electronic device that collects, stores, processes, and retrieves data. Information output is provided under the direction of stored sequences of instructions known as computer programs. The physical parts of a computer are frequently referred to as **hardware,** and the instructions, or programs, are collectively known as **software.** A computer system consists of the following components:

- Hardware
- Software
- Data that will be transformed into information
- Procedures or rules for the use of the system
- Users

Rapid advances in technology reshape computer capabilities and user expectations. Many changes have occurred since the introduction of the first computers in the 1940s. In general, computers have become smaller but more powerful and increasingly affordable.

HARDWARE

Computer hardware is the physical part of the computer and its associated equipment. The computer hardware comprises many different parts, but the main elements are input devices, the central processing unit, secondary storage, and output devices. Figure 2–1 describes the relationship between these components.

Input Devices

Input devices allow the user to put data into the computer. Common input devices include the keyboard, mouse, trackball, touch screen, light pen, microphone, bar code reader, fax modem card, joystick, and scanner.

FIGURE 2–1 • Basic Components of a Computer

Central Processing Unit

The **central processing unit** (CPU) is the "brain" of the computer. It has the electronic circuitry that actually executes computer instructions. The CPU can be divided into the following three components:

- The **arithmetic logic unit** (ALU) executes instructions for the manipulation of numeric symbols.

- **Memory** is the storage area in which programs reside during execution. Memory is subdivided into two categories: read-only memory and random access memory. **Read-only memory** (**ROM**) is permanent; it remains when the power is off. It cannot be changed by the user. ROM contains start-up instructions that are executed each time the computer is turned on. **Random access memory** (**RAM**) is a temporary storage area that is active only while the computer is turned on. It provides storage for the program that is running, as well as for the data that is being processed.

- The **control unit** manages instructions to other parts of the computer, including input and output devices. It reads stored programs one instruction at a time and directs other computer parts to perform required tasks.

The CPU is located inside the system cabinet or housing, the large metal box that many people think of as the computer, although it just houses the CPU, the real computer, as well as the other components. Figure 2–3 later in the chapter shows some things that may be inside a system cabinet.

Secondary Storage

Secondary storage provides space to retain data in an area separate from the computer's memory after the computer is turned off. Common mechanisms for secondary storage include **hard disk drives, floppy diskettes,** and **compact discs.**

Output Devices

Output devices allow the user to view and possibly hear processed data. Terminals or video monitor screens, printers, speakers, and fax modem boards are examples of output devices.

COMPUTER CATEGORIES

Computers vary in size, purpose, capacity, and the number of users that can be accommodated simultaneously. The four main categories of computers are supercomputers, mainframe computers, minicomputers, and microcomputers. Table 2–1 supplies a brief description of each type, as well as its advantages and disadvantages.

Supercomputers are the largest, most expensive type of computer. They are complex systems that can perform billions of instructions every second. Prohibitive cost limits use primarily to government and academic settings.

Mainframes, large computers capable of processing several million instructions per second, are used for processing large amounts of data quickly. Mainframe computers support organizational functions, and therefore have been the traditional equipment in hospital environments. Software for mainframes supports many customized functions, and this level of specialization results in its high cost.

A **minicomputer** is a scaled-down version of a mainframe computer. Minicomputers are slightly less costly than mainframes but are still capable of supporting multiple users as well as the computing needs of small businesses. Because they have become more powerful, minicomputers may now be used in hospitals.

Microcomputers are also known as **personal computers (PCs).** This computer category provides inexpensive processing power for an individual user. A PC may stand alone or be connected to other computer systems through a dial-up connection. Improved reliability, availability, and manageability allow PCs to assume responsibilities once associated with mainframe computers. Some variations of the microcomputer are the notebook and handheld computers. These devices offer portable computer capability away from the office or desktop. The **laptop** or **notebook** computer is a streamlined version of the personal computer, using batteries or regular electric current. These devices may be more costly than comparable desktop computers. **Handheld** or **wireless** computers are special-use devices that offer limited features in comparison to PCs. Some of these devices have been adapted to accept handwriting as input. **Personal digital assistants (PDAs)** are specialized handheld devices used primarily to keep appointment calendars, addresses, and phone numbers.

Table 2-1 **Types of Computers**

Type	Description	Advantages	Disadvantages
Supercomputer	Designed and used for complex scientific calculations	Performs complex calculations very quickly	Expensive Limited functionality
Mainframe	Used to support organizational information systems Multiple processors Varies in size	High-speed transactions Supports many terminals and users simultaneously Large storage capacity	Expensive Software expensive and inflexible
Minicomputer	Smaller version of mainframe Designed for multiple users Supports corporate computing for smaller organizations	Less expensive version of the mainframe Supports many terminals and users simultaneously	Relatively expensive
Personal computer (PC) or microcomputer	Single-processor machine intended for one user	Inexpensive processing power May be connected to other systems through telephone dial connections	High support costs Slower response and fewer capabilities than larger systems
Portable: laptop or notebook computer	Streamlined version of a PC that weighs less than 10 pounds	Provides portable computer capability	Limited battery life More expensive than PC May not offer same features and software as PC May be more difficult to use, e.g., awkward keyboard
Handheld/wireless	Special-use device, e.g., documentation, inventory	Provides portable computer capability at the patient's location ↑ Availability of information ↑ Productivity	Limited features available Lack of standards to facilitate use Software may be difficult to master May not hold up to rough use
Personal digital assistant	Handheld device primarily used to keep appointment calendars, addresses, telephone numbers	Small, lightweight Data can be transferred to a PC	Limited capability at present

PERIPHERAL HARDWARE ITEMS

Peripheral hardware, or more simply a *peripheral,* is any piece of hardware attached to a computer. Examples of peripheral devices include:

- Monitors
- Keyboards
- Terminals
- The mouse and other pointing devices
- Secondary storage devices such as floppy diskettes and compact discs
- Backup systems
- External modems
- Printers
- Scanners

The **monitor** is the screen that displays text and graphic images generated by the computer. PC monitors use television technology to generate colors by combining amounts of red, green, and blue. *Refresh rate* and *resolution* are terms that refer to monitor characteristics. The **refresh rate** is the speed with which the screen is repainted from top to bottom. Early monitors had a slow refresh rate that caused the screen to flicker. Higher refresh rates eliminate flicker. **Resolution** is the number of **pixels,** or dots, that appear horizontally and vertically on the screen, making up the image. Resolution is expressed as the number of horizontal pixels by vertical pixels. Higher resolution numbers provide a better screen image. Some monitors, called touch screens, are sensitive to contact. This allows users to enter data and make selections by touching the screen.

Keyboards are input devices with keys that resemble those of a typewriter. Keyboards allow the user to type information and instructions into a computer.

A **terminal** consists of a monitor screen and a keyboard. It is used to input data and receive output from a mainframe computer. Unlike a personal computer, the terminal itself does not process information, thus giving rise to the expression "dumb terminal."

The **mouse** is a device that fits in the user's hand and can be moved around on the desktop to direct a pointer on the screen. It is often used to select and move items by pressing and releasing a button. A mouse pad optimizes function by providing a surface area with the proper amount of friction while minimizing the amount of dirt that enters the mouse.

Some other examples of pointing devices include joysticks, touchpads, and trackballs. A **joystick** allows the user to control the movement of objects on the screen, and is primarily used with games. A **touchpad** is a pressure- and motion-sensitive surface. When a user moves a finger across the touchpad, the on-screen pointer moves in the same direction. A **trackball** contains a ball that the user rolls to move the on-screen pointer. Trackballs work well when available space is limited, as with laptop computers.

Secondary storage devices are generally provided via the hard disk drive, a CD-ROM drive (compact disk–read only memory), or a floppy diskette drive. The **hard disk drive** allows the user to retrieve, or read, data as well as save, or write, new data. Data is stored in the hard drive magnetically on a stack of rotating disks known as platters. The amount of information that can be stored on disk is known as its **capacity.** Capacity is measured in bytes. In general, hard disk drives offer a larger capacity than do CD-ROM disks and floppy diskettes. Home and office PCs now offer hard disk drives with a capacity that is measured in **gigabytes.** One gigabyte is equivalent to 1,073,741,824 characters.

The traditional **CD-ROM drive** allows the user to read, but not change, information stored on compact discs (CD). Newer CD-ROM drives may use technology that allows the user to read or write to a CD. A CD is the same type of disc on which music is recorded, but it usually stores more forms of data than just sound. The CD provides improved storage capacity and access rate over traditional magnetic floppy diskettes, or disks, which are the storage medium used by the **floppy disk drive.** A floppy disk is a thin plastic platter within a plastic cover. Earlier diskettes were larger in size and had a flexible cover. Currently, the most common diskettes have a 3.5-inch-square plastic outer cover. Most hard drives, CD-ROM drives, and floppy disk drives are located internally within the system cabinet, but they may also be located externally and connected using cables.

Additional secondary storage can be provided through the use of other devices internal or external to the cabinet. These may include tape drives, optical disk drives, magnetic disk or tape drives, and RAID, to be explained shortly.

A **tape drive** copies files from the computer to magnetic tape for storage or transfer to another machine. A **file** is a collection of related data stored and handled as a single entity by the computer. The tape drive uses tiny electromagnets to write data to a magnetic media by altering the surface. **Optical disk drives** rely on laser technology to write data to a recording surface media and read it later. The advantage of this technology is its large storage capacity.

A **redundant array of inexpensive or independent disks (RAID)** is precisely what the name indicates: duplicate disks with mirror copies of data. Using RAID may be less costly than using one large disk drive. In the event that an individual disk fails, the remaining RAID would permit the computer to continue working uninterrupted.

A **backup system** is a procedure that creates copies of system and data files. The copies are secondary storage devices separate from the computer. A backup system is an important measure for protection against computer failure or data loss.

A **modem** is a communication device that allows computers to transmit information over telephone lines. Faster modems transfer information more quickly. This, in turn, saves time and telephone charges. Modem speed is measured by the number of bits that can be transferred in one second of time, or **bits per second (bps). A bit** is the smallest unit of data that can be handled by the computer. In actuality, transfer occurs in thousands of bits per second, or **kilobits (kbps).** Many PCs now include modem and facsimile capabilities via a fax modem board. A **fax modem** board allows computers to transmit images of letters and drawings over a telephone line.

A **printer** produces a paper copy of computer-generated documents. Several types of printers are available. Laser printers offer the highest quality print by transferring toner, a powdered ink, onto paper like a photocopier does. Ink-jet printers heat ink and spray it onto paper to provide a high-quality output. Dot matrix printers create letters and graphics through the use of a series of metal pins that strike a ribbon against paper. Color is an option with all three printer types. Prices vary according to quality and the selection of color as an option, but versions of all three types of printers are available for under $1000. Dot matrix and ink-jet printers are relatively inexpensive to operate. Prior to the development of these three printer types, printers resembled typewriters. One option to consider when selecting a printer is a hybrid machine that can be used as a printer, a scanner, a copier, and a fax machine. Users should base their selection on need. Laser printers are the office standard because they are quiet and provide a high-quality print. Ink-jet printers are suitable for interoffice communication but are slow, and their ink may smear when exposed to moisture. Dot matrix printers are noisy and may provide a poor-quality print.

The **scanner** is an input device that converts printed pages or graphic images into a file. The file can then be stored and revised using the computer. For example, a printed report can be scanned, stored in the computer, and sent electronically to another output device.

NETWORKS

A **network** is a combination of hardware and software that allows communication and electronic transfer of information between computers (Ahuja 1996, Marion 1994). Hardware may be connected permanently by wire or cable, or temporarily through modems, telephone lines, or radio signals. This arrangement allows sharing of resources, data, and software. For example, it may not be practical to have a printer for every PC in the office. Instead several PCs are connected to one printer through a network. Common use of hardware requires consideration of overall needs, convenience of location, priority by user and job, and amount of use. Figure 2–2 depicts a network.

Networks range in size from **local area networks (LANs)** with a handful of computers, printers, and other devices, to systems that link

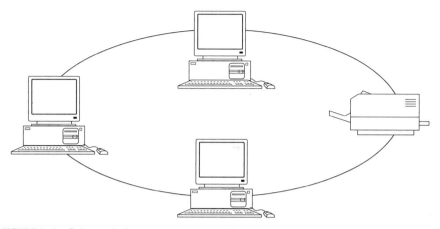

FIGURE 2–2 • Schematic Representation of a Network

many small and large computers over a large geographic area (Maran 1996). For example, LANs provide support for **client/server** technology. In client/server technology, files are stored on a central computer known as the **server.** Any type of computer may act as a server, including mainframes, minicomputers, and PCs. **Client** computers can access information stored on the server. One major advantage of a LAN is that only one copy of a software program is needed for all users, since it can be stored on the server. The client computers then access the server to use the software. This contrasts with the need to supply a separate copy of a software program for each PC user. The primary disadvantage to client/server technology is vulnerability. If the server fails, the network fails. Multiple servers circumvent this problem. Larger, more expansive systems are known as **wide area networks (WANs).**

Thin Client Technology is a relatively new computing model that allows PCs to connect to a server using a highly efficient network connection (Collett 1999). This configuration allows users to perform operations using software that is stored on the server. All system processing occurs on the server, rather than on the client or local PC, as seen in traditional client/server technology. One advantage to this model is that it is not necessary to physically visit each PC whenever installations or software upgrades must be made, as all changes can be made just to the server. In addition, since all software processing occurs on the server rather than the individual PCs, it is not necessary for the PCs to have high memory and processing capabilities. These minimal client requirements have resulted in the name "thin client," as opposed to the "fat clients" seen in traditional client/server technology. In fact, older PCs with less capability can be used, which may result in an incremental savings to the organization when considering the additional cost of the server and thin client software. A disadvantage to using this approach is that little software is currently available that will take advantage of the benefits of thin client technology. Since several developers have recently released software to support the thin client approach, it is expected that use of this technology will expand.

The largest and best known network in the world is the **Internet,** also known as the **Net.** The Internet actually consists of thousands of inter-connected networks. The Internet was once limited to individuals affili-ated with educational institutions and government agencies, but access is now available to the public. Variations of Internet technology are avail-able via intranets and extranets ("Beyond browsers" 1996, Metcalfe 1996). Both intranets and extranets employ software and programming languages designed for the Internet. **Intranets** are private company net-works that are protected from outside access. **Extranets,** on the other hand, apply Internet technology to create a network outside of the com-pany system for use by customers or suppliers.

HOW COMPUTERS WORK

Computers receive, process, and store data. They use binary code to rep-resent **alphanumeric** characters, which are numbers and alphabetic characters. **Binary code** is a series of 1s and 0s. All 1s are stored on the disk as magnetized areas and 0s are stored as areas that have not been magnetized. Each 1 or 0 is called a **bit.** Eight bits make up one **byte.** The unique code for each character is eight bits long. In the code for nu-meric characters, each position corresponds to a specific power of 2. Box 2–1 provides a binary representation of the number 13.

Computer programs, or software, use binary code to provide the in-structions that direct the work computers do. Personal computers and laptop computers differ slightly from super-, mainframe, and minicom-puters in the structure of their CPU. Although the CPU in larger comput-ers generally comprises one or more circuit boards, a PC has a **micro-processor chip,** which contains the electronic circuits of the CPU etched

---

Box 2–1 Binary Representation of an Arabic Number

The arabic number 13 is represented using the binary system as 00001101. Each bit (0 or 1) represents a particular power of 2, depending on its position. If the position is taken by a 0, then it has no value. If a position is taken by a 1, it has the value of the associated power of 2. The arabic number represented is the total of the powers of 2 represented by the 0s and 1s.

Binary represention of 13:	0	0	0	0	1	1	0	1	
Powers of 2 by bit location:	2^7	2^6	2^5	2^4	2^3	2^2	2^1	2^0	
Arabic value of position:	128	64	32	16	8	4	2	1	
Actual value of bit:	0 +	0 +	0 +	0 +	8 +	4 +	0 +	1	= 13

FIGURE 2–3 • Internal View of a PC

on a silicon chip, mounted on a board, otherwise known as the **mother-board.** All electrical components, including the main memory, connect to this board. Figure 2–3 depicts the internal components of a PC. The motherboard also provides slots for network interface cards and peripheral device interface cards. The **network interface card** physically connects a computer to a network, controlling the flow of information between the two. Likewise, **peripheral device interface cards** connect equipment such as printers to the computer and control the exchange of information. The slot arrangement on motherboards allows users to change or add computer system components easily. Portable or laptop computers can be connected to networks or peripheral devices through the use of a **PCMCIA (Personal Computer Memory Card International Association) card.** These cards can be inserted into a slot, in the case of the laptop computer, to add increased functionality such as additional memory or network connections.

PC processor speed is measured in **megahertz.** One megahertz represents one million signal voltage cycles per second. The processor speed determines how rapidly instructions are handled. In general, each new PC model offers a faster CPU speed.

Whenever the power to a PC is turned on, the computer performs a start-up test. The program code for this test is stored in permanent memory and is known as **BIOS (basic input/output system).** The BIOS confirms that information about component parts is present and that this information coincides with existing hardware.

SELECTION CRITERIA

Equipment selection should be based on needs and expectations. When selecting a computer system and related hardware, it is important to consider the following:

- *The types of applications required.* For example, some people use primarily word processing programs, while others need applications to perform numeric calculations.
- *The program execution time and computer capacity needed to process jobs.* Complex jobs require higher processor speed and more memory for timely execution.
- *The number of workers who need computer access at any one time.* Single-user access demands can be met by a PC. Multiple demands for access may be better served by a network.
- *Storage capacity.* Storage needs are determined by the amount of information that must be kept and the length of time that it must be retained.
- *Backup options.* When information stored and processed on computers is critical to conduct daily business, another copy should be available to restore normal services after a crash.
- *Budget considerations.* The cost of hardware and software for various options should be considered in relation to the benefits and limitations associated with each.

These factors will help to determine whether a mainframe, minicomputer or microcomputer, or network is the best option, as well as the required hardware features. Advance planning ensures that current and future computer needs are well served.

User Needs

Human factors should be considered in every work environment but sometimes do not receive sufficient attention (Davis and McGuffin 1995, McCune 1996). **Ergonomics** is the scientific study of work and space, including details that affect worker productivity and worker health (Anderson 1992). Poor placement of computer equipment can lead to a number of somatic complaints including headaches, eye strain, irritation, stress, fatigue, and neck and back pain. **Repetitive stress injuries (RSIs), or repetitive motion injuries,** have also been reported. Repetitive motion injuries result from using the same muscle groups over and over again without rest (Black and Matassarin-Jacobs 1997). One well-known example of a repetitive motion injury is **carpal tunnel syndrome.** Carpal tunnel syndrome occurs when the median nerve is compressed as it passes through the wrist along the pathway to the hand. This compression results in sensory and motor changes to the thumb, index finger, third finger, and radial aspect of the ring finger. Other repetitive motion injuries may involve the neck and shoulders. Good ergonomics can save money by avoiding workers' compensation claims and keeping employees productive. Box 2–2 lists measures that can reduce discomfort when working with computers. Another aspect of ergonomics addresses worker concerns about alleged health risks associated with computer use. The list of alleged health risks includes, but is not limited

Box 2–2	Measures to Reduce Computer-Related Discomfort

- Educate all workers on the need for good body mechanics when working with computers.
- Adjust desk, chair, monitor, and keyboard height for each user.
- Use an adjustable keyboard tray to lower the keyboard to a comfortable typing height.
- Provide chairs with good lumbar support.
- Reduce head and eye movement by reducing the distance between keyboard and monitor. Use copy holders adjacent to monitor screens.
- Position monitors just below eye level to avoid neck strain, especially for bifocal wearers.
- Use wrist rests to avoid repetitive stress injuries.
- Break up repetitive motion with other activities to avoid repetitive stress injuries.
- Periodically look away from the monitor to distant objects to avoid eye focusing problems.
- Minimize screen glare by purchasing non-glare monitors or placing monitors at right angles to windows. Provide blinds or draperies, or adjust area lighting.

SOURCE: Davis, P. T. and McGuffin, C. R. (1995). *Wireless local area networks,* New York: McGraw-Hill. Adapted with the permission of The McGraw-Hill Companies.

to the following: cataracts, conception problems, miscarriage, and/or birth defects. Research has not established any clear links between computer use and these risks. Table 2–2 lists several examples of commercially available ergonomic devices. Controversy exists regarding the degree to which these devices benefit the user and prevent injury.

Physical Constraints

Space is a chronic problem in health care settings. For this reason workstation planning is less a function of good ergonomics and more a function of finding a place to put the equipment. Ergonomics rarely receives high priority in planning. Provisions should be made for adequate numbers of computers in the clinical setting, located in quiet areas such as conference rooms.

Another major constraint to the installation of computers and networks in any institution centers on wiring and cabling. Adding power lines and cables for network connections to a current work space may prove to be more expensive than building a new work area.

SOFTWARE

Software is a set of instructions that tells the computer what to do. **Programs** and **applications** are forms of software. All software is written in **programming languages.** Each programming language provides a detailed

Table 2–2	Examples of Ergonomic Devices

Device	Purpose
Glare filter	Reduces eyestrain related to glare or light reflected from a monitor. Improves resolution and increases contrast leaving the colors brighter and the text easier to read.
Wrist rest or support	Provides a cushioned surface designed to align the upper extremity in a more neutral, natural posture and minimize pressure points. Limits wrist movements to minimize pressure on the median nerve, which can lead to carpal tunnel syndrome.
Back rest	Maintains the back's natural curves and promotes neutral posture minimizing back pain.
Foot rest	Encourages proper posture and supports the lower back by keeping the pelvis properly tilted. Increases circulation to the legs.
Ergonomic keyboard	The modified keyboard shape is designed to better fit the shape of the hands to reduce movement and tension. Relieves the symptoms of RSI and carpal tunnel syndrome.
Document holder	Places documents either at the same height and distance as the monitor or between the keyboard and monitor to minimize the need for eye and head movement between the document and monitor screen.

set of rules for how to write instructions for the computer. Numerous programming languages exist. A few examples are listed here. COBOL (Common Business Oriented Language) remains popular for business applications. MUMPS (Massachusetts General Hospital Utility Multi Programming System) is commonly used for health care applications. BASIC (Beginners All-Purpose Symbolic Instruction Code) is widely found in home computing. Java is a popular language for the development of programs for use on the Internet. Visual Basic is a programming language used for the development of graphical user interfaces. Structured Query Language (SQL) is an example of a programming language that allows the user to query or search a database for specific information.

Several categories of software exist. Each has a different purpose. Some major software categories include operating systems, application software, and utility programs.

Operating Systems

The most essential type of software is the **operating system.** The operating system is a collection of programs that manage all of the computer's activities, including the control of hardware, execution of software, and management of information. Control of hardware refers to the ability of different parts of the computer to work together. Operating systems allow users to manage information through the retrieval, copying, movement, storage, and deletion of files.

The operating system also provides a **user interface.** The user interface is the means by which the individual interacts with the computer. For many years PC users were required to enter specific text commands. The introduction of Microsoft Windows signaled a move to a **graphical user interface (GUI)** for PC users. A GUI provides a set of menus, windows, and other standard screen devices that are intended to make using a computer as intuitive as possible ("Glossary" 1996). GUIs decrease the amount of time required to learn new programs and eliminate the need to memorize computer commands. Work is currently underway to develop natural interfaces. Natural user interfaces are expected to free the user from conventional constraints such as mechanical keyboards, pointing devices, and GUIs, therefore making computers easier to use. Voice and vision recognition and synthesis are needed for natural user interfaces. Both require further work in **artificial intelligence** (Hughes 1995). Artificial intelligence is the development of technology that possesses a demonstrated ability to emulate human reasoning (Anderson 1992, "Glossary" 1996).

Operating systems exist for all categories of computers. MS-DOS (Microsoft Disk Operating System) and Windows represent two popular PC operating systems. Earlier versions of Windows needed MS-DOS to operate and were not true operating systems. Windows 95, 98, 2000, and NT are actual operating systems. LINUX is another operating system. **Macintosh computers** or **Macs** have their own operating systems. Macs are commercial computers that offer a graphical interface and are available for home and office use. Macs are produced by the Apple computer company. Fewer software programs are available for Macs, but adaptations are available that permit Macs to run PC software. **UNIX** is an operating environment developed in the 1970s, and is frequently found on large, commercial mainframe computers.

Application Software

Application software is a set of programs designed to accomplish a particular task such as word processing, financial management, or drawing. Application software builds on the foundation provided by the operating system. Box 2–3 lists some common types of application software and their functions.

Another factor that facilitates computer use is the development of software tutorials and on-line help. Most software packages now offer tutorials for review prior to application use, making software much more accessible to first-time users. Help screens are available while the program is running.

Utility Programs

Utility programs help to manage the computer and its data. Early operating systems offered few utility options such as optimization of the hard

Box 2–3	Common Types of PC Software Applications

- *Word processing.* Allows the creation of documents, utilizing features such as spelling and grammar correction, thesaurus, and graphics or pictures.

- *Desktop publishing.* Offers expanded features that may not be found commonly in word processing programs. Useful for the creation of newsletters and other publications.

- *Presentation graphics.* Supports the preparation of slides and handout materials.

- *Spreadsheet.* Performs calculations, analyzes data, and presents information in tabular format and graphical displays.

- *Database.* Helps to manage large collections of information, such as payroll information, phone directories, and product listing. Performs calculations and produces reports from the stored information. Allows the user to find specific information.

- *Specialized software*

  Project Management. Supports the management of projects with identification of tasks and time frames for completion, including PERT charts.

  Personal Information Managers. Enhance personal productivity with time management tools, including an appointment calendar, telephone directories, and reminder lists.

  Personnel Scheduling. Automates the process of scheduling staff.

---

disk, system backup, or virus checks. To fill this need, a separate category of software evolved. Many utility programs are now included as part of the operating system. However, users may still choose to install and use utility programs that are independent of their operating systems.

ROLES OF SUPPORT PERSONNEL

Even though PCs have brought computers closer to users, many people remain blissfully ignorant of computer technology beyond what they absolutely need to know. As a result, support is extremely important to maintaining user productivity. For example, PC support costs for large organizations typically range to thousands of dollars for each computer. Support costs may include time spent planning system upgrades, installation of upgrades for operating systems and various applications, troubleshooting, and user education. With help from support personnel, users can benefit from computers without knowing or understanding how they work.

In addition to personnel that support the computer user, other essential positions are needed by hospitals and health care organizations that use computers and information systems. A **healthcare information system (HIS)** consists of a computer, including associated hardware and software that is dedicated to the collection, storage, processing, retrieval, and communication of information relevant to patient care within a health care organization (Collen 1983). Staff is needed to create and maintain networks, customize and maintain software, and provide administration and leadership related to the HIS.

Superuser

The superuser has additional computer experience over the average employee and serves as a local resource person. In the hospital setting, the superuser is generally someone who knows the clinical area well and is able to answer most questions from users about the hospital computer system. In some cases the superuser may be involved in user training.

Help Desk Technician

The help desk technician is usually the first line of user support within an organization. A formal process exists for users to contact the help desk, usually by phone or pager. All problems are logged to ensure that proper follow-up and resolution have occurred. If the problem cannot be solved by the help desk staff, it is redirected to the appropriate person.

Microcomputer or PC Specialist

The PC specialist provides users with necessary PC information and training, thus enabling them to perform routine tasks. These specialists often have technical training or an associate or baccalaureate degree in computer science or a related area. While PC specialists provide valuable services, their salaries tend to be lower than those of other support personnel.

Analyst

Health care information system analysts are responsible for a wide range of activities related to the successful automation of information management. They may be clinicians who became involved in system selection and training. Many learned their role on the job and furthered their education by taking computer or information science classes. Analysts interview staff, determine user needs, write specifications for software performance, participate in some computer programming and debugging, implement new automated functions, and document program specifications and changes. Analysts who lack a clinical background may not be paid well initially, but with experience and additional preparation, their earning potential increases.

Clinical Liaison

Clinical liaisons are clinicians who represent the interests and needs of the users, and work with the information system team to address these issues during system design and implementation. They may or may not have formal computer or information system training. Liaisons some-times continue their clinical role while fulfilling this responsibility.

Programmer

Programmers actually write the code, or instructions that tell the computer what to do. They often lack a clinical background. For this reason, analysts are responsible for communicating user needs to programmers. In some institutions, one individual may serve as both analyst and programmer.

Network Administrator

Network administrators are responsible for the planning, management, and expansion of networks. Network administrators must decide whether to contract with outside agencies for network services and support or to educate in-house personnel for these functions. Unfortunately, many organizations lack a mechanism to coordinate equipment selection among different departments, but expect the network manager to get the resulting hodge-podge of equipment linked together. Organizations should involve network administrators in equipment decisions when the ultimate goal involves the creation or expansion of a network. It is possible to become a certified network engineer by taking several courses and subsequently demonstrating competence to manage different types of networks. Network administrators can access all data no matter who owns it. The salaries of network administrators are typically higher than previously discussed personnel.

Trainer

Trainers are responsible for educating clinical users in one or more applications, and may also be required to define and monitor user competencies. Trainers may or may not have a clinical background, but have knowledge of the specific computer application that they are teaching. This role may be filled as a permanent position or may be done by other information systems or clinical staff, as needed.

Security Officer

Security officers are responsible for ensuring that measures exist to protect information privacy. This usually includes a process for assigning and monitoring system access identification codes and passwords. In some cases the security officer may be responsible for protecting the physical equipment and data stored there.

Chief Information Officer (CIO)

This individual should have a broad view of the needs of the institution and the design, implementation, and evaluation of information systems.

Responsibilities include planning, policy development, budgeting, information security, and overall management of the enterprise's information systems. In some agencies the information services (IS) department is responsible for all computers and computer training. The CIO is at the top of the compensation heap for computer-related positions. Preparation is usually at a master's or doctoral degree level.

Webmaster

This individual is responsible for design, maintenance, and security of materials placed on the Internet, intranet, and/or extranet.

CASE STUDY EXERCISES

You are appointed to the hospital's information technology committee as the representative for your nursing unit. The charges of the committee include the following:

- Identify PC software that is needed to accomplish unit work, such as word processing, spreadsheets, and databases.
- Determine criteria for the selection and placement of hardware on the units.

Discuss these issues and how they affect patient care and work flow.

• • •

Your committee is charged with setting up a computer system that will automate transcription of physician orders and reporting of results. Identify the support personnel that you need at this point and write job descriptions for each identified position.

SUMMARY

- Computers are machines that process data under the direction of a program, or stored sequence of instructions.
- The major hardware components of computers are input devices, the central processing unit (CPU), secondary storage, and output devices.
- There are four categories of computers: supercomputers, mainframes, minicomputers, and microcomputers (including personal computers).
- Peripheral hardware items, such as the keyboard, mouse, monitor, modem, and printer, help the user put data into the computer, read output, and communicate with other users.
- Networks are linked systems of computers. Local area networks, wide area networks, and the Internet are all types of computer networks.

- Networks may use various technologies including cabling, radio signals, client/server, and thin client.

- In choosing a computer system, one must consider current and future information processing needs, budget, and human use factors.

- Good ergonomics may reduce physical discomforts and injury associated with computer use.

- Software is the set of instructions that make a computer run and control its resources. Operating systems, applications, utility programs, and programming languages are all types of software.

- Many institutions employ support personnel to help people use computers effectively, and to maintain and upgrade hardware and software.

REFERENCES

Ahuja, V. (1996). *Network and Internet security.* New York: Academic.

Anderson, S. (1992). *Computer literacy for health care professionals.* New York: Delmar.

Beyond browsers. (7 October 1996). *InformationWeek,* 65–66.

Black, J. M., and Matassarin–Jacobs, E. (1997). *Medical surgical nursing: Clinical management for continuity of care,* 5th ed. Philadelphia: Saunders.

Collen, M. F. (1983). General requirements for clinical departmental systems. In J. H. Van Bemmel, M. J. Ball, and O. Wigertz (Eds.), *Proceedings of the Fourth World Conference on Medical Informatics* (pp. 61–64). Amsterdam: Elsevier Science.

Collett, S. (1999). Microsoft nod gives thin clients a boost. *Computerworld, 33*(19), 69.

Davis, P. T., and McGuffin, C. R. (1995). *Wireless local area networks: Technology, issues, and strategies.* New York: McGraw-Hill.

Glossary: A guide to health data terms. (1996). *Health Data Management, 4*(12), 49–53.

Hughes, J. F. (1995). Introduction to interactive multimedia training systems. Section 4, Natural user interfaces. On the Web at: *http://www.surrey.ac.uk/Education/Telemat/Rev2/4nui2.html.*

Marion, W. (1994). *Client/server strategies: Implementations in the IBM Environment.* New York: McGraw-Hill.

McCune, J. C. (1996). Why you should care about ergonomics. *Beyond Computing, 5*(3), 34–37.

Metcalfe, B. (21 October 1996). Private information highways will avoid all congestion on the 'Net.' *Infoworld,* 18(43), 41.

Viewing the display screen. (1996). On the Web at: *http://www.combo.com/ergo/dscreen.html.*

3

Ensuring the Quality of Information

After completing this chapter, you should be able to:

- Describe the difference between the terms *data, information*, and *knowledge*.

- Define data integrity and its relevance for health care.

- Discuss the relevance of data management for data integrity.

- Discuss strategies to ensure the accuracy of data.

- Differentiate between on-line and off-line data storage.

- Explain how storage conditions can affect data integrity.

- Debate the relative benefits of outsourcing data storage.

- Discuss the factors that should be addressed when planning for data retrieval.

- Identify characteristics associated with quality information.

Data is a collection of numbers, characters, or facts that are gathered according to some perceived need for analysis and possibly action at a later point in time (Anderson 1992). Examples of data include a client's vital signs. Other data examples are the length of hospital stay for each client; the client's race, marital, or employment status; and next of kin. Sometimes this type of data may be given a numeric or alphabetic code, as shown in Table 3–1.

A single piece of data has little meaning. However, a collection of data can be examined for patterns and structure that can be interpreted (Saba and McCormick 1996, Warman 1993). **Information** is data that has been interpreted. For example, individual temperature readings are data. When they are plotted on a graph, the client's change in temperature over time and comparison to normal values become evident, thus becoming information. Table 3–2 provides examples of data and information. While it is possible to determine whether individual values (data) fall within the normal range, the collection of several values over time creates a pattern that in this case demonstrates the presence of a low-grade fever (information).

Knowledge is a more complex concept. Knowledge is the synthesis of information derived from several sources to produce a single concept or idea. It is based on a logical process of analysis and provides order to thoughts and ideas and decreases uncertainty (Ayer 1966, Engelhardt 1980). Validation of information provides knowledge that can be used again. Historically nursing has acquired knowledge through tradition, authority, borrowed theory, trial and error, personal experience, role modeling, reasoning, and research. Today, computers are used to facilitate the data collection and analysis associated with research. In other words, computers provide a tool that facilitates the acquisition of knowledge. An example of knowledge can be seen in the determination of the most effective nursing interventions for the prevention of skin breakdown. If a research

Table 3–1	Example of Coded Data: Employment Status Codes	

Code	Status	Explanation
1	Employed Full-Time	Individual states that he or she is employed full-time.
2	Employed Part-Time	Individual states that he or she is employed part-time.
3	Not Employed	Individual states that he or she is not employed full-time or part-time.
4	Self-Employed	Self-explanatory
5	Retired	Self-explanatory
6	On Active Military Duty	Self-explanatory
7	Unknown	Individual's employment status is unknown.

study produces data related to the prevention of skin breakdown achieved through specific interventions, this data can be collected and analyzed. The trends or patterns depicted by the data provide information regarding which treatment is more effective than others in preventing skin breakdown. The validation of this information through repeated studies provides knowledge that nurses can use to prevent skin breakdown in their clients.

Because data are building blocks in the formation of knowledge, it is essential that data be managed well. This means ensuring the quality of the data and maintaining its integrity.

DATA INTEGRITY

Data integrity refers to the ability to collect, store, and retrieve correct, complete, and current data so that it is available to authorized users

Table 3–2	Examples of Data and Information		

Time	Temperature	Pulse	Respirations
7 am	37.8 C	88	24
12 n	38.9 C	96	24
4 pm	38 C	84	22
8 pm	37.2 C	83	20

The values in the table above represent data: a client's vital signs over the course of a day. Each individual value is limited in meaning. The pattern of the values represents information, which is more useful to the health care provider.

when needed. Data integrity is one of the most important issues related to computing and information handling in health care because treatment decisions are based on information derived from data. If the data is faulty or incomplete, the quality of derived information may be poor, resulting in decisions that may be inappropriate and possibly harmful to clients. For example, if the nurse interviewing a client collects data related to allergies but fails to document all reported allergies, the client may be given drugs that cause an allergic reaction. In this case, the data was collected but not stored properly.

Ensuring Correct Data Collection and Entry

Computer systems facilitate data collection but may increase the potential for entry of incorrect data through input errors. These errors may include hitting the wrong key on a computer keyboard, selecting the wrong item from a screen using a light pen or mouse, or failing to enter all data collected. Several measures can be taken to decrease the likelihood of input errors, including educating personnel, conducting system checks, and verifying data.

Educating Personnel Staff who are proficient in the use of the computer system are less likely to make data collection and entry errors (Eastwood 1995, Faaoso 1992). All personnel should attend classes that emphasize appropriate system access, input device use, potential harmful effects associated with incorrect data, data verification techniques, and error correction. Upon the completion of classes, all employees should demonstrate competence in system use. Even after staff have shown competence, continuing education should occur on a routine basis and as indicated by problems such as increases in data errors.

System Checks to Ensure Accurate Data Entry and Data Completeness Data entry systems should be easy to use and provide periodic checks to ascertain that data is correct and complete. A **system check** is a mechanism provided by the computer system to assist users by prompting them to complete a task, verify information, or prevent entry of inappropriate information. Computer systems facilitate data collection and verification in several ways. Examples of computer-generated prompts and system safeguards include the following:

- Requesting information about a client's allergies when no entry has been made regarding allergies. In the absence of an entry regarding allergies, the system may not accept medication and radiology orders.
- Informing the user that an order already exists when the user attempts to enter a duplicate order. The system requests verification before processing the duplicate order. This can prevent unintentional repetition of expensive diagnostic tests. For example, a physician previously ordered a complete blood count (CBC) to be drawn today. An-

other physician has ordered a hemoglobin and hematocrit (H & H), also to be drawn today. When the order for the H & H is entered into the computer, the system will alert the user that this is a duplicate order, since the H & H is part of the CBC.

- Producing printouts alerting the nurse that a prescribed medication has not been documented as given. This improves the quality of client care and documentation.

Data Verification Techniques Another means to ensure data accuracy is to provide clients with opportunities to verify data that is collected during the admission and assessment processes (Brennan 1996). The active participation of the client in the data verification process is a relatively new concept in relation to computer systems. This verification may be accomplished through one of the following methods:

- Verbal confirmation
- Asking clients to review data on selected screens
- Asking clients to review printouts of entered data

Each of these methods has potential problems. For example, with verbal confirmation clients may answer "yes" without actually hearing or understanding what was said to them. Screen review is difficult for the visually impaired, or may be done too quickly for the client to scan all information. Finally, reading printouts is impractical for the visually impaired or illiterate. It also creates the additional problem of papers that must be disposed of with consideration for their confidential nature. All methods may be problematic for the individual who does not speak English.

While the initial data collection and entry process provides an excellent opportunity to verify data accuracy and completeness, it should not be the only time that this is done. Health care consumers should be able to review their records at any time and furnish additional information that they feel is important to their care.

How to Minimize Fraudulent Information Another concern in the concept of data integrity is the entry of fraudulent information. Fraudulent information can lead to financial loss to the provider and/or third-party payer, as well as treatment errors. At present, admitting clerks and physician office staff ask for the client's insurance card at the time of treatment. This request should also include proof of identification, preferably photo identification, as a means to decrease claims filed under another person's identity. Clients should be informed of the purpose of this request and sign a statement indicating that they are aware that insurance fraud is a criminal act and that use of another person's insurance data may result in bodily harm secondary to treatment decisions based on someone else's health record.

DATA MANAGEMENT

The changing health care delivery system provides the driving force for improved data management. Computers are an essential tool in this process. **Data management** is the process of controlling the storage, retrieval, and use of data to optimize accuracy and utility while safeguarding integrity.

Several levels of personnel are involved in data management. System analysts help the users to specify the data that is to be collected and how this will be accomplished. Programmers create the computer instructions or program that will collect the required data. They also build the **database,** a file structure that supports the storage of data in an organized fashion and allows data retrieval as meaningful information. Some facilities may also employ a **database administrator** (DBA), who is responsible for overseeing all activities related to maintaining the database and optimizing its use.

A **relational database** is designed using data that is represented as tables. This type of database is easily updated and can provide specific information to answer a query. A **data warehouse** provides an even more powerful method of managing and analyzing data. A data warehouse is a repository for storing data from several different databases so that it can be combined and manipulated to provide answers to complex analytic questions (Benander and Benander 2000).

Cost is another consideration in the management of data. Storage and management of paper and film records is labor-intensive and expensive. Retrieval of paper and film records must be done manually, and information may not be available when and where it is needed. Physical records are also subject to loss. One current solution is **document imaging,** which involves scanning paper records to computer disks or other media, to facilitate electronic storage and handling (Chunn 1996, Rardin 1996). Converting paper records to other storage media may facilitate management, but a better solution is to move away from paper, with data entered directly to automated records. Although automated solutions may also be costly, they will provide increased efficiency and improved access.

Automation of health care records creates new issues related to data storage (DePompa 1996, Kaufmann 1996). Recent estimates project that PC, network, and mainframe storage requirements will grow 50 percent per year. Along with an increase in volume and types of materials for storage, data storage and retrieval requires special conditions to ensure data integrity.

Data Storage

At present there are two basic types of data storage: on-line and off-line. **On-line storage** provides access to current data. On-line storage is rapid, using high-speed hard disk drives. **Off-line storage** is used for data that is needed less frequently, or for long-term data storage, as may be seen with old client records. Off-line storage can be done on any secondary storage device. Access to data stored off-line is slower than with on-line storage. Immediacy of need for particular data is a key factor in determining whether it is stored on-line or off-line. Table 3–3 describes various types of storage media, along with their advantages and disadvantages.

To protect computerized information, organizations need a storage strategy that addresses the following issues (Kaufmann 1996):

- *Environmental conditions and physical hazards.* These include temperature, humidity, shock, and dust control, and protection from damage by fire, water, or electromagnetic fields. Some media are more sensitive to environmental factors than others. Strict environmental controls protect the storage media and the data it contains.

- *Control of equipment and media.* This refers to who may access computer equipment and data and is supported through a combination of physical and logical restrictions. Physical restrictions maintain a secure locked environment for the computer hardware and operations areas. Logical restrictions limit data access to only those staff who require this information. For example, admission clerks might be restricted from accessing clinical information such as test results, but might be able to access demographic and insurance information.

- *Contingency planning.* A secondary or backup copy of the data is created as a safeguard in the event of loss or damage to the primary data. This backup copy should be stored at another location separate from the computer, reducing the danger that a disaster will affect both the computer and the storage area.

- *Storage period for each record type.* The minimum length of time that client records must be stored is dictated by state laws. An organization may choose to retain records indefinitely, but cost and physical storage constraints must be considered.

- *Plans to transfer data to new media before degradation occurs.* For example, data stored on magnetic tape may degrade after 15 years. If the organization intends to retain records indefinitely, the data must be transferred to other media.

Outsourcing Data Management and Storage

Internal data storage is costly in terms of human resources and space that can be allocated for other purposes. Storage costs include the purchase price for devices and the costs of media, maintenance, and environmental control. These costs may consume one-third of the IS budget (Enticknap 1996). Storage can be handled internally or outsourced. **Outsourcing** is the process by which an organization contracts with outside agencies for services. Outsourcing provides a means to cut costs that would otherwise

Table 3–3   **Storage Media**

Type	Description	Advantages	Disadvantages
Magnetic tape or cartridges	The magnetic field on the media surface is altered using tiny electromagnets to "write" the data	Traditional mainframe storage media Inexpensive Available in several formats Can store large amounts of information Easy to duplicate and move to another location Reusable 10- to 15-year life	Slow May be difficult to use Backup requires verification Tape drives require maintenance Can be damaged by exposure to dust, electromagnetic fields, moisture Store under climate-controlled conditions, 20–22C
Optical media	A laser is used to alter the recording surface, which is then read as data	Faster than tape High data capacities 2 major types: WORM (write once read many) and rewritable WORM: • does not use previously written sectors • difficult to alter—provides good data protection • identification is stamped into disks at production • sets aside corrupt data sectors • accessible repeatedly over 30-year shelf life	Readable only in specific drives Disk swap time is the most consuming part of retrieval; use of high-capacity disks ↓ number of swaps and ↑ retrieval performance
CD-ROM	Inexpensive optical variant	Large storage capacity Requires little storage space	Slow Not feasible for large-scale data storage
Magneto-optical	Uses a special alloy layer modified by a magnetic field later read by laser	Durable and transportable Rewritable 30-year shelf life	Slow search time

Table 3–3 Storage Media (Continued)			
Type	**Description**	**Advantages**	**Disadvantages**
DVD-ROM disks	Uses video compression	Higher data capacity than CD-ROM Suitable for video images and audio Offers backward compatability for CD-ROM	Has difficulty reading current CD format
RAID	Uses two or more hard drives connected together to mirror data on duplicate drives	Very safe storage method	Requires purchase of twice the needed storage
Removable hard drives	Easily removable from computer "docking bays"	Quick	Limited storage compared to optical media Questions surround long-term reliability

be required for the physical space, special conditions, and support personnel needed to maintain storage media and data.

Outsourcing companies specialize in all aspects of data management for multiple customers, providing services at a lower cost than if the customers performed the tasks themselves. It is important to review the contract to ensure that the outsourcing company can meet all of the institution's requirements for data storage and retrieval.

Data Retrieval

Data retrieval is a process that allows the user to access previously collected and stored data. Data retrieval most commonly occurs as a function of a software application in conjunction with secondary storage media. Recent developments in technology have cut storage costs and improved access and capacity. In addition to new options in storage media, a variety of automated devices are now available that provide access to stored data. Automated magnetic tape appears to be the most economical choice for large archives (Chunn 1996, Kaufmann 1996).

The significance of data retrieval may be seen in the development of an automated client record that covers the client's life span. While these advances are critical to the development of a birth-to-death health record, many providers are still in the first phases of developing systems for each client visit and have limited archival access. Furthermore, present hospital data storage systems save data but often lack the ability to manipulate data to demonstrate patterns. For example, it should be possible to easily extract demographic data on the population served, individual and aggregate responses to specific treatment modalities, or abnormal lab values for a given client.

The following factors should be considered when planning for data retrieval:

- *Performance*. Performance refers to the ability of the system to respond to user requests for data retrieval. Some of the specific factors that define performance include acceptable retrieval response time and the ability to accommodate numerous simultaneous requests for data.

- *Capacity*. Capacity is the number and size of records that can be stored and retrieved.

- *Data security*. Data must be protected against unauthorized access and retrieval.

- *Cost*. The costs include hardware, software, and support personnel. Data storage and retrieval costs overlap in many cases.

Retrieval needs are frequently underestimated. For example, some systems sharply limit the amount of archival data available to users and may impede treatment. Determination of system performance requirements helps data management personnel and administrators choose storage and retrieval strategies for user needs. Generally, record demand is highest soon after data is collected, with the number of access requests and need for rapid retrieval diminishing with the passage of time.

Data Exchange

In the past, data retrieval was primarily performed for use within a single institution. Changes in the health care delivery system now mandate exchange of client information between institutions. For example, a client may have surgery at a major medical center, but have follow-up appointments at a satellite location. The client's record must be accessible to clinicians at both sites. Several other factors contribute to the need to send client records in a timely fashion from one provider to another and to submit reimbursement claims in a timely fashion. These factors include, but are not limited to, a highly mobile population and consumer demands for efficiency. As the number of automated client record systems increases, so does the need to establish standard record structure and identifiers for individual data items to facilitate **electronic data interchange (EDI)**. EDI is the communication of data in binary code from one computer to another.

Although EDI facilitates record exchange, there are problems associated with it. A major problem is that different computer systems use different formats for data. The data format from the sending system may not be understood by the receiving system. One solution to this problem is the development of a standard data format for EDI. At present no agreement exists among health care groups in the United States about a common EDI standard. Several groups are currently working toward a common standard. One proposed solution is **Health Level 7 (HL7).** HL7 is both the name of the group and a standard for the exchange of clinical data. HL7 has an extensive set of rules that apply to all data sent.

CHARACTERISTICS OF QUALITY INFORMATION

If the recommended procedures for data collection, validation, storage, management, and retrieval are followed, then the end result is quality information. The significance of quality information is its potential impact on client care. High-quality information is needed by clinicians to make appropriate clinical decisions. In addition, quality information supports the ability of researchers to contribute to nursing science. The following characteristics describe quality information (Burke 1992, Kahn 1995, Tozor 1994, Zorkoczy and Heap 1995):

- *Timely.* Information is available when it is needed. The ability to access the client's insurance information at the time of an outpatient visit allows timely verification of coverage for specified procedures.
- *Precise.* Each detail is complete and clear. An example of a lack of precision is the client's report of previous "abdominal surgery." Precise data would be the identification of the specific surgical procedure, such as appendectomy.
- *Accurate.* Information is without error. An example of inaccurate data is documentation of the wrong leg in a below-the-knee amputation.
- *Numerically quantifiable.* The ability to measure data improves quality. An example is seen with the ability to measure and stage a decubitus ulcer, which aids the subsequent assessment of its status by other professionals.
- *Verifiable by independent means.* Two different people can make the same observation and report the same result. If two people listen to a client's apical heart rate simultaneously, they should both report the same rate.
- *Rapidly and easily available.* For example, the nurse can quickly retrieve a client's allergies from a past medical record stored by the computer system when a critically ill patient arrives in the emergency department.
- *Free from bias, or modification with the intent to influence recipients.* Data should be based on objective rather than subjective evaluation. Documenting that a client is depressed represents subjective interpretation. A better approach is to document observations about the client's activity level and interactions with others. These are quality data.
- *Comprehensive.* Required information is present. When a nurse asks a client for a list of current medications, it should include medication name, dosage, and frequency taken.

Box 3–1	Threats to Information Quality, Availability, and Confidentiality

Threats to Information Quality

- *Alteration of files.* The accidental or intentional addition or change of data erodes the quality of the information. Accidental changes are known as data corruption, while intentional changes are viewed as forgery.

- *System alteration.* When systems are changed, the way that data is processed may be affected. For example, the addition of a new function may result in the loss of data due to planning or programming deficiencies.

- *Introduction of viruses.* Viruses are unwanted programs, created with malicious intent, that can damage or destroy data. Viruses may be inadvertently introduced to a computer by infected disks, or downloaded from another system.

Threats to Information Availability

- *Destruction of hardwre, software and/or data.* This may occur through natural or man-made disasters, or lack of attention to environmental conditions and security.

- *Interruptions in power or radio frequency disruption.* Interruptions in the processing of data may result in data loss.

- *Sabotage.* Sabotage is the intentional destruction of hardware, software, or data. Potential sabotage should be considered in the design of security measures.

Threats to Confidentiality

- *Eavesdropping.* Eavesdropping may involve unauthorized access to information, either looking at the system directly or reading confidential printouts. Security measures must limit computer access to authorized persons and provide appropriate guidelines for the handling and disposal of confidential printouts.

- *Unauthorized reception of wireless network technology transmissions.* The reception of radio frequency transmission used in some wireless networks may provide another opportunity to eavesdrop. The use of technology safeguards including coding data and changing frequencies may minimize this threat.

Source: Gordon, J. (1993). Data encryption and its applications to computer security. In J. E. Ettinger (Ed.), *Information security: Applied information technology* (pp. 115–128). London: Chapman & Hall.

- *Appropriate to the user's needs.* Different users have different data needs. The appropriate data must be available for each user. For example, the nurse must be able to access data related to a client's previous diabetic teaching.

- *Clear.* Information is free from ambiguity, reducing the likelihood of treatment errors. An example is seen in the client's report of an allergy to eggs. Upon questioning, the nurse determines that the client only dislikes eggs and does not wish to be served them, but has never had a truly allergic response.

- *Reliable no matter who collects it.* There may be certain data that multiple professionals collect. Client allergies may be documented by the nurse, physician, and pharmacist. All documentation of allergies should agree.

- *Current.* All files should contain the most current information available to the health care team. For information to be kept current, a regular system for updating must be put in place. Having current information available on the computer will help avoid errors that could be harmful to clients. For example, data retrieved at an outpatient setting should include all recent inpatient data that is pertinent, not just the most recent outpatient data.

- *In a convenient form for interpretation, classification, storage, retrieval, and updates.* The user must be able to access and use the data without difficulty.

Quality is also an issue when large amounts of data on different computer types and using different formats must be extracted for storage or analysis (Bort 1995). Format variations can accentuate inaccuracies and erode data quality, particularly as the number of databases and the age of the stored data increase. For example, a client may have been registered and treated at one hospital a number of times, using a slightly different version of the client's name for each registration. For example, one registration may have been created using a client's legal name, another using a nickname, and another omitting a middle initial. There may have also been a change in address during this period. It can be difficult in this instance to verify that all records belong to the same person. Until recently each record had to be examined individually for error. Software tools can now perform this task. The data source that is most likely to be correct is used for this purpose. Box 3–1 lists a summary of threats to quality, availability, and confidentiality of information.

CASE STUDY EXERCISES

Agnes Gibbons was admitted through the hospital's emergency department in congestive heart failure. During her admission she was asked to verbally acknowledge whether her demographic data were correct. Ms. Gibbons did so. Extensive diagnostic tests were done including radiology studies. It was later discovered that all of Ms. Gibbons' information had been entered into another client's file. How would you correct this situation? What departments, or other agencies, would need to be informed of this situation?

• • •

A non–English-speaking Vietnamese male was admitted through the emergency department with suspected tuberculosis (TB). The system carried information under his name. Mr. Nguyen nodded his head when the admitting clerk pointed to the demographic screen. Mr. Nguyen was tested and treated for TB. When the public health nurse went to Mr. Nguyen's address for follow-up, the man there was not the Mr. Nguyen who had been treated for TB. How would you address this problem? Explain your rationale.

• • •

You volunteered to serve on a committee to identify information from prior admissions that would be helpful to staff caring for current inpatients. What information, if any, would you select for ready access, and how long would you recommend that it remain active in the system? Remember that your system has limited capacity so that items must be carefully selected and prioritized. Identify the priority assigned to each item and provide your rationale for this priority.

SUMMARY

- Data is a collection of numbers, characters, or facts that are gathered according to some perceived need for analysis and possibly action at a later point in time.
- Data has little meaning itself, but a collection of data can be examined for patterns and structure that can be interpreted. At this point data becomes information.
- Knowledge is the synthesis of information derived from several sources to produce a single concept or idea.
- Data can be managed using a database application.
- A data warehouse is a collection of several databases that can be manipulated to provide complex data analysis.
- Information quality is ensured when measures to protect it are an integral part of its collection, use, storage, retrieval, and exchange.
- Data integrity strategies should provide safeguards against data manipulation or deletion, and entry of fraudulent facts.
- Data storage measures should provide safe, accessible storage to authorized persons through a plan that considers provider, client, and third-party payer needs; physical threats to information and media; performance requirements; pros and cons of on-site versus off-site storage; technological advancements; and future needs.
- Performance, capacity, data security, and cost should be considered when planning for data retrieval.
- Electronic data interchange standards provide timely access to providers at distant sites and computer systems.
- Quality information is essential to the delivery of appropriate client care.

REFERENCES

Anderson, S. (1992). *Computer literacy for health care professionals.* New York: Delmar.

Ayer, A. J. (1966). *The problem of knowledge.* Baltimore, MD: Penguin.

Benander, A., and Benander, B. (2000). Data warehouse administration and management. *Information System Management. 17*(1), 71.

Bort, J. (1995). Scrubbing dirty data. *InfoWorld, 17*(51), 1, 57–58.

Brennan, P. (1996). *Nursing informatics: Technology in the service of patient care.* Continuing education activity of West Virginia University Hospital, Morgantown, WV.

Burke, J. G. (1992). *System analysis, design, and implementation.* Boston: Boyd & Fraser.

Chunn, T. (1996). A storage comparison: Electronic archiving of radiology images. In *Document Information Management and Workflow Solutions in the Healthcare Enterprise,* a special supplement to *ImagingWorld, Healthcare Informatics & InfoCare* magazines. S23–S25.

DePompa, B. Sharing the cost of recovery. *InformationWeek,* 146–150 (9 September 1996).

Eastwood, A. (1995). End-users: The enemy within? *Computing Canada, 21*(1), 41.

Engelhardt, H. T., Jr. (1980). Knowing and valuing: Looking for common roots. In H. T. Engelhardt and D. Callahan (Eds.), *Knowing and valuing: The search for common roots* (Vol. 4, pp. 1–17). New York: Hastings Center.

Enticknap, N. Living space. *Consumer Weekly,* 381 (25 April 1996).

Faaoso, N. (1992). Automated patient care systems: The ethical impact. *Nursing Management, 23*(4), 46–48.

Gordon, J. (1993). Data encryption and its applications to computer security. In J. E. Ettinger, (Ed.), *Information security: Applied information technology* (pp. 115–128). London: Chapman & Hall.

Kahn, M. G. (1995). The computer-based patient record and Robert Fulghum's 16 principles. *M.D. Computing, 12*(4), 253–258.

Kaufmann, J. (1996). The technologies and processes of optical storage security. *Enterprise Systems Journal, 11*(7), 58, 60–61.

Rardin, K. D. (1996). Information warehousing within the CPR. In *Document Information Management and Workflow Solutions in the Healthcare Enterprise,* a special supplement to *ImagingWorld, Healthcare Informatics & InfoCare* magazines, S5–S6.

Saba, V., and McCormick, K. (1996). *Essentials of computers for nurses.* New York: McGraw-Hill.

Tozor, G. V. (1994). *Information quality management.* Cambridge, UK: Blackwell.

Warman, A. R. (1993). *Computer security within organizations.* London: Macmillan.

Zorkoczy, P., and Heap, N. (1995). *Information technology: An introduction,* 4th ed. London: Pittman.

4

Electronic Communication and the Internet

After completing this chapter, you should be able to:

- Define *electronic communication.*
- Explain the Internet and World Wide Web.
- Identify the process required to access both the Internet and World Wide Web.
- Discuss services available on the Internet and World Wide Web.
- Relate the advantages and disadvantages that the Internet and World Wide Web have over traditional means of communicating information.
- Identify examples of Internet and World Wide Web resources that may be useful to nurses and other health care professionals and consumers.
- Compare and contrast a Web page and a Web portal.
- Discuss the terms *search index, search engine,* and *search unifier.*
- Compare and contrast the purpose and use of intranets and extranets to the purpose and use of the Internet.
- Discuss the advantages and disadvantages of the Internet as a platform for health care applications.
- Understand the concepts of e-business and e-commerce and their role in the health care arena.

Computers can expedite the location and retrieval of information (Shelly, Cashman, Waggoner, and Waggoner 1996, Simpson 1995). This ability is particularly useful when material is difficult to obtain or quickly outdated. Electronic communication and Internet technology have the potential to support health care knowledge needs. **Electronic communication** is the ability to exchange information through the use of computer equipment and software. This is generally done through fixed network connections or the use of a **modem.** A modem is a communication device that transmits data over telephone or cable lines from one computer to another. This process allows individual users to communicate and share hardware, software, and information and is otherwise known as **connectivity. On-line** is a term that indicates a connection to various computer resources, such as the Internet and World Wide Web, which provide forums that encourage electronic communication and have revolutionized the way that information is shared.

The **Internet (Net)** is a worldwide network that connects millions of computers together (Goldberg 1996, Shellenbarger and Thomas 1996, Tomaiuolo 1995). This technology first began as a government project to encourage researchers at different academic sites to share their findings. It now links government, universities, commercial institutions, and individual users. The Internet is not under the control of any government or single organization, although the Internet Society guides its development. The Internet Society is a nonprofit, professional organization that focuses on standards, education, and policy issues surrounding the use of the Internet for the use and benefit "of all people throughout the world" (Internet Society 1999).

The Internet expands the range of available health care information through e-mail, discussion lists, File Transfer Protocol (FTP), Telnet, and World Wide Web resources. Many materials are no longer published on paper but are available electronically. Some examples include research reports, practice guidelines, educational materials, and conference proceedings.

The **World Wide Web (Web** or **WWW)** is an information service for access to Internet resources by content instead of file names. An easy-to-use graphical user interface (GUI) makes it simple to learn and use. The Web supports text, images, and sound as well as links to other documents. Users may search by specific words or move from one link to another. Links are displayed by highlighted keywords, text, or images. Selection of information in highlighted areas is accomplished through a click of the mouse button.

THE INTERNET

The Internet is the largest, best-known wide area network in the world. Its exact size is difficult to estimate because of its rapid growth, but its users number in the millions. One major factor in the growth of the Internet is the development of companies known as **Internet service providers (ISPs)** that furnish Internet access for a fee (Goldberg 1996). Some well-known examples of ISPs include America On-Line (AOL), Microsoft Network, Prodigy, CompuServe, and Delphi. Many local ISPs exist as well. Internet access through an ISP requires computer access, a modem, and communication software. An emerging technology for Internet users is the use of television cable connectivity, replacing traditional transmissions via telephone connections. Internet transmissions over cable connections are a great deal faster than those using telephone technology. ISPs provide software and directions on how to access the Internet and a special **SLIP/PPP** account that provides Internet and World Wide Web access. SLIP/PPP refers to the Serial Line Internet Protocol (SLIP) and Point-to-Point Protocol (PPP). Both protocols allow passage of data through communication lines. Customers generally pay their ISP a monthly fee. In some cases there is an additional charge for access time. Most ISPs provide a local telephone number for customer use. The majority of information on the Internet is available without charge. ISP access can be obtained without a fee if the user is willing to tolerate advertisement. The quality of free ISP service varies. Users may need to click on sponsor banners to maintain the connection. It may be difficult to download large files with free ISP accounts because the connection may be severed, technical support is limited, and it may be difficult to establish a connection because free services are oversubscribed.

The Internet offers many types of services and resources, including the following (Baxter 1996, Johnson 1996, Shelly et al. 1996, Welz 1997):

• *Electronic mail or e-mail.* **E-mail** is the use of computers to transmit messages to one or more persons. Delivery can be almost instantaneous. Text messages may be accompanied by attachment files. E-mail may be sent anywhere in the world as long as the individual has an Internet address. Like street addresses, Internet addresses are specific to a location and type of institution or ISP.

- *File transfer.* This capability allows users to move files from one location to another. The benefit of file transfer is that users can capture, view, edit, or use work developed by others rather than starting anew.
- *Database searches.* This feature allows users to conduct comprehensive literature searches over a shorter period of time than could be accomplished via a manual approach. More than 200 universities and public libraries offer on-line databases for review. In this instance, on-line refers to databases that are available through Internet connections.
- *Remote log-on.* This feature allows use of computer facilities at other locations to access directories, files, and databases. This ability is accomplished through the Telnet protocol. Some systems such as the Virginia Henderson International Nursing Library require an account, identification, and a password for user access.
- *Discussion and news groups.* The Internet provides a place where specialty interest groups can address concerns, discuss solutions, and exchange information in a timely fashion.
- *Internet Relay Chat (IRC).* This feature allows interactive discussions. At present most chats are typed. The Internet does have the capability to support voice chats, although both users must be on-line at the same time and have software to support voice chats.

E-mail

E-mail is one of the most frequently used Internet applications. It is commonly found in private organizations, colleges, universities, corporations, and private homes. It is a powerful connectivity tool and is often the feature that first attracts users to the Internet. E-mail encourages networking among peers, yields helpful tips and shared resources, and saves time and money that would otherwise be spent in individual problem-solving. E-mail is a convenient way to contact employees, colleagues, students, and recruiters. It allows users to participate in educational offerings and send announcements and resumes. Box 4–1 lists some advantages and disadvantages associated with e-mail. The next few paragraphs explain the composition and management of e-mail.

Every e-mail message has a header and message text (Goldberg 1996, Hoffman 1996, Staggers 1996, Wink 1995). The **header** lists who sent the message, when, to whom, and at what location, and the address to which a reply should be directed if different from the sender's address. Message copies may also be directed to others. Messages can be composed on-line or in advance. In this case, on-line refers to the period that one computer is actively connected to another. Composing messages ahead of

Box 4–1   E-Mail: Advantages and Disadvantages

Advantages

- *Eliminates telephone tag.* Provides the ability to leave a written message.
- *Convenient.* Can be sent or retrieved from multiple locations, including work, home, or while traveling. Can be used on a 24-hour basis.
- *Easy to prepare and send.* Electronic mail requires less effort to prepare, address, and send than the traditional means of dictation and mailing.
- *Saves time and money.* Eliminates postage and paper expenses.
- *Delivery can be almost instantaneous.* Eliminates the time lag associated with traditional mail.
- *Messages are time- and date-stamped.* Provides documentation of the actual time of the mail transaction. Can also provide a log of when the message was received, read, and answered.

Disadvantages

- *Interpretation of messages without the benefit of voice inflection.* Unlike telephone conversations, e-mail eliminates the additional information that may be communicated through verbal cues.
- *High volume of messages sent and received.* E-mail's popularity and ease of use make it easy to generate large numbers of messages, including copies, forwarded messages, and "junk mail."
- *Viral contamination with e-mail attachments.* Attached files that contain a virus may contaminate the recipient's computer.
- *Security concerns related to maintaining confidentiality.* E-mail is easily intercepted and forwarded, and may be read by unintended parties. Employers have the right to read e-mail transmitted using company resources. In addition, deleted messages may be retrieved during system backups.

---

time may decrease costs for connection time and improve the organization of expressed thoughts. Mail received may be read while on-line or downloaded to the recipient's computer for later review.

An **e-mail package** is a computer program that assists the user to send, receive, and manage e-mail messages. One such package is the UNIX mail program for mainframe computers. However, because many individuals find the UNIX mail program difficult to use, Elm and Pine were developed as friendly alternatives. Popular commercial e-mail packages include Microsoft Mail, Lotus CC: Mail, Eudora, and Da Vinci E-Mail. Despite its popularity in other settings, e-mail is not universally available for all employees in health care institutions at this time.

As e-mail popularity grows, so do concerns related to its use. These concerns include threats to data integrity, confidentiality, and verification that messages emanate from the identified source (Bort 1996, Edwards 1996, Leinfuss 1996, Staggers 1996). Data integrity may be threatened by **computer viruses.** Viruses are malicious programs that can disrupt or destroy data. While viruses are not usually spread through e-mail, they may be attached to files sent with e-mail messages. The threat of viruses can be minimized by scanning all attachment files prior to use. When content needs to be kept secure and confidential, **encryption** is recommended. Encryption uses mathematical formulas to code messages. Message recipients decode content with an encryption key. This feature can be found with many commercial e-mail packages. Methods to validate e-mail author identity do exist but are not widely used at this time. Two specific validation methods include **public key infrastructure** (PKI) and digital credentialing. PKI provides a unique code for each user that is imbedded into a storage device. User information is stored in a database by the organization that created the code. Identity is confirmed when the storage device and a password or other form of ID match information stored in the database (Guenther 1999). The digital credential is a unique identifier issued to the physician for use in e-mail communication. It is routed through a firewall to the Intel Internet Authentication Service (ITAS), which validates user identity and creates an audit trail. The digital credential represents a collaborative effort by Intel and the American Medical Association. The digital credential does not now require biometic measures to verify identity. It may also be available as a service to other health care workers (Brakeman 2000).

Other issues surrounding e-mail focus on its increasing volume, the time required to shift through e-mail messages, unwanted or "junk" e-mail, and accurate interpretation of messages. Box 4–2 provides some informal rules to guide e-mail use.

Like other Internet services, e-mail is based on a client/server system. In client/server technology, files are stored on a central computer known as a server (Cini 1996, Hoffman 1996, Siwicki 1996). In this case the server receives mail from other Internet sites and stores it until it is read, answered, or deleted. The client computer requests mail access from the server and generates new mail that will be handled by the server.

File Transfer

File transfer is the ability to move files from one location to another across the Internet (*Dictionary of Computing* 1996, File Transfer Protocol 1997). Users may download archived files that they find interesting or give their files to others. Transferred files can include graphics, text, or shareware applications. The actual movement of data is accomplished through the **File Transfer Protocol (FTP).** FTP is a set of instructions that controls both the physical transfer of data across the network and its appearance on the receiving end. The benefit of file transfer is that users can preview work developed by others rather than starting anew. FTP may be available with World Wide Web software. Internet etiquette calls for FTP execution after peak business hours to prevent slow response times.

Box 4–2	Informal Rules for E-Mail Use

- Change passwords for e-mail access immediately after they are first assigned, and frequently thereafter.
- Limit copies to the people that need the information. This keeps the number of messages manageable.
- Choose an accurate description for the subject line. This practice helps recipients to determine which messages should be read first.
- Give e-mail messages the same consideration given to business correspondence. E-mail may be seen by parties other than intended recipients. In an e-mail message, nothing should be written that one would not publicly post.
- Make messages clear, short, and to the point.
- Avoid the use of all capital letters. This is difficult to read, and may be perceived as shouting, according to e-mail etiquette.
- Limit abbreviations to those that are easily understood.
- Read mail, file messages in categories, and delete messages no longer needed on a regular basis. This frees storage space and helps to optimize system function, as well as making it easier to find and retrieve messages later.
- Consider using mechanisms to prevent unwanted mail.

The World Wide Web

The World Wide Web is an information service that can access data by content and support a multimedia approach. It was first developed at the European Center for Particle Physics in Geneva for scientists to publish documents while linked via the Internet. The Web's graphical user interface makes it the most user-friendly service on the Internet, as well as the fastest growing. The Web provides a forum for the exchange of ideas, free marketing, and public relations. It now serves as a platform for a growing number of businesses. Box 4–3 lists advantages and disadvantages associated with using the World Wide Web.

Figure 4–1 displays information uploaded to the Web by the American Nurses Association about its subsidiary and affiliate groups. Web pages frequently change as content is revised and new technologies are incorporated. This results in a different appearance for the page the next time the user accesses it. The use of new technology and software in Web page design may leave some users unable to access certain features or content. Periodic browser updates and the use of additional applications that can be downloaded from the Web or purchased in stores help to address this situation. It may also be necessary to evaluate, upgrade, and replace hardware and software to access and use desired Web features and applications.

Box 4–3 **The World Wide Web: Advantages and Disadvantages**

Advantages

- Browser software is available for all types of computers, including mainframes and Mac- and IBM-compatible personal computers.
- Browser software is easy to use.
- Supports text, pictures, video, and sound.
- The amount of information available on the Web is constantly expanding.
- Decreases Internet overload because it links to other documents instead of including them as attachments.
- Eliminates need to hold a line open while a document is read because the document is transferred to the host computer and the connection is terminated.
- Facilitates document transfer.
- May support voice communications.

Disadvantages

- No one person or group controls the Web, just as no one controls the Internet. This results in a wide variation of quality and accuracy of material.
- The quality of available information varies widely.
- Documents may not supply sufficient depth in content.
- Not all Web pages display a date of authorship.
- Web sites may change without a "forwarding address" being provided.
- The Web is vulnerable to hacker attacks.
- The large amount of available information may be overwhelming.
- Employers may be concerned over wasted company time and lost productivity as people explore the Web.

Products such as Web television and network computers make on-line access both easier and more accessible to a larger number of people (McCollum 1996). Web television eliminates the need for a computer and basic computer skills to access the Web. The network computer provides a simple, inexpensive device for Web access. There are no hard drives for storing data or programs. Applications and information are downloaded from the Web as needed.

One particularly popular Web feature is the **home page,** the first page seen at a particular Web location. The home page presents general information about a topic, person, or organization. Pages are written in **HyperText Markup Language (HTML).** A markup language includes text as well as special instructions known as tags for the display of text and other media. HTML also includes highlighted references to other documents that the user may choose if additional information about that topic

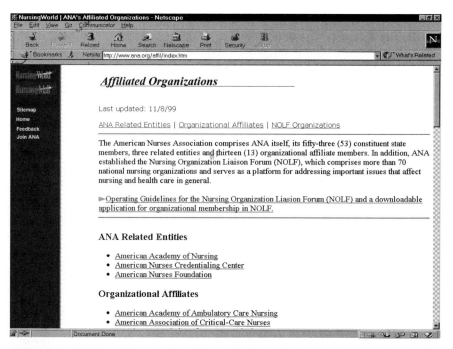

FIGURE 4–1 • "Affiliated Organizations" (reprinted from the American Nurses Association Web Site, *http://www.ana.org/affil/index.html/* by permission of the American Nurses Association)

is desired. World Wide Web software interprets HTML tags for display. Tags specify formatting information such as the type of heading, font size, and alignment of type. Tags also indicate the location of other media such as graphics or even music. HTML can include links to other documents and may incorporate text, graphics or video, and sound files.

Portal is a term that refers to some Web sites. Portal sites require registration and collect information from the user that can be used to personalize features for individual users. Services such as e-mail, news search capability, and on-line shopping may also be available. Portals organize data with different formats from multiple sources into a single, easy-to-use menu (Wilder, Davis, and Dalton 1999). Portals started as entry points to the Web that added additional features to attract and maintain user interests. America On-Line and Yahoo represent general portal sites. There are also special interest or niche portals. Some examples of nursing portals include Nursing Net (*http://www.nursing.net*), the Thornbury Nursing Portal (*http://www.nursing-portal.com*), and Nurses and Nursing (*http://www.virtualnurse.com*). WebMD, HealthGate, OnHealth, and HealthCentral provide services for physicians, consumers, nurses, and office managers (Hussey 2000). CVS and PlanetRx represent two pharmacy portals. Both of these sites provide information for consumers and fill prescriptions over the Internet. Portals are constantly evolving. Basic portals furnish information in a static fashion. More sophisticated sites are interactive, allowing users to complete and submit forms on-line, complete health assessments, and perform other activities. There are variations on the portal theme. **Active portals** focus on a specific topic and use a customized search agent that automatically updates searches. **Enterprise portals** provide access to information quickly and easily, extending user access across departments and organizations (Saunders 1999).

Links, also known as hypertext, are words or phrases distinguished from the remainder of the document through the use of highlighting or a different screen color. Links allow users to skip from point to point within or among documents, escaping conventional linear format. Clicking on links with the mouse establishes a **TCP/IP** connection between the client and server, which sends a request in the form of a **HyperText Transfer Protocol (HTTP)** command. **TCP/IP (Transmission Control Protocol/Internet Protocol)** are the most commonly used rules for exchanging information among the networks (Tabar 2000). The TCP/IP connection is closed after the information is sent, while the user is seamlessly transported to another area of the document or another Web site.

HTTP supports hypermedia information systems, including the Web. The initial portion of Web site addresses, "http," refers to this protocol. Links are maintained via a **uniform resource locator (URL),** a string of characters similar to a postal address. The URL identifies the document's Web location and the type of server that it resides on, such as HTTP or other Web server, FTP, or news server. Addresses that include an "s" (https) indicate secured sites, such as those that request entry and submission of credit card numbers.

Box 4–4 lists some steps required to create, post, and maintain a home page. Web sites may consist of a single page or hundreds of pages of information. They vary in complexity from simple text to sites with elaborate graphics, sound, and videos. The person responsible for putting a Web site together and maintaining it is known as the Webmaster.

Nurses may use the World Wide Web to learn more about any of the following topics:

- *Undergraduate, graduate, and doctoral nursing programs.* Many schools have Web pages that provide information about their philosophy, curriculum, and application process. In some cases potential candidates can complete an application on-line.

- *Professional associations.* Many groups, including the American Nurses Association, maintain Web sites that provide information about the purpose of the group and advantages of membership. This increases visibility for the group and serves as a recruitment strategy to attract new members.

- *Nursing informatics.* Announcements of upcoming meetings and calls for papers about nursing informatics can be found on the Web.

Box 4–4

Steps in Creating, Posting, and Maintaining a Home Page

Content and Design Considerations

- *Determine purpose and content.* A well-designed Web page starts with good planning.

- *Consider copyright issues.* Request permission prior to using materials developed by others. Register original work with the U.S. Copyright Office and place a copyright notice with year next to protected material. Develop a written agreement that identifies copyright ownership when working with a Web designer.

- *Select a Web-authoring tool.* A variety of tools can be used to create Web pages, including word processors, browsers, and dedicated Web-authoring tools. The complexity of design, user comfort, and experience are factors in tool selection. Basic knowledge of html markup commands is helpful but not essential.

- *Determine page layout.* Avoid the tendency to crowd pages with too much information and too many images. Limit introductory page information so that essential data is visible without scrolling. Review existing Web pages for pleasing appearance and useful features.

- *Choose links.* Links can make the site more interesting and useful. Organize links to help users find what they are looking for. Use specific link references rather than the phrase, "click here."

- *Include contact information.* Contact information, such as name, organization, credentials, an e-mail link and a postal address, provide the appearance of credibility and a means to establish contact.

- *Update/revision information.* A date helps the user to determine whether posted information and links are current. Updates and revisions also maintain interest, giving users a reason to come back. Consider the addition of icons to identify new or recently revised materials.

- *Download time.* Lengthy download times can frustrate users, causing them to move to other sites.

- *Check the page for errors.* Spelling, grammar, and content errors reflect poorly on the author or site. Review all materials prior to posting.

Posting Considerations

- *Test the page prior to posting.* Ensure that it looks and performs as conceived. Pages that do not load properly or that have a sloppy appearance make a poor impression.

- *Gather information on Internet service providers and Web servers.* Compare service, cost, and support when selecting an ISP and home for Web pages.

- *Establish Internet access.* Internet access is essential for periodic review of Web materials and to receive mail generated by the site.

- *Find a Web server.* Many ISPs and Web sites offer space for home pages. Determine which service provider can best meet the requirements for the page being posted.

- *Obtain a Web or domain address.* An address provides a location to post pages. A domain name refers to one or more IP addresses. Domain names are used in URLs. Suffixes provide information about the type of affiliation. Memorable names help users to find and return to pages.

- *Review and revision procedures.* To remain timely, pages should include review or revision dates.

SOURCE: Adapted from Shellenbarger, T., and Thomas, S. (1996). Creating a nursing home page on the World Wide Web. *Computers in Nursing, 14*(4), 239–245.

- *On-line nursing journals.* Some traditional journals offer electronic versions of their publications in addition to the printed version, while others restrict efforts to the electronic format.
- *Continuing education offerings.* Program announcements and even entire courses may be found on the Web.
- *Disease-specific information and recommended treatment modalities.*
- *Consumer education.* The American Heart Association and the National Cancer Institute are among the growing list of groups that maintain Web sites.

Appendix C provides a list of nursing Web sites and related sites of interest.

Browsers

A **browser** is a retrieval program that allows access to hypertext and hypermedia documents on the Web by using HTTP. The computer acting as server interprets the client's HTTP request and sends the requested document back for display. Browsers can also use Telnet FTP protocols. Browsers may be obtained from an ISP or a computer store, or bundled with other software loaded on PCs at the time of sale. The National Center for Supercomputing Applications (NCSA) developed Mosaic, the first Web browser. Web use increased after the introduction of Mosaic. Additional browsers and versions of Mosaic now exist, although Netscape Navigator and Microsoft's Internet Explorer dominate the market. Browsers use the URL to request a document from the server.

Browsers are available for many types of systems and frequently offer features that extend their utility (Dern 1996, Dickey 1996, Grow 1996). However, there are still many things that browsers do not do. **Helper programs** and **plug-in** programs evolved to fill this void. Helper and plug-in programs are computer applications that have been designed to perform tasks such as view graphics, construct Web pages, play sounds, or even remotely control another PC over the Internet. The main difference between helper and plug-in programs is that the first does not require the browser to be running in order to function while the second does require the browser to be running. Both are typically available on the Web at no cost and are often written in **Java.** Java is a programming language that enables the display of moving text, animation, and musical excerpts on Web pages. Java is popular for the following reasons:

- Applications will run on any Java-enabled browser.
- Actual code can reside on the server until it is downloaded to the client computer as it is needed.
- Java reduces the need to purchase, install, and maintain on-site software.

Microsoft's ActiveX is an alternative to Java for the development of Internet-enabled tools and technologies.

Search Tools

Several types of **search tools** are available to help users find information on the Web (Baxter 1997a, Rodgers 1996). The distinction among the types of tools is sometimes blurred (Vidmar 1999). Some sites, such as Yahoo, index links by broad subject categories. **Search indexes** are appropriate when general information is requested. **Search engines** use automated programs that search the Web, compiling a list of links to sites relevant to keywords supplied by the user. The search may also include Usenet discussions. Search engines are indicated when it is necessary to find a specific topic. LookSmart and AltaVista are examples of search engines. Each search tool maintains its own list of information on the Web and uses its own method to organize materials. Because of this variation in organization, searches conducted with different engines yield different results. Although subtle differences exist among each, all permit the user to enter a search word or phrase. Web sites that contain the search item are then displayed. The number of hits or Web sites that carry this word or phrase varies according to the search engine used and the time the search is done, since new sites are constantly being indexed. Enclosing key phrases in quotation marks is recommended as a way to obtain better results with some, but not all, search tools, otherwise all documents containing portions of the key phrase will be identified. Help pages are available to aid the user in conducting searches. Medical World Search (*http://www.mwsearch.com*) is a search tool for selected medical sites. It uses indexing and a thesaurus of uniform health care terms, which users can view prior to conducting a search.

Until recently, retrieval of comprehensive results meant repeating a search several times with a different search engine each time to identify all relevant sites. **Search engine unifiers** provide a more efficient approach. Search unifiers shorten search time by using several engines at one time. Some examples of search unifiers include Dogpile (*http://www.dogpile. com*), Savvysearch (*http://www.savvysearch.com*), and MetaCrawler (*http:// www.metacrawler.com*).

Listservs

A **Listserv** is actually an e-mail subscription list. A mailing list program copies and distributes all e-mail messages to subscribers. All mail goes through a central computer that acts as the server for the list. Some groups have a moderator who first screens messages for relevance. Listservs are sometimes referred to as discussion groups, mailing lists, or electronic conferences (Baxter 1997b, Dysart 1996, Goldberg 1996, Tomaiuolo 1995). Listservs provide information on thousands of topics. A complete list of listservs may be obtained by sending the request "lists global" to any listserv or by searching the Liszt Select directory of mailing lists at the following Web site: *http://www.liszt.com*. Appendix C identifies specific listservs and their addresses.

To subscribe to a listserv, individuals must send the e-mail message "sub" or "subscribe," followed by their first and last name. Exact commands may vary slightly. Most listservs provide help and instructions upon request. Subscribers may participate in discussions or just monitor them. Listserv participants should read their mail frequently and skim messages for subjects of interest to keep up with discussions. Subscribers may terminate their participation at any time by sending an "unsubscribe" message.

News Groups

Usenet news groups are another popular Internet feature. Usenet groups are similar to listservs in content and diversity (Dysart 1996, Goldberg 1996, Hoffman 1996). More than 20,000 discussion groups exist, each dedicated to a different topic. These groups provide a forum where any user can post messages for discussion and reply. Users do not subscribe to these groups, nor do they receive individual messages. Instead, they may participate at any time free of charge. Internet service providers (ISP) do not carry every news group. ISP administrators decide which news groups will be available to their customers, and how long messages will be stored. Only messages that are currently stored on the user's ISP computer may be read. Older messages are automatically deleted. Special programs called **news reader software** are needed by the individual users to read messages posted on the news group. Many different news readers are available. News readers come bundled with Web browsers. Some examples of nursing Usenet groups include

- *sci.med.nursing.* This is a general forum for the discussion of all types of nursing issues. A review of discussion topics reveals current concerns in the profession by country and practice area. Individual nurses may request assistance with particular problems and receive help from people across the globe.
- *alt.npractitioners.* Issues pertaining to nurse practitioners provide the focus for this group.
- *bit.listserv.snurse-l.* This is a group for International Nursing Students.
- *environmental-health-nursing.* Environmental health and nursing is the organizing theme for this group.

No single person is in charge of universal Usenet procedures, but informal rules and etiquette for participants have developed. The first rule is that all new users should read the **frequently asked questions (FAQ)** document before sending any messages of their own. The FAQ file serves to introduce the group, update new users on recent discussions, and eliminate repetition of questions. Additional Usenet guidelines call for

- *Short postings.* This helps to maintain interest while preventing any individual or subgroup from monopolizing the group.

- *No sensationalism.* The intent of Usenet groups is the sharing of information, not gossip.
- *No outright sales.* Usenet originated in academia and relies on a cooperative environment. Advertising, by custom, is kept at a minimum.
- *Respect for the group focus.* Posting messages that are not relevant wastes time and resources.

News groups may be discovered through any of the following methods: searching the Web by topic; word of mouth from individuals with like interests; conferences; professional publications; or searching through lists of all available news groups. If no news group exists for a given topic, instructions on how to start one can be found on the Internet.

Bulletin Board Systems

Bulletin Board Systems (BBSs) offer a computerized dial-in meeting and announcement system that allows users to make announcements, share files, and conduct limited discussions ("The jargon of the Internet" 1996, Shelly et al. 1996). The traditional BBS differs from listserv and usenet groups in that it does not require Internet access, just a computer and modem. Once very popular, BBSs have largely been replaced by Web sites. A moderator determines what messages will be placed on the BBS.

Access to Health Care Information and Services

Internet and Web resources provide another means to increase access both to information for professionals and health care consumers and to select health care services (Anderson 1999, James-Catalano 1997, Joch 2000a, McCormack 1999, Milholland 1996). Much of this information is free. Federal agencies, health care institutions, physicians, nurses, psychologists, dentists, on-line journals, drug companies, equipment manufacturers, and discussion groups all offer information and advice. Information may be located by symptom, disease, drug interaction, nutrition, common injuries, or support group. Users can post inquiries, read documents of commonly asked questions and answers, or search by keyword or subject. Some services, such as consults and disease management, involve costs. Third-party payers may not pay for Web-based services.

Professional Information Sharing The Internet encourages timely sharing of information among professionals, health care organizations and alliances, vendors, federal agencies, schools, and students. It decreases geographic isolation and allows professionals in remote areas to keep informed of the latest discoveries, treatment modalities, regulations, trends, drugs, and adverse reactions or interactions. Nurses benefit from communication with experts, listservs and discussion groups, on-line literature searches, and access to Web sites. These resources offer tutorials, multimedia instruction, on-line journals, and continuing education. Electronic communication disseminates information quickly, allowing clinicians to learn about revisions in practice guidelines and new study findings. The Internet provides teleconferencing capability for distance learning and continuing education. Electronic communication facilitates networking among nurses, saves labor through the sharing of useful tips and policies, and facilitates collaborative research and writing.

Information for Consumers The rapid development and dissemination of new knowledge today means that the consumer may hear about discoveries and treatments before the professional does. Consumers may even consult the same source as their health care providers. On-line resources can aid in diagnosis, present new treatment options, and help consumers locate support groups. The Web also presents another medium for health teaching. Despite the value of on-line resources, however, these materials cannot be considered as a replacement for actual health care. Most Web sites of health care providers guide users to follow-up care. Questions about professional liability for information found on the Web are unresolved at this time.

The number of client education materials and support groups is growing as more people access the Internet and Web. The Internet and Web offer a way to reach large numbers of people easily and inexpensively. In addition, materials can be updated easily and printed. Some examples of Web sites that furnish client education materials include the American Heart Association and American Cancer Society. Figure 4–2 shows a page from the American Heart Association Web site explaining heart attack.

Some practitioners even provide information on the Web as a public service. AmericasDoctor.com (*http://www.americasdoctor.com*) "Ask a doc" feature invites people to ask medical questions. Users are first asked if they accept a disclaimer, then to identify the topic that their inquiry falls into and their geographic location. This information directs inquiries to physicians in the appropriate area of specialization and provides a mechanism for referrals to a local facility. Another site specific for pediatric questions is DrPaula.com (*http://www.drpaula.com*). Other sites such as Your Family Doctor (*http://www.consult.iperweb.com/*) and Virtual Doctor (*http://www.virtualdoctor.net*) charge a consultation fee. Several sites furnish the opportunity to ask a nurse a question. One example is seen at the University of Missouri neurosurgery Web site (*http://www.surgery.missouri.edu/ns/Services/nurse.html*), where advanced practice nurses answer questions posted by health care consumers.

Evaluation of On-Line Information The Internet may offer a wealth of information, but not all of it is valid or current. Some information on the Web can even be harmful. The lack of a controlling body over the Internet makes it impossible to regulate the quality of information prior to its posting. For this reason health care professionals and consumers must be wary. On-line resources should be evaluated with the same criteria ap-

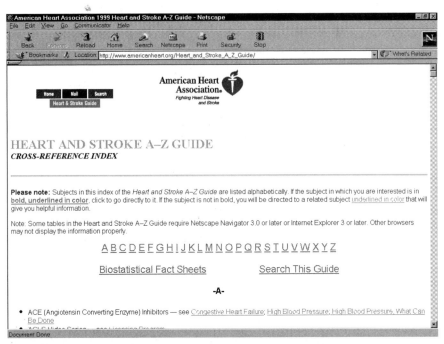

FIGURE 4–2 • "Heart and Stroke A–Z Guide" (reproduced with permission, American Heart Association World Wide Web Site, *Heart and Stroke Guide Section*, © www.americanheart.org, 2000, www.americanheart.org, 1999, copyright American Heart Association. From the AHA Web site, *http://www.americanheart.org/Heart_and_Stroke_A_Z_Guide/*

plied to other sources of information. Large professional associations, such as hospitals, universities, government, and official health organizations, tend to have the most reliable sites. A number of groups are looking at the quality of posted materials, including most professional organizations, the Health Internet Ethics (Hi-Ethics) Alliance, and The Health on the Net Foundation (HON). Hi-Ethics is an alliance of 20 health information Web sites whose mission is to develop standards designed to ensure that consumers are provided with health information that is reliable, safe, and trustworthy. Hi-Ethics will look at the following four areas: content, advertising, privacy, and commerce. HON now indexes sites that comply with the criteria that it has established to help ensure the quality of health. These criteria can been found on the HON Web site (*http://www.hon.ch/HONcode*). Some points for evaluation follow:

• *Credentials of the source.* Inability to validate the authenticity of the source is one negative aspect associated with the Internet. This validation can be difficult unless the source can be traced back to a reputable university or other agency. Many messages and Web sites identify a person or persons to contact for further information. When facts and studies are cited the original source should be stated so users can review it and draw their own conclusions.

- *Accuracy.* Since no single person controls information that is placed on the Internet, mere existence of information does not indicate that it is accurate. Postings should identify contact persons or cite references that may be checked to allow evaluation of posted information.

- *Date of issue or revision.* One problem with the Internet and World Wide Web is that not all pages contain dates indicating when material was written, revised, or reviewed, making it difficult to determine whether information is current.

- *Bias of the posting organization or person.* Commercial uses of the Internet are growing daily. The consumer must consider whether information is biased in favor of a particular product or commercial service. One means to consider bias is to look for a site listing of funding and advertising policy.

On-Line Publications and Journals

Soaring costs for paper, layout, printing and distribution, and the time that it takes to get materials to press make publication an expensive process (Siwicki 1996, Shelly et al. 1996). Publication via the Internet offers several advantages over traditional approaches, including the following:

- *A shorter time frame between writing and publication.* This is particularly important when material is quickly outdated, as occurs in health care. Individuals can place information on the Internet as soon as it is written rather than wait until a formal article or manuscript is accepted for publication.

- *Lower printing and distribution costs.* Electronic publication eliminates the need for paper, postage, and handling costs. Instead, documents are transferred from computer to computer in binary code. This transfer process is known as **electronic document interchange (EDI).** EDI also lowers publication costs because information is typed only once. An example of EDI is seen when an author submits an article for publication via file transfer protocol.

- *Revisions can be made quickly and distributed instantly.* For example, recommended treatment modalities are often changed with the latest research findings. Texts, professional standards of practice, nursing procedure manuals, and advice for consumers must reflect current recommendations. The electronic format also eliminates the need to replace and discard large volumes of out-of-date print materials.

- *Facilitation of joint authorship.* Colleagues at any location can share ideas and revise manuscripts without actually meeting in one physical location or spending scarce resources for travel or telephone charges.

- *Rapid identification of knowledge deficits.* Frequently asked questions on the Internet may indicate areas where research is needed. Surveys can be conducted quickly via e-mail and other electronic means.
- *Multimedia capability.* The inclusion of sound, voice, and still images and video permit a comprehensive simulation of clinical problems and aid in student learning.
- *Immediate access to materials.* Persons who need or want information late in the evening or at night do not need to wait until a library is open.

Several nursing and allied health journals are currently available on-line. Some are published in both print and electronic format, while others are available only electronically. The existence of on-line journals may be researched through many of the same methods discussed earlier to find discussion groups and Web sites. Appendix C lists URLs for nursing and allied health journals available on-line.

Marketing Services

Web sites are a cost-effective public relations tool in health care. This is particularly true for sites that attract return visitors through the incorporation of interactive features. The Internet and Web can provide a competitive edge in the health care delivery system in the following ways:

- *Job postings.* Both employers and persons who are job hunting can use the Web to advertise positions and find new opportunities. Several sites offer help in locating job opportunities. The American Journal of Nursing Career Guide (*http://www.nursingcenter.com/career/ajn.cfm*) and Springhouse Publishing (*http://www.springnet.com*) maintain two such sites. Several employment services make it possible to complete resumes on-line, and some employers incorporate employment applications into their Web sites for electronic completion.
- *Virtual tours of educational institutions.* Some schools use their Web sites to introduce their facility and key people as well as allow the potential student to view available resources and complete an application on-line.
- *Support groups.* Emotional support and information is available for professionals and health care consumers. For example, the listserv AANurses (*AANurses@ontos.usa.com*) is a support group for nurses, while the news group alt.support.arthritis is a support group for the lay population. The presence of these resources on the Internet makes them readily available to a large number of people 24 hours a day.
- *Advertisement of services and consumer education.* Many health care providers furnish information about their services, assist with finding a physician or dentist, and provide general health care information

via Web sites. Figure 4–3 depicts the home page for a health system that uses the Web in this way.

- *Dissemination and revision of product information.* Pharmaceutical companies and hospital equipment suppliers may also maintain Web sites that provide additional information about their products.

- *On-line risk assessments.* Some health care providers post tools that users may complete to determine their risk for developing a particular health problem. Basic advice for follow-up care may be provided along with names of area providers.

- *Completion of forms.* The time spent in the health care delivery system can be shortened when on-line prescreening forms are completed at the same time that appointments are requested (Brakeman 2000).

E-health

The Internet offers the potential to increase access to health care information, empower consumers, educate practitioners, and transmit information quickly and cheaply (Blodgett 1996, Marietti 2000, Milholland 1996, Paone 1995a). It is already used for business transactions, electronic prescriptions, on-line hospital registration, consumer education via Web sites, continuing education, and communication among profession-

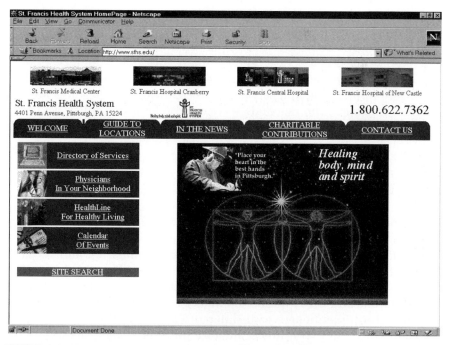

FIGURE 4–3 • Reproduced by permission of St. Francis Health System

als. Numerous terms have been coined recently to describe these applications including e-business, e-commerce, and e-health or e-healthcare. **E-business** and **e-commerce** are not specific to health care. Both of these terms refer to services, sales, and business conducted over the Internet (Tabar 2000). Benefits associated with e-business and e-commerce include real-time responses to inquiries, clinical alerts, and the ability to submit claims quickly. **E-health** brings information, products, and services on-line. **E-care** is a broader term used to refer to the automation of all parts of the care delivery process across administrative, clinical, and departmental boundaries. E-care can include purchasing and patient management. The Internet has even been proposed as the infrastructure to achieve the computerized client record by providing a network to link all health care providers together, as well as payers and clients. Examples of e-health include wellness tips found on Web sites, e-mail reminders of appointments, follow-up e-mail from health care practitioners to consumer questions, electronic prescriptions, centralized storage of health records on the Web, regional telemedicine networks on the Web, consults, and long-term management of chronically ill patients. Another major application is electronic submission of claims and payment. Electronic claims submission reduces time and costs for claims submission and results in fewer rejections. Other aspects of e-health include on-line purchases of supplies (Joch 2000b).

The Internet provides easy access to health-related information, including medical literature, location of clinical trials, and support groups for persons with particular health problems. An increasing number of providers and third-party payors are taking advantage of the power of the Internet to market their services and publish up-to-date patient education materials, wellness newsletters, and eligibility information in a cost-effective fashion. At the same time the number of individuals seeking on-line health care information and services is also growing. The result is an empowered consumer who demands services now found on other Web sites but slow to arrive in health care. These include personalized, service-oriented features, such as scheduling, reminders for care, physician messaging, personal Web pages for the storage of health care information, and remote monitoring. The majority of these features streamline care, improve the quality of service, and improve patient tracking.

Another service that ultimately benefits the consumer is the electronic prescription. Electronic prescriptions eliminate the problem of lost or unreadable prescriptions while providing access to Web-based personal health information, drug interaction warnings, formularies, and verifications that reduce the incidence of medication errors. Handheld prescribing devices facilitate the electronic prescription process. The use of the Web to store health care information makes it available from different locations and to practitioners with different computer systems. A number of current sites allow consumers to store information and modify it for access when it is needed. One Web-based application that holds great promise for improved patient outcomes and lower long-term costs is disease management (Joch 2000a). Chronic illness now accounts for the majority of health care costs. Web-based management provides a way to monitor large numbers of patients efficiently on a daily basis. Client participation is stimulated through the development of health goals and recording improvements. A device may be used to measure overall health. In this case, readings are obtained and sent for review by a health care practitioner. Devices have been used for asthmatics and persons with congestive heart failure. Technology can warn practitioners of abnormal findings that require intervention. The simplicity of the Web allows the addition of features easily and relatively inexpensively.

E-health is changing the relationships between health care professionals and consumers as well as the way that the health care industry is conducted (Douglad 1999, Gillespie 2000, Goedert 2000, Hagland 2000). Browsers and the Web provide a truly user-friendly environment that allow users to focus on their needs rather than the technology (Kohn 2000). The Web provides the framework to expedite the delivery of services and revolutionize the way that care is delivered. Web portals help to create virtual communities both for professionals and consumers. Educated consumers come for treatment armed with knowledge that empowers them and may lead them to question treatment modalities. Some authorities on Internet health care applications expect that consumers will drive the market for on-line services (Dyer 1999, Fell 2000).

Current trends in health care delivery include use of on-line services for purchasing, referrals, submission of claims, and storage of patient information. There is a shift away from heavily modified information systems maintained by the individual organization toward Web-based applications supported by vendors. These are known as **application service providers** or **ASPs.** ASPs are ready for immediate use and available at a lower initial cost (Stammer 2000). ASPs can facilitate administrative and clinical functions.

CONCERNS RELATED TO THE USE OF THE INTERNET

The single largest concern related to Internet use in health care is the security of client data, followed by worries over slowdown, collapse, and the ability to transact business smoothly (Goldberg 1996). Lesser concerns include viral contamination and a lack of adherence to Internet standards among some products.

Firewalls

The open design of the Internet invites security abuse, particularly for private networks with Internet access. At least 20 percent of all organizations with an Internet connection have had a security breach. For this reason, private networks need a gateway to intercept and examine Internet messages before they are permitted to enter the private network (Ahuja 1996, "Attack of the Internet intruders" 1996, Paone 1995a, b, Semeria 1996). A **gateway** is a combination of hardware and software used to connect local area networks with larger networks. A **firewall** is a type of gateway designed to protect private network resources from outside hackers, network damage, and theft or misuse of information. A firewall should be transparent to users. A firewall does not preclude the need for a security plan or periodic security testing. Outside intruders may still be able to penetrate firewall protection.

Not all threats to a network arise from outside sources. Firewalls alone do not protect against internal attacks or prevent viral contamination. Strong security policies for employees can minimize these threats as long as users are aware of the policies, their responsibilities, and the implications for policy violations. Another key factor in network protection is knowledge. Network administrators must educate themselves about attacks on Internet sites and protective measures recommended by the federally funded Computer Emergency Response Team (CERT) Coordination Center and Usenet groups.

Web Security

Most organizations focus security efforts on their internal networks, for the obvious reason that any disruption in computer operation affects service. As a consequence of this action, Web sites receive less attention. This omission leaves Web sites vulnerable to attack because of their visibility and the fact that they have been easy targets. However, disruption of Web sites may impact business operation as well. For example, hacker changes to Web pages may prove embarrassing, endanger consumers who follow altered advice, and/or result in libel charges. This recognition brings with it a heightened awareness of the need to safeguard Web sites as well as internal networks. At the same time, Webmasters are being encouraged to put their organizations on the Web so the world can get to them, but they must also protect the organization from intruders (Behan 1999).

The following measures can protect Web sites and their information (Dorobek and Jackson 1996):

- *Construct a separate firewall for the Web server.* Firewalls provide the same level of protection for Web servers as they do for private networks with Internet access. Some, if not all, hacker attacks can be prevented with a firewall for each Web server.

- *Limit access to Web page content or configuration.* The risk of internal attacks or accidental damage is directly related to the number of persons with authority to change Web information or setup.

- *Isolate Web servers.* Web servers should not have direct connections to other agency systems, nor should they be located at a site subject to attack. This action minimizes the chance of Web site damage.

- *Heed security advisories.* Updates on hacker attacks and warnings on new breach techniques are posted by several sites on the Web including the WWW Security FAQ and commercial sites such as *Symantec.com.* Webmasters should anticipate attack and take proactive measures.

- *Discontinue unused services.* Unused services may serve as a portal for attack.

- *Install alarms to hail attacks.* Webmasters or network administrators need to install alarms and tracking mechanisms to alert them to attack early as a means to minimize Web site damage.

Organizational Policy

Organizations with an Internet connection need policies that address the following areas (Leinfuss 1996, Smith and Kallman 1996):

- *E-mail privacy.* The organization has the legal right to read employee e-mail unless stated otherwise. Employees should be aware of their organization's e-mail policy.

- *Encryption.* Potentially sensitive data should be coded or encrypted to prevent unauthorized people from reading it. One example of sensitive data that would require encryption for transmittal over the Internet is HIV status.

- *Transmission of employee data or photographs.* Employers should obtain consent prior to the transmittal of employee pictures or personal data over the Internet.

- *Intellectual ownership.* Guidelines should establish how issues of intellectual ownership are determined for network postings and other communications. In other words, it is important to resolve who owns the information: the employee who developed it or the employer.

- *Free speech.* The organization's stance on ideas or images that it considers offensive or inappropriate should be plainly delineated.

- *Acceptable Internet uses in the workplace.* Permissible Internet uses must be identified and communicated to employees. Violations of accepted use may constitute grounds for dismissal. One means to enforce this policy is the inclusion of a section on acceptable Internet use in the employee's annual performance evaluation.

- *Citation of sources and verification of information downloaded from the Internet/Web.* Authors of materials on the Internet and Web deserve the same recognition as authors of any other media. Failure to cite sources is plagiarism. Guidelines for the citation of on-line resources can be found at the American Psychological Association and the Modern Language Association Web sites as well as at most college and university sites.

- *Acknowledgment of receipt of Internet policies.* Employees should sign a statement that they have read and understand the organization's Internet policies at the time of hire and upon yearly review.

Overload

The Internet consists of many interconnected networks. Actual collapse is improbable, although vendor and facility outages and problems will likely continue as the number of users increases. Many first-time providers are undercapitalized or have poorly trained staff, so that periodic overload or slow service can be expected. These problems raise interesting questions about maintaining data availability and integrity for the health care institution that uses the Internet to transport health data.

The majority of overload and collapse problems result from technical problems such as traffic jams, transmission difficulties, and poor Web site design (Anthes and Wagner 1996, Dern 1996, Metcalfe 1996a). These problems may occur on the user's network or an outside network. The popularity of the Internet makes it difficult to accommodate the needs of all of the users. For this reason work is in progress to launch another version of the Internet. Internet2 (Internet2/2000 mission and goals) is a collaborative effort of universities, government, industry, and various research and educational groups. The purpose of the Internet2 effort is to build and operate a research network capable of enhancing delivery of education and other services, including health care. This includes the development and support of advanced applications and standards. Another project that is working on ways to improve Internet speed and efficiency is the Next Generation Internet launched by the Clinton Administration (Baldwin 1999).

Viral Contamination

Viruses may be spread when files are imported for use without subjecting them to a viral scan (Goldberg 1996, Tomaiuolo 1995). The danger of viral contamination cannot be eliminated, but it can be reduced through the following measures:

- *Strict policies on Internet use.* These policies should include scanning all files prior to use, including FTP files. Viruses may be included in materials available for public consumption.
- *Using the latest version of antiviral software.* New viruses are created daily. Older releases of antiviral software cannot recognize new viruses.

THE DEVELOPMENT OF INTRANETS

Intranets are private computer networks that use Internet protocols and technologies, including Web browsers, servers, and languages, to facilitate collaborative data sharing (Metcalfe 1996a). They were first developed in response to concerns over slowdowns, security breaches, and fears of Internet collapse. Intranets sit behind firewalls or other barriers and are not normally available to people outside of the organization.

Purpose

The major reason to use intranets in health care is that they allow disparate information systems to communicate (Kohn 1996, Littauer 1997, McCormack 1996, Morita 1997, Siwicki 1996). This represents a major accomplishment that has yet to be fully realized, either with or without intranets. Intranets can save money by providing an easy-to-use, familiar interface that is intuitive and therefore requires little training. Intranets are also an effective tool for marketing and advertising. Intranets in health care enterprises may also be used for mail and messaging, conferencing, and the infrastructure for the computerized client record after security, ownership, and legal issues are settled. It is difficult to predict the full impact of intranets upon health care at this time. Network management through the Web from any site promises to eliminate the need for expensive, on-site network management around the clock. Intranets offer a number of advantages, as shown in Box 4–5. Most organizations use the corporate intranet first for publishing (Wilkins and Hovhanesian 1999). This cuts down on paper and distribution costs, makes materials availability more quickly and widely, and helps to ensure version control. It also acclimates employees to using the intranet as the single source of information. This type of intranet application may be used to distribute

---

Box 4–5   Advantages of Intranets

- Easy to use
- Familiar approach for users
- Limited training required
- Relatively inexpensive
- Support multiplatform approach and open systems approach
- Fit well with client/server architecture
- Provide paperless distribution of internal documents
- Improve interdepartmental communication
- Provide inexpensive access to corporate data
- Supplement existing network with links to other sites/systems
- Permit rapid retrieval of information, which may save lives if health care agencies use intranets
- Allow health care agencies to focus on data presentation

policy and procedure manuals or other reference materials. As intranet use evolves, additional features may be added, such as the ability for employees to view and enroll in benefits, request vacation days, and apply for internal jobs. Intranets can even be used to hold on-line meetings, saving travel time and costs.

Problems

The following have been identified as intranet problem areas:

- *Inadequate security.* This situation is expected to improve as vendors develop new products to meet consumer demand (Lopez 1997, Weston and Nash 1996). This is a major concern in health care, where confidential client information is transmitted.

- *A lack of written policies.* Issues of ownership, appropriate use, and conditions that may lead to termination of employment must be established (Nash 1996).

- *System design and demands.* The same server may be used for Internet and intranet connections. This may decrease initial cost but it cannot keep pace with the demands posed by both Internet and intranet use (Desai 1997, Kohn 1996, McCormack 1996). Additional equipment and/or software may be required.

- *A lack of available intranet management tools (Littauer 1997).* This type of software facilitates tracking of individual users as well as overall traffic patterns. It is expected that more tools of this type will be available soon.

EXTRANETS

Extranets represent another variation of Internet technology ("Beyond browsers" 1996, Metcalfe 1996b). **Extranets** are networks that sit outside the protected internal network of an organization, and use Internet software and communication protocols for electronic commerce and use by outside suppliers or customers. For example, a vendor may develop an extranet that customers can use to obtain prices and place orders for merchandise. Security measures can be used to restrict access and secure information, making extranets more private than the Internet. Extranets are not the same as portals, although there are similaries between the two. Portals can be created on intranets, extranets, or the Internet.

CASE STUDY EXERCISES

As the representative for your medical center's Better Care Initiative, a project with the purpose of identifying ways that services can be delivered in a more efficient manner, you have suggested that the Internet be made available to clinicians at the point of care. You must develop a report listing the potential uses of the Internet, as well as potential problems that might occur.

• • •

One of your clients has a rare genetic defect. The client is requesting additional information about this from you, but no reference books on the unit describe this condition. Discuss strategies for how you might obtain this information using the Internet and electronic communication.

SUMMARY

- Electronic communication is the ability to exchange information through the use of computer equipment and software, using network connections or a modem.

- The Internet is a network of networks, connecting computers worldwide. It offers a wealth of information about many topics, and can be extremely useful for the exchange of health care information.

- The World Wide Web (Web or WWW), a popular Internet feature, allows users to find information more easily by conducting word searches using browser software or locating a specific Web site or address. It is characterized by a graphical user interface that makes it easy to use.

- A popular Web feature is the home page, the first page seen at a particular Web location. The home page provides general information about a topic, person, or organization.

- Links are words, phrases, or pictures that are distinguished from other parts of a WWW home page, usually by color, and enable users to move directly to another Web location.

- Nurses, other clinicians, and consumers may use the Web to obtain information regarding clinical topics, diseases, treatments, and health care agencies.

- Electronic mail, or e-mail, is the use of computer technology to transmit messages from one person to another. Delivery can be almost instantaneous. The Internet allows e-mail to be sent anywhere in the world, as long as the recipient has an Internet address.

- File transfer is the ability to move files from one location to another across a network.

- Other forms of electronic communication include listservs (electronic mailing lists) and usenet groups (message discussion groups). These forums provide information and support.

- E-commerce, or e-business, uses Internet technology to provide health care organizations with mechanisms to safely and quickly exchange information with other business entities.

- E-health refers to on-line availability of health information, products, and services.

- E-care is a broad term used to refer to the automation of all parts of the care delivery process, including purchasing and patient management.

- Security is a major concern surrounding the use of the Internet and electronic communication. Firewalls and encryption are two prevalent strategies for safeguarding information.

- Internet technology is used internally in an organization in systems known as intranets, or external to the organization in systems known as extranets.

- Application service providers (ASPs) represent an alternative to institutional purchase and customization of information systems and software applications. ASP advantages include lower initial expenses, reduced wait time, and easier upgrades.

REFERENCES

Ahuja, V. (1996). *Network and Internet Security.* Chestnut Hill, MA: Academic.

Anderson, J. G. (1999). The business of cyberhealthcare. *MDComputing, 16*(6), 23–25.

Anthes, G. H., and Wagner, M. (1996). Internet outages spark disaster fears. *Computerworld, 30*(27), 14.

Attack of the Internet intruders. (February 1996). *Data Communications,* 20.

Baldwin, G. (1999). New Internet technologies getting closer and closer. *Health Data Management, 7*(10), 14, 24.

Baxter, B. (1996). Nursing the Net. *Nursing96, 26*(12), 26.

Baxter, B. (1997a). Nursing the Net: Traveling the Web with search engines. *Nursing97, 27*(4), 30–31.

Baxter, B. (1997b). Nursing the Net: Using E-mail and listservs. *Nursing97, 27*(1), 31–32.

Behan, M. (1999). Internet security: Making your e-business a safe business. *Beyond Computing,* 8(5), 34–39.

Beyond browsers. (7 October 1996). *InformationWeek,* 65–66.

Blodgett, M. (1996). Health care's on-line remedy? *Computerworld, 30*(27), 14.

Bort, J. (1996). The key to security. *Infoworld, 18*(36), 1, 51–52.

Brakeman, L. (2000). Number of Internet users tops the 100 million mark. *Managed Healthcare, 10*(1), 48, 2p.

Cini, A. (1996). How to play and win the Intranet game. *Internetwork*, *8*(1), 30–32, 34–35.

Dern, D. (1996). Beefing up browsers. *Communications News*, *33*(10), 46–47.

Desai, V. (1997). Web-based management: Welcome to your next nightmare. *Internetwork*, *8*(1), 40–42.

Dickey, S. (1996). To standardize or not to standardize. *Midrange Systems*, *9*(17), 16, 18, 20.

Dictionary of Computing, 4th ed. (1996). New York: Oxford University Press.

Dorobek, C. J., and Jackson, W. (1996). DOJ incident exposes Web insecurities. *Government Computer News*, *15*(23), 1, 100.

Douglad, J.V. (1999). Healthcare adopts e-commerce. *MDComputing*, *16*(6), 13.

Dyer, K.A. (1999). Cybermedicine enters the new millennium. *MDComputing*, *16*(6), 49–50.

Dysart, J. (1996). Using Usenet. *Beyond Computing*, *5*(9), 42–44.

Edwards, M. J. (1996). E-mail virus wall: Medicine for Internet-borne viruses. *Infoworld*, *18*(36), N/2, N/4.

Fell, D. (31 March 2000). Health care and the Internet. Paper presented at *Health Care 2000 Forum: A New Beginning*, Monroeville, PA.

File Transfer Protocol. (1997). *The Practical Internet Guide*. On the Web at: *http://www.practinet.com/iguide/pftp.htm*.

Gillespie, G. (2000). Hanging an electronic shingle. *Health Data Management*, *8*(1), 26, 28, 30.

Goedert, J. (2000). A real shot in the arm. *Health Data Management*, *8*(2), 34, 36,38.

Goldberg, B. (1996). Surfing the Internet. *Enterprise Systems Journal*, *11*(7), 44, 46, 48–49.

Grow, K. (1996). The ActiveX files. *Internetwork*, *8*(1), 36–37.

Guenther, K. (1999). Wanted: A new healthcare e-dentity. *Health Management Technology*, *20*(10), 67, 2p.

Hagland, M. (2000). Electronic prescribing gold rush. *Healthcare Informatics*, *17*(2), 20, 22.

Hoffman, P. E. (1996). *The Internet Instant Reference*, 3rd ed. Alameda, CA: Sybex.

Hussey, J.S. (2000). Healthcare on-line. *Healthcare Informatics*, *17*(2), 100.

Internet2 Mission and goals. (Downloaded 3 March 2000). Available on-line at: *htttp://www.internet2.edu/html/mission_and_goals.html*.

Internet Society. (17 September 1999). *Internet Society Mission Statement*. On the Web at: *http://www.isoc.org/isoc/mission*.

Jacobs, P. (1996). Site management pains. *Infoworld*, *18*(44), 63–64.

James-Catalano, C. (1997). Doctor's advice. *Internet World*, *8*(2), 30, 32.

The jargon of the Internet. (1996). *Health Data Management*, *4*(12), 61–62.

Joch, A. (2000a). Can the Web save disease management? *Healthcare Informatics*, *17*(3), 59–60, 62, 64.

Joch, A. (2000b). The web reinvents procurement systems and virtual medical superstores help healthcare keep prices low. *Healthcare Informatics, 17*(2), 58, 60.

Johnson, D. L. (1996). Modems: The gateway to cyberspace. *Computers in Nursing, 14*(4), 215–217.

Klaus, C. W., & Ranum, M. J. (1996). Does scanning for vulnerabilities mean your firewall is safe? *Infoworld, 18*(31), 79–80.

Kohn, D. (1996). "Intranets" ease costs of healthcare communications. *Health Measures, 1*(3), 42.

Kohn, D. (2000). Caught in the Web by the killer app! An update. *Journal of Healthcare Information Management, 14*(1), 7–15.

Leinfuss, E. (1996). Policy over policing. *Infoworld, 18*(34), 55–56.

Littauer, B. (1997). Why you need a full view of your Intranet. *Internetwork, 8*(1), 8.

Lopez, S. J. (1997). The Internet paradigm will dominate in 1997. *Internetwork, 8*(1), 6.

Marietti, C. (2000). A common thread. *Healthcare Informatics, 17*(2), 12.

McCollum, T. (1996). The future is now. *Nation's Business, 84*(12), 16–19, 22–24, 26, 28.

McCormack, J. (1996). Live on the Internet: Surgery. *Health Data Management, 4*(11), 21–22.

McCormack, J. (1999). The top 10 ways the Internet is changing Health Care I.T. *Health Data Management, 7*(12), 34–36, 38, 39.

Metcalfe, B. (1996a). The Internet is collapsing: The question is who's going to be caught in the fall. *Infoworld, 18*(47), 62.

Metcalfe, B. (1996b). Private information highways will avoid all congestion on the Net. *Infoworld, 18*(43), 41.

Milholland, D. K. (September 1996). New information technologies suggest new roles for nurses. *The American Nurse*, 2–3.

Morita, R. (1997). Taking management to the Web. *Internetwork, 8*(1), 8.

Nash, K. S. (1996). Policing the net. *Computerworld, 30*(27), 1, 89.

Paone, J. (1995a). Cyberspace invaders. *Internetwork, 6*(6), 33–34, 46.

Paone, J. (1995b). Guarding the Internet door. *Internetwork, 6*(12), S1, S3–S4.

Rodgers, B. L. (1996). Searching the Web. *Computers in Nursing, 14*(4), 246–247.

Saunders, J. (1999). Corporate portal opens data door. *Computing Canada, 25*(43), 23, 2p.

Semeria, C. (1996). Internet firewalls and security. *Enterprise Systems Journal, 11*(7), 32, 34, 36, 37–38.

Shellenbarger, T., and Thomas, S. (1996). Creating a nursing home page on the World Wide Web. *Computers in Nursing, 14*(4), 239–245.

Shelly, G. B., Cashman, T. J., Waggoner, G. A., and Waggoner, W. C. (1996). *Using computers: A gateway to information.* Danvers, MA: Boyd & Fraser.

Simpson, R. (1995). Getting wired for success. *Nursing Administration Quarterly, 19*(4), 89–91.

Siwicki, B. (1996). Intranets in health care. *Health Data Management, 4*(8), 36–38, 41–42, 44–47.

Smith, J. J., and Kallman, E. A. (1996). Managing the net. *Beyond Computing, 5*(3), 14–15.

Staggers, N. (1996). Connecting points: Electronic mail tips and tricks. *Computers in Nursing, 14*(5), 264–266.

Stammer, L. (February 2000). ASPs will transform healthcare into a truly Internet-friendly business. *Healthcare Informatics, 17*(2), 46, 48.

Sykes, R. (1996). On-line: Can we chat? *Infoworld 18*(47), 7W/4.

Tabar, P. (2000). The latest word. *Healthcare Informatics, 17*(3), 75–132.

Tomaiuolo, N. G. (1995). Accessing nursing resources on the Internet. *Computers in Nursing, 13*(4), 159–164.

Vidmar, D.J. (1999). Darwin on the Web: The evolution of search tools. *Computers in Libraries, 19*(5), 22, 5p.

Welz, G. (1997). Multimedia comes of age. *Internet World, 8*(2), 45–49.

Weston, R., and Nash, K. S. (1996). Intranet fever. *Computerworld, 30*(27), 1, 15.

Wilder, C., Davis, B., and Dalton, G. (8 February 1999). Data gateway. *InformationWeek*, 18–20, 22.

Wilkins, A., and Hovhanesian, J. (1999). The virtual workplace. *Healthcare Informatics, 16*(11), 65–66, 68.

Wink, D. M. (1995). Electronic communication: An introduction to nursing on the Internet. *Nurse Educator, 20*(6), 9–13.

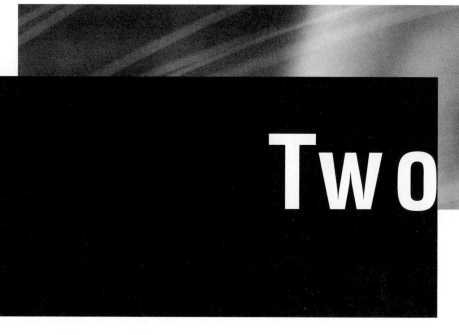

Two

Health Care Information Systems

5

Health Care Information Systems

After completing this chapter, you should be able to:

- Identify the various types of information systems used within health care institutions.

- Define the following terms: *hospital information systems*, *clinical information systems*, *nursing information system*, and *administrative information systems.*

- Explain the functions of a nursing information system.

- Differentiate between the nursing process and critical pathways/protocol approaches to the design of a nursing system.

- Review the key features and impacts on nursing associated with order entry, laboratory, radiology, and pharmacy information systems.

- Describe the functions of patient registration and scheduling systems.

- Explain the purpose of decision support and expert systems.

A n **information system** can be defined as the use of computer hard-ware and software to process data into information to solve a prob-lem. The term **hospital information system (HIS)** refers to a group of systems used within a hospital or enterprise that supports and enhances patient care. The HIS comprises two major types of information systems: clinical information systems and administrative information systems. Ac-cording to Axford and Carter (1996), **clinical information systems (CISs)** are large, computerized database management systems. Clinicians use these systems to access client data that is used to plan, implement, and evaluate care. Clinical information systems may also be referred to as client care information systems. Some examples of CISs include nursing, labora-tory, pharmacy, radiology, and medical information systems. **Administra-tive information systems** support client care by managing financial and demographic information and providing reporting capabilities. This cate-gory includes client management; financial, payroll, and human resources; and quality assurance systems. Figure 5–1 shows the relationships between various components of a hospital information system.

Clinical and administrative information systems may be designed to meet the needs of one or more departments or functions within the orga-nization. These can be implemented as stand-alone systems, or may work with other systems to provide information sharing and seamless function-ality for the users. Any one health care enterprise may use one or several of the clinical and administrative systems, but will probably not use all of them.

CLINICAL INFORMATION SYSTEMS

Although many clinical information systems are designed for use within one hospital department, the data collected by each system is frequently used by clinicians from several areas. For example, the nurse may docu-

FIGURE 5–1 • Relationship of the Hospital Information System Components

ment a client's allergies in the initial assessment. This data may be used by the physician, the pharmacist, and the radiologist during the client's hospital stay. The goal of CISs is to inform clinicians regarding treatments and tests in ways that keep them from overspending on unnecessary services, while still delivering the appropriate medical response (Morrissey 1996). The following descriptions of CISs address those that are most frequently seen in the hospital setting.

Nursing Information Systems

A **nursing information system** supports the use and documentation of nursing processes and provides tools for managing the delivery of nursing care (Hendrickson 1993). An effective nursing information system must accomplish two goals. The first goal is that the system should support the way that nurses function, allowing them the flexibility to use the system to view data and collect necessary information, provide quality client care, and document the client's condition and the care that was given. Necessary information includes past medical history, allergies, test results, and progress notes, among other things. The second goal of an effective nursing information system is that it should support and enhance nursing practice through improved access to information and tools. These include on-line literature searches such as the Cumulative Index of Nursing and Allied Health Literature (CINAHL) and MedLine, and automated drug information and hospital policy/procedure guidelines. Consideration of these two goals in the selection and implementation of a nursing system will ensure that it benefits nursing. The challenge for nursing is to identify and implement technology and information systems solutions that provide more breadth, depth, flexibility, and standardization (Hughes 1997).

Generally there are two approaches to nursing care and documentation using automated information systems. These are the traditional nursing process approach and the critical pathway, or protocols, approach. The traditional nursing process approach allows documentation of nursing care using well-established formats, such as admission assessments, problem lists, and care plans. A more recent approach uses critical pathways as guidelines for multidisciplinary care and documentation. These protocols suggest specific treatments related to the client's diagnosis and outline the anticipated outcomes. The advantages of using a nursing information system are listed in Box 5–1.

Nursing Process Approach The nursing process approach to automated documentation is based on the paper forms traditionally used by nurses. Often the nursing diagnosis serves as the organizational framework. Many current information systems follow this format.

- *Documentation of nursing admission assessment and discharge instructions.* A menu-driven approach to the admission assessment assures capture of essential information. A **menu** lists related commands that can be selected from a computer screen to accomplish a task. For example, the menu may include selections such as past medical history, advanced directives, organ donation status, psychosocial history, medications, and review of body systems. This approach can also be used to ensure that all necessary information is covered in the client's discharge instructions, including follow-up appointments and diagnostic studies; diet and activity restrictions; wound care; and

Box 5–1 | **Advantages of a Nursing Information System**

- Increased time spent with clients
- Access to information
- Improved quality of documentation
- Improved quality of client care
- Increased nursing productivity
- Improved communications
- Reduced errors of omissions
- Reduced medication errors
- Reduced hospital costs
- Increased nurse job satisfaction
- Compliance with JCAHO* regulations
- Development of a common clinical database
- Improved client perception of care
- Enhanced ability to track client's record
- Enhanced ability to recruit/retain staff
- Improved hospital image

SOURCE: Saba, V., and McCormick, K. (1998). Essentials of Computers for Nurses, 2nd ed. New York: McGraw-Hill. With permission from The McGraw-Hill Companies.

medication information such as drug names, instructions for administration, and common side effects that the client should report. The system should generate printed copies of these instructions for clients to review upon discharge and for their use at home.

- *Generation of a nursing worklist that indicates routine scheduled activities related to the care of each client.* These activities can be grouped according to scheduled time or skill level.

- *Documentation of discrete data or activities such as vital signs, weight, and intake and output measurements.* The automation of this type of data promotes accuracy and allows the data to be readily available to all care providers at any time.

- *Documentation of routine aspects of patient care, such as bathing, positioning, blood glucose measurements, notation of dietary intake, and/or wound care in a flowsheet format.*

- *Standardized care plans that the nurse can individualize for clients as needed.* This feature saves time yet allows flexibility to address the client's needs while promoting quality care.

- *Documentation of nursing care in a progress note format.* The nurse may accomplish this through narrative charting, charting by exception, or flowsheet charting. Regardless of the method, automated documentation can improve the overall quality of charting by prompting the nurse with predefined selections. Box 5–2 describes three of these traditional formats and some typical automation approaches.

- *Documentation of medication administration.* This complex procedure may require several steps, described below.

  1. The system can generate a medication list, indicating which medications are scheduled for administration during the nurse's shift. This list may also include unscheduled or prn medications for each client, as well as instructions related to administration. For example, the list might include a reminder to check the client's pulse before giving digoxin, and to hold the medication if the pulse falls below a standard rate or the physician's ordered parameter. The nurse may use this list to write notes and check off medications as they are given if a portable device is not available for direct documentation into the system.

  2. The nurse can then access the medication administration record (MAR) in the information system to document medications that were given or held. An automated MAR helps the nurse document administration of medications in a manner that satisfies regulatory and nursing policy requirements. The system prompts the nurse to enter other related information, such as injection site, pulse, or pain scale value. If a medication is not given, the system prompts the nurse to enter the reason.

  3. The system can generate a report indicating medications that were not charted as a reminder to the nurse.

Box 5–2 **Automation of Traditional Nursing Documentation Methods**

Many traditional forms of nursing documentation have been automated by various nursing information systems. Some of these formats are listed below.

- *Narrative charting.* Traditionally, nurses complete charts using narrative text. In a nursing information system, this may be accomplished using free text entry or menu selections.

- *Charting by exception.* Client-specific documentation addresses only the client's exceptions to normal conditions or ranges. Automated documentation should provide all normal standards and allow the nurse to easily document any exception observed. This may involve menu selections or free text entry.

- *Flowsheet charting.* Routine aspects of care are documented in tabular form. This format is most effective when presented in a PC-based graphical user interface. A pointing device such as a mouse is used to make menu selections or text entries. One form of flowsheet charting is the automation of medication administration records (MARs).

4. The system can issue a warning when medications are charted as given two or more times for the same time slot, and request verification or correction of the same.

5. Some systems allow automatic patient billing for medications and related supplies such as intravenous (IV) tubing and IV dressing changes based on documented care.

Critical Pathway/Protocols Approach The critical pathway or protocol approach to nursing documentation is becoming more prevalent in automated nursing information systems, particularly with the onset of managed care. This approach is often used in a multidisciplinary manner, with many types of care providers accessing the system for information and to document care. Nurses, nursing or patient care assistants, dietitians, social workers, respiratory therapists, physical and occupational therapists, case managers, and physicians all use these systems for documentation. Critical pathway systems include the following features:

- *The nurse, or other care provider, can select one or more appropriate critical pathways for the client.* If more than one path is selected, the system should merge the paths to create one "master" path or protocol.

- *Interaction with physician orders.* Standard physician order sets can be included with each critical pathway, and may be automatically processed by the system.

- *Tracking of protocol variances.* The system should identify variances to the anticipated outcomes as they are charted, and provide aggregate variance data for analysis by the providers. This information can be used to fine tune and improve the critical pathways, thereby contributing to improved client outcomes.

Clinician Information Systems

Clinician information systems are information systems that may be used by any clinician. These users may include nurses, physicians, pharmacists, social workers, respiratory therapists, dieticians, physical therapists, and any other clinician requiring access to the patient record. Clinician information systems may allow the user to document client condition and response to treatment, or they may limit the user to viewing client information without the capability of entering data. Internet technology is changing the way that users interact with clinician information systems. For example, physicians may be able to access client data from remote sites such as their home or office using the Internet.

Monitoring Systems

Monitoring systems are devices that automatically monitor biometric measurements in critical care and specialty areas, such as cardiology and obstetrics. These devices may send information to the nursing documentation system. For example, a monitoring system would enter measurements such as blood pressures directly, eliminating the need for the nurse to enter this data manually. Box 5–3 describes some additional features of monitoring systems.

Order Entry Systems

With **order entry systems,** the nurse or health care provider can alert all departments to carry out physician orders. For example, when a physician orders a barium enema, the order entry system can automatically notify the dietary department to hold the client's breakfast, the pharmacy to send the appropriate medications, and the radiology department to schedule the test. These systems prompt the clinician to provide the information necessary for carrying out the order.

Another feature of an order entry system is duplicate checking. When an order is entered, the system checks to see if a similar order has been placed within a specified time frame. If this is the case, the system can alert the user with a message, or automatically combine the two orders, permitting only one execution of the order.

The order entry system can reflect the current status of each order. For example, the status may be listed as pending, complete, or canceled. This allows the user to see a comprehensive list of the client's orders at any point in time.

Laboratory Systems

Laboratory information systems (LIS) can provide many benefits, including a shorter turnaround time for results, prevention of duplicate testing, decreased likelihood of human error, and identification of abnormal results according to age, sex, and hospital standards. In addition, mi-

---

Box 5–3 **Some Common Features of Monitoring Systems**

- *Alarms alerting the nurse of significant abnormal findings.* Sophisticated systems provide different alarms indicating various abnormalities. For example, the nurse may be able to hear a specific alarm sound that indicates which cardiac arrhythmia the client is experiencing.

- *Portable monitoring systems.* These allow easy transportation of the client throughout the facility without loss of data or functionality.

- *Records of past abnormal findings.* The system maintains a record of all past abnormal findings during this monitoring episode. The system allows the user to find trends in data using graphical displays and focus on specific details.

- *Downloading capabilities.* The system may be able to transfer patient data to a separate system in another facility to provide a continuous patient record.

crobiology culture and sensitivity testing can provide treatment suggestions for the physician.

Automatic generation of specimen labels should occur when an order is placed either directly into an LIS or passed to an order entry system. Labels may include client demographic identifiers, the name of lab studies to be performed, and collection instructions such as tube color, amount needed, and directions such as "Place on ice." Labels may be configured to print immediately at the client location for stat or nurse-collected specimens, or in the lab in batch mode for lab-collected specimens. Batch mode allows the labels to be printed in groups for standard collection times, either on demand or at predefined times.

When specimens are processed by the laboratory instrumentation, the results are automatically transmitted to the LIS. The results can be viewed directly from the LIS or transmitted to another information system, such as the nursing or medical information system. Lab values are available immediately upon completion of the testing process. If desired, printed paper copies of the results may be produced immediately at predefined locations, such as the nursing unit or physician's office, or can be printed in cumulative format for permanent chart copies. Another feature of many lab systems is automatic client billing for tests completed. This information may be communicated to the client billing system.

In one emerging technology, results are transferred from a hand-held test device directly into the lab system (Watson 1995). This type of device allows testing to be performed at the bedside, allowing almost immediate turnaround for results. Use of this technology in an intensive care area may improve client care by providing important lab values very quickly.

Another feature of some laboratory systems is the ability to use rules-based testing. A **rule** is a predefined function that generates a clinical alert or reminder. **Arden syntax** is the standard language used in the health care industry for writing rules. A rules-based LIS could automatically order a second test based on the results of an initial test. For example, if a client has an abnormal CBC value, the system will perform a differential, which is a more specific second test. Rules-based testing could also eliminate unnecessary testing after several consecutive normal results have been obtained, as when physicians order daily lab work. These measures save costs and the staff time of assessing the need for and performing the tests.

Radiology Systems

A **radiology information system** (RIS) provides scheduling of diagnostic tests, communication of patient information, generation of patient instructions and preparation procedures, transcription of results and impressions, and file room management such as tracking of film location. Orders may be entered directly into the radiology system or transmitted from an order entry system. Radiology clerical staff use order information to schedule patients for testing. Once the test is complete, the radiologist interprets the findings and dictates a report. This report can be transcribed using the radiology system or a separate transcription system. The radiology system generates billing information that can be sent to the billing system. The reports are then stored within the radiology system. They may also be faxed to the physician's office or viewed through the clinician or nursing information systems.

One example of how a radiology system might be used is seen with magnetic resonance imaging (MRI) orders at St. Francis Health System in Pittsburgh, Pennsylvania. As the first step in placing an MRI order, the system generates a questionnaire that asks questions pertinent to the MRI procedure. For example, it asks whether the client is cooperative or claustrophobic, and if there are any metal foreign bodies related to previous surgeries or injuries. The nurse reviews these questions with the client, then enters the answers to each question and the order requested into the system. A radiologist reviews the order request and the questionnaire answers, and determines if the client is appropriate for testing. This procedure allows scheduling of appropriate patients only, and eliminates the time-consuming and costly scheduling and attempted testing of inappropriate clients.

More recent developments in radiology information systems include digital, filmless images as a replacement for traditional radiology films. These **picture archiving and communication systems (PACS)** allow images to be electronically transmitted and viewed using sophisticated, high-resolution monitors. The enhanced quality of these images over traditional films may result in fewer repeat procedures and improved diagnostic capability. The use of digital filmless imaging is also an integral component in the evolution of the electronic client record. Use of this technology may allow hospitals to do away with radiology images captured on film. This reduces or eliminates the large expense of radiology films, as well as handling and storage of the x-rays. In addition, PACS can provide the physician with a radiology image viewed on a computer screen within seconds after the completion of the procedure (Hensley 1999). Another benefit of a PACS is that more than one physician can view an image simultaneously in multiple locations (Ball and Collen 1992).

Other benefits of this technology are seen when these images are transmitted to high-acuity areas, such as emergency departments and intensive care units, where quick turnaround and immediate availability of images are critical to providing optimum client care. The use of this technology can also facilitate client care in remote rural health care facilities where a radiologist may not be on-site. Images can be transmitted to a major medical center for evaluation by radiologists and other physicians. Benefits are realized in terms of cost, since it is not necessary to staff a radiologist, and improved client care when a radiologist is on staff but not available.

Pharmacy Systems

Pharmacy systems offer many benefits that promote cost containment and improve the quality of care. These systems can be used by a variety of health care professionals who perform activities related to the ordering, dispensing, and administration of medications. A hospital pharmacy may use an information system to access client data such as demographics, health history and diagnosis, and medication history, or to track client allergies and potential drug interactions. These systems can identify allergy and interaction problems more quickly and accurately than people working in an unautomated, hectic situation. They also provide automatic alerts that can save lives.

Another benefit offered by pharmacy systems is the tracking of medication usage, costs, and billing information. Automation of these functions generally improves accuracy and is more cost-effective than manual methods. In addition, this information can be manipulated and analyzed more easily for executive decision making when it is available as a computer file.

Physicians and other direct care providers may also use pharmacy systems. These systems provide on-line access to client and drug information that is critical in the drug prescription process. Pharmacy systems can provide easy access to clients' health and medication history, as well as their allergies and demographic information. Access to formulary information and on-line drug reference information helps physicians determine the most effective drug and the appropriate doses for clients. In addition, these systems can provide comparisons of costs and drug effectiveness, particularly important in the managed care arena.

Automatic Medication Dispensing in the Pharmacy Pharmacy systems can automatically dispense each client's medications in unit dose format, creating labels for each dose with the client's name and other demographic identifiers. The actual dispensing of the medications may be accomplished either with or without the intervention of the pharmacist. Some systems automatically dispense ordered medications in unit dose packages, which the pharmacy staff place in the client's medication drawer. This process can be streamlined by using robotic systems, which both collect the appropriate medications and place them in the drawers (Rozonkiewiecs and Walters 1995).

Automatic Dispensing Systems on the Nursing Unit Another aspect of pharmacy systems is the use of automatic dispensing systems for use by the nurse. These systems provide a medication dispensing unit in the clinical area, generally for use by nurses who administer medications. The system is usually secured by requiring a user ID and password for access to the system and the actual medications. Features include menu-driven prompts for identifying the client, medication, dose, and number of unit doses removed. The user can also be prompted to count the current number of doses on hand when removing narcotics or other controlled substances. Automatic dispensing systems provide accurate records of medicines given in terms of what was taken from the unit and the date, time, and user who performed this activity. These records can be accessed centrally in the pharmacy to determine when supplies in the clinical area dispensing units must be replenished. In addition, this information can be used to efficiently and accurately bill clients for medications used.

Prevention of Medication Errors An increasing awareness of the frequency and potential severity of medication errors in the hospital setting is the motivating force behind recent legislation and enhancements to information technology. The potential for medication errors has increased dramatically because of the large number of drug names in use, which number more than 15,000 (Gorman 1999). Combining pharmacy information systems with bar code technology, as described in Box 5–4 can drastically reduce medication errors. Information systems can provide checkpoints at each phase of the medication ordering and administration process (Waldo 1999).

Other Clinical Systems

A number of other clinical systems address the needs of specific departments within the health care setting. Box 5–5 lists some of these systems.

Box 5–4 **Using Information Systems to Reduce Medication Errors**

Order entry and pharmacy systems, along with automated medication supply management systems, can be used to assist health care providers in reducing the occurrence of medication errors. These systems interact to provide checks and alerts throughout the medication ordering and administration process, as described in the following example:

- A physician enters a medication order into the order entry system.

- The information is automatically transmitted to the pharmacy system.

- The pharmacy system checks the patient's history and alerts the physician to any drug interactions or allergies. The physician can change the order at this time, if indicated.

- The order creates a requisition in the pharmacy that contains a bar code indicating the correct medication, as well as a bar code identifying the patient.

- A robot in the pharmacy fills the medication order by matching the medication bar code on the requisition to the bar code on the medication. The medication is transported to the nursing unit.

- The nurse scans a bar code on the patient's identification band and the bar code on the medication, and administers the medication only if there is a match.

- The nurse documents the medication administration in the automated medication administration record.

Box 5–5	**Other Common Clinical Systems**

- *Medical records/abstracting systems* facilitate the abstracting, or coding, of diagnoses and chart management processes. Client records may also be stored on optical disk.
- *Operating room systems* may be used to schedule procedures, manage equipment setup for individual physicians, facilitate inventory control, and provide client billing.
- *Emergency department systems* provide ready access to independent systems such as poison control. They also allow the nurse to print specific discharge and follow-up instructions based on the client's diagnosis.
- *Home care systems* allow the health care provider to access information on clients and outpatient resources, and to document care provided.

The rapidly changing health care environment has resulted in several requirements on the part of the clinical information system vendor. The vendor's initial support services and ability to provide ongoing support are critical success factors as the health care paradigm continues to shift (DePietro, Tocco, and Tramontozzi 1995).

ADMINISTRATIVE SYSTEMS

Various administrative systems may be used in health care organizations to support the process of providing client care. Box 5–6 provides a brief review of many of these systems.

Box 5–6	**Administrative Information Systems Used in the Hospital Setting**

- Financial systems provide the facility with accounting functions. Accurate tracking of financial data is critical for enabling the organization to receive reimbursement for services.
- Payroll and human resource systems track employee time and attendance, credentials, performance evaluations, and payroll compensation information.
- Contract management systems manage contracts with third-party payers.
- Risk management systems track and plan prevention of unusual occurrences or incidents.
- Quality assurance systems monitor outcomes and produce reports that are used to guide quality improvement initiatives.
- Physician office systems support patient registration, scheduling, and billing in the physician's office.
- Executive information systems provide administrators with easy access to summarized information related to the financial and clinical operations of the organization.
- Materials management systems facilitate inventory control and charging of supplies.

Registration Systems

The client registration system is critical to the effective operation of many other systems within the health care setting. This system is used to collect and store client identification and demographic data that is verified and updated at the time of each visit. For this reason, these may also be known as admission/discharge/transfer (ADT) systems. Clinical information systems utilize this data for the management of client care and billing purposes. The information is shared with those clinical systems that communicate directly with the registration system.

An important aspect of a registration system used in a multientity health system network is the development of a unique client identifier. This number or identification code is used to identify the client in all information systems across the organization and across all entities. This enables accurate client identification, supporting the development of a longitudinal client record that contains all clinical information available for the client.

Scheduling Systems

A scheduling system allows a health care organization to schedule patients and resources efficiently. Patient demographic information must be available in the system either by direct entry or through electronic communication with a registration system. For the system to be used to schedule patient appointments, it must contain information regarding available resources. This resource information may include the following:

- Referral and authorization by patient's insurance
- Department
- Equipment
- Dates and times
- Room
- Staff
- Permits and preps
- Charging and billing information

The system uses predetermined rules for determining how resource and patient information should be used to schedule a particular type of appointment. This provides users with the capability to schedule a patient via one transaction. In addition, scheduling across all facilities in an enterprise can be accomplished using one system. The benefits associated with using a scheduling system include increased staff productivity, increased patient satisfaction, and cost savings to the organization (LeDonne 1997).

DECISION SUPPORT AND EXPERT SYSTEMS

Decision support and expert systems use data from both the clinical and the administrative information systems, and can provide information related to clinical and administrative users. According to Turley (1993), little agreement exists on the definition of the terms *decision support systems* and *expert systems* except for the distinction of how much authority is placed in the computer system.

Decision support systems aid in and strengthen the selection of viable options using the information of an organization or field to facilitate decision making and overall efficiency. Decision support software organizes information to fit new environments. It provides analysis and advice to support a choice. The final decision rests with the practitioner. Software can be off-the-shelf or homegrown. **Off-the-shelf** software is commercially available. The advantage to the consumer is that someone else has borne the cost for its development and testing. It is, however, geared to a general market and may not meet the needs of a particular party. **Homegrown** software has been developed by the consumer to meet specific needs usually because no suitable commercial package is available. The customer bears the cost of its development, testing, and communication with other software applications. Decision support software can provide a competitive edge and facilitate the move to managed care. Tools range from clinical practice guidelines to financial applications. An example of a decision support application is a program that assists nurses performing a skin assessment to review available alternatives from which the best may be selected to maintain skin integrity.

Research demonstrates that clinical decision support systems can save health care dollars by aiding in diagnosis, allowing physicians to write prescription orders electronically, and providing access to practice guidelines and subsequently decreasing the length of hospital stay. For example, electronic prescriptions provide the following benefits (Cross 1996, Zurier 1995):

- Elimination of phone authorization for refills
- Review of clients' drug histories prior to ordering drugs
- Reminders to order home medications for the hospitalized client
- Alerts about drug interactions
- Checking of formulary compliance and reimbursement
- Provision of a longitudinal prescription record

Electronic prescriptions require direct links between physician offices, hospitals, pharmacies, and third-party payers. Some state laws must also be changed to accommodate electronic prescription writing.

Expert systems use artificial intelligence to model a decision that experts in the field would make. Unlike decision support systems that provide several options from which the user may choose, expert systems convey the concept that the computer has made the best decision based on criteria that experts would use.

CASE STUDY EXERCISES

You are a nurse participating in the customization and implementation of a medication documentation system. Define the data that must be included in the medication order entry process and the medication administration record documentation process.

•   •   •

You are participating in the customization and implementation of the radiology system. Define the data that must be included in the order entry process. Define the information that the nursing staff would like to view or print from the radiology system.

SUMMARY

- A hospital information system comprises clinical and administrative systems.
- Well-designed clinical information systems can improve the quality of client care.
- Clinical information systems can extend the capabilities of health care providers.
- A nursing information system using the nursing process approach should support the use and documentation of nursing processes, and provide tools for managing the delivery of nursing care.
- The critical pathway/protocol approach to nursing information systems provides a multidisciplinary format for planning and documenting client care.
- Other clinical systems, including order entry, radiology, lab, and pharmacy systems, give the nurse and other heath care providers the support and tools to more effectively care for clients.
- Administrative systems support the process of client care by managing nonclinical, client-related information, including demographics and insurance.
- Information systems enable decision makers to examine trends and make informed choices during these times of health care reform.

REFERENCES

Axford, R., and Carter, B. (1996). Impact of clinical information systems on nursing practice. *Computers in Nursing, 14*(3), 156.

Ball M., and Collen M. (1992). *Aspects of the computer-based patient record.* New York: Springer.

Cross, M. (1996). Kicking the prescription pad habit. *Health Data Management, 4*(10), 82–86.

DePietro, S., Tocco, M., and Tramontozzi, A. (1995). Pharmacy systems: Keeping pace. *Healthcare Informatics, 12*(12), 29–44.

Gorman, C. (1999). Mixed-up medusa. *Time, 154*(24), 117.

Hendrickson, M. (1993). The nurse engineer: A way to better nursing information systems. *Computers in Nursing, 11*(2), 67–71.

Hensley, S. (1999). Leaders of the PACS in radiology. *Modern Healthcare, 29*(48), 54–58.

Hughes, S. (1997). Time for new thinking. *Healthcare Informatics,* May, 57–68.

LeDonne, J. (1997). Rehab facility saves $300,000 a year, reduces FTEs, with scheduling system. *Health Management Technology, 18*(7), 30.

Morrissey, J. (1996). Clinical systems add market momentum. *Modern Healthcare, 26*(19), 114–132.

Rozonkiewiecs, M., and Walters, J. (1995). Robots in the Rx: Automatic medication distribution. *Healthcare Informatics, 12*(12), 20–26.

Saba, V., and McCormick, K. (1996). *Essentials of computers for nurses.* New York: McGraw–Hill.

Turley, J. P. (May 1993). The use of artificial intelligence in nursing information systems. On the Internet at: *http://www.vicnet.net.au/vicnet/hisa/MAY93/MAY93-The.html.*

Waldo, B. (1999). Closing the loop on medication errors. *Health Management Technology, 20*(11), 68.

Watson, S. (1995). Network support critical in choosing a lab system. *Health Data Management, 3*(7), 57–65.

Zurier, S. (1995). Telemedicine is bringing electronic doctors closer. *Government Computer News, 14*(21), 56+.

6

Strategic Planning

After completing this chapter, you should be able to:

- Define *strategic planning*.

- Describe how strategic planning is related to an organization's mission, goals, and objectives.

- Identify the participants in the strategic planning process.

- Understand the relationship between strategic planning for information systems and planning for the overall organization.

- Explain the importance of assessing the internal and external environments during the planning process.

- Discuss how potential solutions are derived from data analysis.

- Review the benefits of using a weighted scoring tool when selecting a course of action.

- Understand the importance of developing a timeline during the implementation phase of strategic planning.

- List tools or processes that may be used to evaluate the outcome of and provide feedback to the planning process.

- Discuss the relationship between strategic planning and information technology.

Strategic planning is the development of a comprehensive long-range plan for guiding the activities and operations of an organization. This process includes defining the corporate mission, specifying achievable goals and objectives, developing strategies, and setting policy guidelines (Wheelen and Hunger 1995). The organizational strategic plan should in turn guide the planning for all areas within the organization. For many businesses, including health care delivery, technology is transforming the strategic landscape and must be factored into the organization's strategic plan (Gilks 2000).

THE MISSION

The **mission** is the purpose or reason for the organization's existence, and represents the fundamental and unique aspirations that differentiate the organization from others. This mission is often conveyed in the form of a mission statement that tells the organization's personnel and customers "who we are" and "what we do." An example of a mission statement is seen in Box 6–1.

The purpose of the St. Francis Health System is clearly evident in its mission statement, which states that "the essence of our Mission and Philosophy is best depicted in our logo—St. Francis and the words 'Healing Body, Mind and Spirit.'" This medical center's unique purpose is to provide healing for the mind and spirit, in addition to the expected purpose of physical healing. Its mission statement communicates this purpose effectively to both employees and customers.

The **scope** of an organization's mission defines the type of activities and services it will perform (Carson 1995). Therefore, the scope should be clearly identified in the mission statement so that employees and customers understand which aspects of organizational operation are most important. For example, a broad scope for a health care enterprise might

Box 6–1 **Mission Statement of St. Francis Medical Center, Pittsburgh, PA**

The Mission of St. Francis Medical Center is the same as the Mission of St. Francis Health System, which is:

1. To establish and maintain a hospital and other health care facilities for the care of persons suffering from illnesses or disabilities which require that the patients receive hospital or long-term care, without distinction as to their religious beliefs, race, national origin, age, sex, disability or economic status.

2. To carry on any educational activities related to rendering care to the sick and injured or the promotion of health which, in the opinion of the Board of Directors, may be justified by the facilities, personnel, funds or other requirements that are or can be made available, including, but not being specifically limited to, the conduction of schools for the education of registered nurses and practical nurses with power to grant diplomas to graduates and residency programs for physicians in training.

3. To promote and carry on scientific research related to the care of the sick and injured insofar as, in the opinion of the Board of Directors, such research can be carried on in or in connection with the hospital.

4. To participate, as far as circumstances may warrant, in any activity designed and carried on to promote the general health of the community.

In working toward the fulfillment of these objectives, as members of the health care team, we strive to give generously of our efforts and work harmoniously together for the love of God and of our neighbor. As a result, we find that our own lives and the lives of those with whom we come in contact are being enriched and blessed.

The essence of our Missions and Philosophy is best depicted in our logo—St. Francis and the words "Healing Body, Mind and Spirit."

SOURCE: Reprinted by permission of St. Francis Health System, Pittsburgh, PA.

be to "provide health care." The problem with such a broad scope is that the target client population is not identified, nor are the types of services that will be provided. A narrower scope provides the amount of detail necessary to appropriately guide administrators and managers in decision making. The scope of the St. Francis Medical Center is also seen in the mission statement, which states, "the patients receive hospital or long-term care, without distinction as to their religious beliefs, race, national origin, age, sex, disability or economic status." The medical center's unusual commitment to caring for the indigent population is clearly described in the mission statement. This scope is the basis for the development of certain goals and objectives that guide the decision makers in strategic planning.

GOALS AND OBJECTIVES

Identification of an organization's goals and objectives is a critical factor in fulfilling the mission. The goals and objectives explain how the mission will be realized. A **goal** is an open-ended statement that describes in general terms what is to be accomplished. Examples of goals include maintaining quality client care while promoting cost-effective operations, striving to increase market share by attracting a larger percentage of clients than their competitors, and broadening the scope of services offered. The ability to achieve defined goals is especially important in the rapidly changing health care environment as hospitals merge into large enterprises and services evolve to meet changing needs.

Objectives state how and when an organization will meet its goals. Some of the primary areas that goals and objectives may address are listed in Table 6–1. For example, objectives that support the goal of broadening the scope of services offered may include the following:

- *Development of clinics that support and promote wellness services.* Traditionally, clinics provide treatments for various medical problems. Expansion of these services to support wellness maintenance may attract a larger market share. Some additional services that may be offered are mammography and blood pressure and cholesterol screening.
- *Expansion of home care services.* These services might be expanded to include routine postsurgical follow-up visits as well as occupational and physical therapy.

DEVELOPING STRATEGIES

An organization's **strategy** is a comprehensive plan that states how its mission, goals, and objectives will be achieved (Wheelen and Hunger 1995). An examination of the mission and goals will help to define the steps that are necessary to attain them. A clear understanding of the endpoint is critical to the effective development of the plan. Expediting the

Table 6–1 Areas of Potential Strategic Planning	
Goals and Objectives	**Strategy**
Efficiency	Redesign workflow so that fewer people may accomplish more work.
Growth	Expand service area to include rural and outlying communities.
Utilization of Resources	Train workers so that they are multiskilled.
Technological Leadership	Use newer technologies to transfer information. Examples include telemedicine, optical imaging, video conferencing, and use of the Internet.

SOURCE: Adapted from T. Wheelen and J. Hunger, *Management and business policy,* 5th ed. (p. 21). © 1995 Addison-Wesley Publishing Company Inc. Reprinted by permission of Addison Wesley Longman Inc.

achievement of the mission and goals is the primary purpose of a strategic plan.

Strategic planning is led by members of the organization's upper management, including the board of directors and chief executive officer (CEO), who is ultimately responsible for the organization's strategic management. The next level of management, those who report to the CEO such as vice presidents, are also major participants in strategic planning. This should include the chief information officer (CIO). The CIO must be able to talk with other executives about how information technology can be used to advance the goals of the entire organization. Other lower-level managers within the organization, such as department heads, are responsible for supporting the planning process by providing information related to the current operations as well as insight into future needs of the organization. This information enables the planning team to balance the present reality against the future vision and goals.

STRATEGIC PLANNING FOR INFORMATION SYSTEMS

Although the broader scope of strategic planning concerns all areas of the health care institution, one important component is the plan for information systems (IS). Without a plan that points information systems in the right direction and helps the organization to use IS to execute its business strategies, the organization will not be able to effectively meet its overall goals (O'Connor 1994, Lederer and Sethi 1998).

The strategic planning process is often initiated by other changes that are taking place within the organization. For example, suppose a health care enterprise plans to purchase a client monitoring system to be used throughout its facilities. Other organizational changes—such as plans for construction and unit relocation, infrastructure upgrades including computer wiring and cabling, and updating the client care information systems in general—may have initiated the plans for obtaining the monitoring system. Once administrators realize the need for strategic planning for the monitoring system, they must identify the goals of the plan. These goals should be developed in accordance with the mission and goals of the organization.

Some of the goals of information systems strategic planning are discussed below. Each goal is followed by a brief explanation of how it applies to the previously described example of selecting a new client monitoring system.

- *To support business and clinical decisions*. Data management supports better decision making by providing timely and accurate information. In the example of planning for a new monitoring system, a driving force behind these plans is the need to provide physicians and nurses with accurate and complete data regarding the client's condition.

- *To make effective use of emerging technologies.* New technologies can create administrative efficiencies and attract physicians and clients. In addition, the organization can participate in data sharing through technologies such as the Internet and e-health. Attention to new clinical advancements should be included in the strategic planning process when selecting a new monitoring system. Add-on features such as the hand-held blood analyzer interface should be investigated. This device allows blood samples to be analyzed at the bedside, and the results to be interfaced with the monitoring system.

- *To enhance the organization's image.* The effective use of information technologies enhances how the organization is perceived by physicians, clients, the community, and other external groups. This is especially critical in these times of competitive health care. For example, achieving state-of-the-art technology for cardiac monitoring will provide efficient and effective client care, which will enhance the organization's image.

- *To promote satisfaction of market and regulatory requirements.* Effective IS strategic planning must include those issues related to meeting market and regulatory requirements, such as e-health, payer requirements, Joint Commission for Accreditation of Hospital Organizations guidelines, client confidentiality, and data security. For example, when selecting a monitoring system, it is also important to determine that the system complies with safety regulations such as protection against damage from defibrillation.

- *To be cost-effective.* Cost-effectiveness is achieved when redundancies are eliminated. In the monitoring system example, this advantage is evident. If all of the critical care and monitored bed areas in the enterprise use the same monitoring system, training is cost-effective, since nurses need be trained on only one system to work in any monitored area of the hospital. Other cost benefits are seen in the need to maintain only one type of backup monitor for replacement of nonoperational equipment, as well as increased efficiency for the biomedical technicians who must maintain the monitoring equipment.

STEPS OF THE STRATEGIC PLANNING PROCESS

The first step of the strategic planning process is the realization that there is a need for change. Each department in the organization should have its own long-range plan, and most departments within the organization are dependent on the management of information systems. As a result, each department comes to the information services department with its own requirements related to strategic planning. It is the responsibility of IS to prioritize and merge these ideas together, developing a master strategic plan for the organization. This task is complicated by the rapidly changing nature of information technology and the emerging role of the Internet in health care delivery (Baldwin 1999). The fast pace of evolving technology requires periodic review and revisions of both the organization's strategic plan and the IS department's strategic plan.

The CIO is ultimately responsible for IS strategic planning (Bunschoten 1996). "The need to create administrative efficiencies through e-commerce, huge mergers and acquisitions, and requests for outcomes reporting" forces CIOs to think in broad terms about ways that information technology can be used to achieve strategic and operational changes (Hagland 2000, p. 76). The CIO generally selects a project manager or chairperson for each major project within the overall strategic plan. The project manager may help to develop an advisory board or strategic planning team. The strategic planning team is generally composed of top-level managers who devise the plan and present it to the CIO, who in turn presents it to the board of directors.

Another level of strategic planning is performed by members of the project implementation team, which reports to the advisory board. This team is composed of representatives from the user departments, including managers and frontline employees who are most familiar with the activities of the department. The project implementation team should also include the analysts and programmers who will implement the system changes. Frequent communication between the advisory board and the implementation team is imperative for the ongoing success of the strategic plan. This plan generally addresses a time frame covering between three and five years into the future.

Identification of Goals and Scope

Once the strategic planning teams have been identified, the actual planning process can begin. The first step is to identify the goals and scope of the project. The goals of the project must meet the needs of the users as well as support the mission and goals of the institution. The identified goals will then provide the direction for the remainder of the planning process.

In the example of selecting a cardiac monitoring system for a health care enterprise, the goals and scope of the project might be to implement a one-vendor solution. This should result in the selection of a single system that will meet the needs of all monitored areas in the organization.

Scanning the External and Internal Environments

The next step in the planning process is to **scan,** or gather information from, the external and internal environments. The **external environment** includes those interested parties and competitors that are outside of the health care institution, such as vendors, payers, competitors, clients, the community, and regulatory agencies. The **internal environment** includes employees of the institution, as well as physicians and members of the board of directors. The purpose of scanning the environment is twofold: to define the current situation and identify areas of need.

Environment scanning is best accomplished by developing a detailed plan for collecting pertinent data. This step is often called the needs assessment. Information related to current trends in both health care and information technology should also be collected. Data may be collected from a variety of sources, including the following (McCormack 1996):

External Environment Scanning

- Published literature and reports
- Information from vendors
- Regulatory and accreditation requirements
- Information related to market trends

Internal Environment Scanning

- Interviews and questionnaires from managers and end users
- Observations of current technology and operations, as well as anticipated technological developments

When selecting a monitoring system, information may be obtained from vendors regarding the technologies that are currently available. All pertinent regulatory and accreditation requirements must also be investigated. A scan of the internal environment may include an inventory of equipment currently in use throughout the enterprise.

Data Analysis

After data has been collected during the internal and external environmental scans, the project implementation team must perform analysis, identifying trends in the current operations as well as future needs and expectations. Current trends in health care should be identified when considering future needs, and may be related to topics such as managed care and other financial health care coverage and reimbursement considerations. Some trends to consider include the merging of hospitals into large enterprises and the growing focus on care outside of the acute hospital setting, which has resulted in an increased number of services related to wellness promotion and home care. Information technology trends such as e-health, the Internet, telemedicine, client-server technologies, and the computerized client record must also be addressed (Morrissey 1996, Morrissey 2000).

In selecting a universal cardiac monitoring system, the features of each vendor's system must be evaluated, including the desirable and undesirable features of each. For example, strengths may include an easy learning curve, vendor support, integration capability, transport monitor capabilities, and screen visibility. Weaknesses may include a large number of screens for each function, busy or hard-to-read screens, slow speed of initial data entry, and unsuitable cabling requirements.

Identification of Potential Solutions

The next step in the planning process involves the identification of potential solutions, which may be in the form of system upgrades or replacements. At this point, the strategic planning team should be aware of the information system needs of the end users.

When identifying potential solutions, health care organizations must address many issues, including the following:

- *Hospitals with differing information systems may be merged together into one enterprise.* In this situation, either each organization continues to use its previous system or one system is chosen for use throughout the enterprise as a means to build a cohesive information systems strategy (Cross 1996). Several factors influence the decision to retain or adopt an information system, including costs associated with the purchase and use of software and hardware; site licenses, consulting fees, contract negotiation, maintenance and support agreements, expenses associated with training personnel to use a new system, and the availability of support staff.

- *Many hospitals use mainframe* **legacy systems,** *older vendor-based systems that have often been highly individualized to meet customer specifications.* As it is necessary to upgrade or replace these systems, CEOs and CIOs must weigh the advantages and disadvantages of alternatives that may better meet the needs of the organization. These might include new versions of vendor software, client/server or thin client technologies, outsourcing services or using an application service provider (ASP). Box 6–2 lists several information technology considerations related to strategic planning. Box 6–3 identifies pros and cons associated with the outsourcing of services.

Selecting a Course of Action

Once all of the potential solutions have been identified, they must be analyzed and compared. One way to accomplish this task is to measure the components of the plan in terms of their ability to meet identified current and future needs. This can be accomplished by listing these needs and weighting them according to their importance. For example, essential features may be given a weighting factor of 5, and desirable but not essential features may be given a weighting factor of 3. Weighting of each desirable system feature should be completed before the various systems are scored.

The next step is to score the features, or requirements, of each potential system. For example, each feature may be given a score from 0 to 5, with 0 indicating that the requirement is not met, and 5 indicating that the requirement is fully met. Finally, the score is multiplied by the weighting factor for each item to determine the weighted score. The overall score is the sum of weighted scores for all items.

Box 6–2 | **Information Technology Considerations for Strategic Planning**

- Does the system use open architecture?
- Is the system based on personal computer (PC), client/server, thin client, or Internet technology?
- Does it utilize a graphical user interface? Is it user friendly?
- Does the software comply with HL7 standards?
- Does the system allow the user to query aggregate data and produce online reports?
- Does it support performance measurement?
- Does it support a customized view?
- Can it support expansion of features, increased numbers of users, and/or records?
- Does it allow the use of evolving technologies, such as smart cards, optical disks, interface engines, wireless technology, integrated services digital network (ISDN) communication, e-health or e-commerce, video conferencing, telemedicine, and fiberoptic networks?
- Does it support a paperless environment?
- Have criteria been developed to measure successful implementation?

SOURCE: Adapted from O'Connor, K. (1994). "Where is your long range plan?", *Healthcare Informatics*, 11*(12)*, 64–68.

Figure 6–1 illustrates using a weighted score as an evaluation tool to select a hospitalwide cardiac monitoring system. This figure lists only a minimal number of the features that would actually be evaluated in this situation.

Evaluation of the various potential solutions should also include a summary of pertinent findings that have been discovered during data analysis. Other factors that should be considered when making a final decision include the following:

- Purchase costs versus outsourcing costs
- Ongoing maintenance and support costs
- Time required for installation
- Number of employees required to install and maintain the system
- Vendor's history and stability
- Service considerations
- Existence of national user groups
- Time and staff resources required for training

The process of strategic planning and selecting a course of action may involve time, money, and personnel resources. Nonetheless, the resources expended during this process are well worth the value of the plan that is produced, since this plan will guide the decision making of the IS department and the health care enterprise.

Box 6–3 **Pros and Cons Associated with the Outsourcing of Services**

Pros

- Allows the organization to focus on its core competencies.
- Can shorten the timeframe to implement new applications or technology.
- Better compliance with project implementation dates.
- Easier to budget and manage because costs for development and implementation are shifted to the outsourcing agency.
- May improve customer satisfaction because services can be delivered at the same or at a higher level as in-house services but at a lower cost.
- Provides leading-edge technical skills when skilled labor resources are not available in-house.
- Contract negotiations aid definition of project scope.

Cons

- Limited control over data security and confidentiality.
- Lack of control over application maintenance and downtime.
- Insufficient advance notice of downtime.
- Lack of control over when updates are implemented.
- Customization may not be available.
- Promises may exceed ability to deliver.
- Costs can be much higher than anticipated.
- Identification and resolution of system problems may be delayed.
- Ability to change outsourcing services may be limited.

Implementation

The next phase in the strategic planning process is implementation of the chosen solution. The first step in the implementation process is to identify the working committee for the implementation phase. Development of a timeline is one of the initial tasks the committee will perform. Once all of the individual components of the timeline have been identified, the tasks can be assigned and initiated. Other tasks during this phase include budgeting, procedure development, and execution of the plan.

When implementing a universal cardiac monitoring system, the working committee may include representatives from the IS, purchasing, and staff development departments, as well as physicians and nurse managers. This group would first develop a timeline, prioritizing the order in which units would begin using the system. They would also be active in developing a procedure and a plan for educating staff in the use of the new equipment. Box 6–4 lists some measures to ensure a successful experience when services are outsourced.

Selection of a Hospital-Wide Cardiac Monitoring System

Monitoring System: _____
Evaluator: _____

Ratings (How well does the system do this?):
  1 = Poor   2 = Fair   3 = Adequate   4 = Good   5 = Excellent

System Feature	Rating	×	Weighting Factor	=	Weighted Score	Comments
Operation						
1. Easy to learn and operate			5			
2. Easy to set up screen			3			
Alarms						
3. Easy to set alarms			3			
4. Alarm limits displayed continuously			5			
Bedside Monitors						
5. Does the bedside unit work exactly the same as the central station and transport monitors?			3			
6. Can you view, control, review, and record any parameter from any bed on the network?			5			
					_____	**Overall system score** (Total of weighted scores):

FIGURE 6–1 • Example of an Evaluation Tool for Cardiac Monitoring Systems

Ongoing Evaluation and Feedback

Strategic planning is an ongoing process (DeJarnett 1999). Frequent evaluation of the current processes as well as the current and future needs must be performed. In this way, the organization is able to remain current with changing technology and health care trends. The process for identifying evaluation tools can be difficult. Measures must be adjusted to environmental changes and competitor actions as a means to help ensure success of strategic plans. One particular type of measure is benchmarking.

Benchmarking is the continual process of measuring services and practices against the toughest competitors in the health care industry.

Box 6–4   **Measures to Ensure a Positive Outsourcing Experience**

- Define information technology functions for possible outsourcing.
- Research vendor availability and capabilities.
- Establish outsourcing goals and objectives.
- Select the vendor that meets the requirements.
- Negotiate a contract that outlines the following:
  - Term of contract and provisions for termination and renewal
  - Management of the relationship
  - Vendor and client responsibilities
  - Liabilities
  - Warranties
  - Ownership issues regarding assets/intellectual property
  - Fee structure
  - The process for staff assignment
  - Performance measures
  - Resources key to success
  - Security safeguards
  - Back-up and disaster recovery measures
  - Service level agreements inclusive of availability, response times, service quality
- Develop and use oversight procedures.
- Insure against losses related to poor work.

An example of benchmarking is to compare the number of IS staff required to support the clinical applications for the enterprise to that of other health care providers with similar demographic and volume statistics. When needs are no longer met, or the organization falls far below the benchmark, the process of identifying potential solutions and selecting the best option is begun again. Clinical examples of benchmarks might include the organization's cost for open heart surgery or length of stay.

CASE STUDY EXERCISES

You are a nurse manager in a hospital that has recently merged with two other hospitals, forming a large health care enterprise. Each of the three hospitals currently uses a different nursing information system. You are a member of the strategic planning committee, which is charged with the task of selecting which of the three systems will be used throughout the enterprise. Describe the process you would use to scan the internal and external environments, as well as the types of data you would collect.

• • •

Develop a tool to evaluate each of the three nursing information systems for the scenario described above.

• • •

Your facility belongs to one of three healthcare delivery systems in the city. Competition is fierce. You have been asked to serve on a committee to study and recommend the retention or deletion of certain clinical services. Develop a plan for how you would do that and for how information services might facilitate that task via the use of benchmarking.

SUMMARY

- Strategic planning is the development of a comprehensive long-range plan for guiding the activities and operations of an organization.
- Strategic planning is one of the most important factors in the selection, design, and implementation of information systems, because it can save valuable resources over time and ensure that the needs of the enterprise are met.
- The strategic plan should support the mission, goals, and objectives of the organization.
- The mission is the purpose for the organization's existence, and represents its unique aspects.
- Strategic planning is guided by upper-level administrators, including the CIO, but requires participation from other levels of management as well.
- Strategic planning involves the following steps: definition of goals and scope, scanning of external and internal environments, data analysis, identification of potential solutions, selection of a course of action, implementation, evaluation, and feedback.
- Strategic planning is an ongoing process.

REFERENCES

Baldwin, G. (1999). The Internet can make strategic I.T. planning precarious. *Health Data Management*, 7(12), 42, 44, 46, 48.

Bunschoten, B. (1996). From the back room to the board room. *Health Data Management*, 4(2), 33–41.

Carson, C. L. (1995). *Healing body, mind and spirit*. Pittsburgh: Carnegie Mellon University Press.

Cross, M. A. (1996). Building an I.S. strategy in the wake of a merger. *Health Data Management, 4*(10), 85–89.

DeJarnett, L. R. (1999). Integrated strategic measures—a new value from your IT investment. *The Executive's Journal, 16*(1), 3, 4p.

Gilks, J. (2000). IT strategy needs a rethink. *CMA Management, 74*(1), 52, 2p.

Hagland, M. (2000). The many hats of a CIO. *Healthcare Informatics, 17*(5), 69–70, 72, 74, 76.

Lederer, A. L., and Sethi, V. (1998). Seven guidelines for strategic information systems planning. *The Executive's Journal, 15*(1), 23.

McCormack, J. (1996). Strategic planning in changing times. *Health Data Management, 4*(12), 6–16.

Morrissey, J. (1996). A broader vision. *Modern Healthcare, 26*(10), 110–113.

Morrissey, J. (2000). Internet dominates providers' line of sight. *Modern Healthcare, 30*(15), 72, 74, 76, 78, 80–82, 84, 86, 88, 90, 92.

O'Connor, K. (1994). Where is your long range IS plan? *Healthcare Informatics, 11*(12), 64–68.

Wheelen, T. L., and Hunger, J. D. (1995). *Management and business policy*, 5th ed. Menlo Park, CA: Addison–Wesley.

7

Selecting a Health Care Information System

After completing this chapter, you should be able to:

- Define the term *life cycle* as it relates to information systems.

- List the phases of the life cycle of an information system.

- Discuss the purpose of the needs assessment.

- Identify the typical membership composition of the system selection steering committee.

- Explain the importance of using the mission statement in determining the organization's information needs.

- Identify several methods for analyzing the current system.

- Discuss the value of using a weighted scoring tool during the selection phase.

- Review the system criteria that should be addressed during the selection process.

- Describe the request for information and request for proposal documents.

- Describe the process for evaluating request for proposal responses from vendors.

The selection and implementation of an information system occurs through a well-defined process known as the **life cycle** of an information system. This term describes the ongoing process of developing and maintaining an information system. This cycle can be divided into four main phases that cover the life span of the information system. These four phases are

1. Needs assessment
2. System selection
3. Implementation
4. Maintenance

Figure 7–1 illustrates the relationship of these phases as circular, since needs assessment and evaluation are ongoing processes. As needs change, the organization may find it necessary to upgrade information systems periodically. The first two phases, needs assessment and system selection, are discussed in this chapter. Details regarding system implementation and maintenance are covered in the next chapter.

It is essential to develop a timeline that delineates the major events or milestones when working through the various phases of the information system's life cycle. For example, while it is desirable to complete the needs assessment and selection processes in less than one year it is necessary to recognize that the process may take a year to complete. Therefore, it is vital to organize responsibilities around a realistic time frame. Figure 7–2 provides a template that may be used to develop a timeline or Gantt chart for the needs assessment and system selection phases of the information system's life cycle.

NEEDS ASSESSMENT

Needs assessment is the first phase in the information life cycle (Zielstorff, McHugh, and Clinton 1988). This process is usually initiated by a person

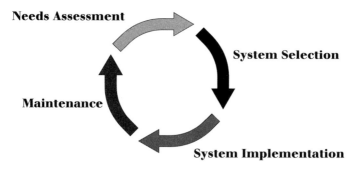

FIGURE 7–1 • The Life Cycle of an Information System

Milestone	Person Responsible	Estimated Start Date	Completion Date
PHASE 1: NEEDS ASSESSMENT			
Develop steering committee			
Perform needs assessment:			
Identify system requirements and weighting of criteria Technical Administrative/general Registration Order entry/results reporting Medical records Accounting			
PHASE 2: SYSTEM SELECTION			
Develop the RFP Organization description System requirements Response evaluation procedures			
Evaluate RFP responses			
Conduct site visits			
Select the system for purchase			
Contract negotiations and contract signed			

FIGURE 7–2 • Sample Template for Developing a Timeline or Gantt Chart

or group with a vision of the future. The needs assessment should analyze the overall needs of the organization with consideration to the strategic plan. After this is done it is appropriate to look at segments within the organization (Oberst 1991). A deficit in the current method of manual or automated information handling is often recognized by people from several different groups or disciplines, such as clinical and administrative personnel who use the information, as well as programmers and other technical staff who manage the information system. Once the deficit or need is realized, a more detailed understanding of the issues must be developed.

After the group discusses the current deficits and needs, they brainstorm to generate a list of possible directions for action. These actions may include minor modifications to the current manual or automated system, major enhancements to the current system, or the purchase of a new automated information system.

The analysis of identified possible actions and the decision-making process must be a collaborative effort, and is often performed by a committee that includes clinical users, information systems specialists, and administration or executive board representatives.

The Steering Committee

The steering committee is an essential component of the assessment and selection processes. Leadership of this group may impact the success or failure of the project. The committee chairperson may be a manager or director of information services, or have an administrative position elsewhere in the hospital. The committee membership must be multidisciplinary, including representation from all departments affected by the new system and incorporating the clinical, administrative, and information system divisions. This strategy is essential for identification of all pertinent issues, and reduces the possibility of overlooking potential problems (Hewlett-Packard 1990). In those health care organizations that include affiliations with other facilities, it is imperative that representation from these areas be included to address any additional needs. A general rule to follow is that any department or area that uses the information or is affected by it must have a voice in the selection process.

The structure of the steering committee must be defined early in the process. When designing the committee, it is important to consider the appropriate size of the group (Hewlett-Packard 1990). The committee should be large enough to make a good decision, but small enough to be effective and efficient. At this point, it is necessary to define who has the authority to make the final decisions. For example, decision-making power may be given to a particular department, shared among a group of administrators from various departments, or shared equally among all members of the steering committee.

One strategy that is effective in larger organizations is to develop a multilevel committee. The upper level or executive board of the committee is responsible for the final decisions regarding selection (Center of Healthcare Information Management 1991). This may be a small group of high-level executives, including the chief executive officer, chief information officer, chief financial officer, vice presidents responsible for major departments, and medical staff leadership. This subcommittee is supported by a larger group of department managers and supervisors. The committee should also include some frontline employees who will actually be using the system. These are the people who will be responsible for doing most of the groundwork and investigation during the assessment and selection processes. For this reason, it is prudent to choose committee members who are able to devote the necessary time and energy to the project. Their managers must be willing to provide them with time away from their normal responsibilities and support their involvement in the project. An effective strategy is to assign tasks to individual members or subgroups based on their expertise and knowledge. Their findings are then presented to the larger committee for discussion and approval.

Consultants

The committee should consider whether and when a consultant should be used. Consultants may be hired for assistance in any phase of the selection process, including assessing the current information system. Consultants may also be used to help with system planning, testing, security, policy and procedure development, and implementation. The effective use of consultants requires clear definition of the contractual relationship and expected outcomes as well as good communication throughout the association. The consultant should be provided with all available data regarding the current system and identified needs. The consultant's role is to analyze this information and make recommendations for action. Box 7–1 lists some of the primary qualities of an effective consultant or consulting service. On occasion problems arise with the use of consultants that may include limited experience and knowledge of the needs and hardware and software applications under consideration as well as a lack of incentive to work toward the most useful and cost-effective solution.

Developing a Common Vision

The needs assessment committee should start the process by examining the vision and mission statements of the organization as well as the strategic plan. This will guide the committee in looking to the future and determining the organization's information needs while continuing to support the mission. From this, goals or a charge should be developed to guide the work of the committee. These goals must reflect the organization's purpose, scope of services, and customers. The primary goal of the committee is to identify how health care delivery can be enhanced to provide optimum client care. This can be accomplished by providing more meaningful and accurate client data. Some additional expectations of an

Box 7–1 Qualities of an Effective Consultant

- Experience, including longevity and diversity
- Knowledge and understanding of the health care industry
- Good consulting skills and a proven methodology
- Good verbal and written communication skills
- Good project management and communication skills
- Clearly defined work plan and deliverables
- Advice that will result in cost savings
- Flexibility and availability
- A fit with the corporate culture

SOURCE: Adapted from Consulting Services *Contingency Planning and Management* (p. 20), July, 1996.

information system might be to save time, increase productivity, contain costs, promote quality improvement, and foster staff recruitment and retention. The committee should consider using brainstorming techniques when defining the expectations of an information system. An open-minded and creative approach will facilitate comprehensive exploration of all possibilities.

Understanding the Current System

A thorough understanding of how information is currently collected and processed is the starting point in performing a needs assessment. This is also known as assessing the internal environment. Methods for accomplishing this include questionnaires and observation of day-to-day activities (Saba and McCormick 1996). The goal is to determine what information is used, who uses it, and how it is used. Every data item used in the current paper or automated system should be analyzed. Some examples of data items include client name, sex, marital status, or diagnosis. Next, the committee must decide what information should be kept, what information is redundant, and what information is unnecessary. They should evaluate the strengths and weaknesses of the current manual or automated information system to determine the needs of the health care enterprise.

Determining System Requirements

To determine the appropriate course of action, the committee must first understand the organization's requirements for operation. One strategy for obtaining this information is to interview staff from each department or work area. The interviewer might ask what information is necessary to conduct business and what information is desired but not essential. These are often called the "musts" and the "wants." Some examples of essential information include client name, admitting physician, and insurance information. It is important to also consider those criteria that may not be necessary at the present time, but might be important in the future, such as voice recognition technology. The information from numerous interviews is then compiled into a list of "musts" and "wants."

The next step is to prioritize or weight the list of "musts" and "wants" from high to low. To accomplish this task, selection committee members should develop a rating scale such as a 1 through 10 scale or rankings of low, medium, and high. Table 7–1 displays an example of some weighted "wants" and "musts" that could be identified when performing the needs assessment. The criteria should also be grouped into functional categories to present a comprehensive picture of the system requirements. Some of the common categories that may be considered are listed below.

Technical Criteria Technical criteria include those hardware and software components necessary for the desired level of system performance. Areas to consider are the following:

- *Type of architecture.* **Architecture** refers to the structure of the central processing unit and its interrelated elements. An **open system** uses protocols and technology that follow publicly accepted conventions and are employed by multiple vendors, so that various system components can work together.

Examples of Criteria

1. The system maintains an open architecture environment that can continue to evolve as new technology becomes available.

Table 7–1 Sample of Criteria Defining "Musts" and "Wants"		
Charting/Documentation Information Criteria	**Must or Want**	**Weight***
Capable of multidisciplinary charting	M	10
Able to chart medications, IVs, and treatments	M	10
Has mechanism to remind the user of undocumented activities, treatments, medications and IVs at intervals specified by department	M	10
Automatically calculates charted IV products into intake and output	W	7
Automatically totals fluid balance by shift and 24-hour period	W	8
Able to easily switch between functions (such as, charting and entering orders)	W	5

* 1–10, where 10 = most important.

2. Features ease of implementation and support of real-time integration to existing and future information systems.

- *Amount of downtime.* **Downtime** refers to the period of time when an information system is not operational and available for use. Some systems have daily scheduled downtimes, during which maintenance and backup procedures are performed.

Examples of Criteria

1. Provides 24-hour system availability with no scheduled daily downtime.
2. Does not have a history of prolonged or frequent unscheduled downtimes.

- *Connectivity standards.* These standards help to maximize the connectivity between application and information files, supporting system integration.

Examples of Criteria

1. Provides for HL7-compliant interfaces.
2. Includes the ability to interface from and to client care instruments such as client monitors.

- *Test environment separate from live environment.* A separate environment for the development and testing of updates and changes to the system must be available, so that the actual system (live system) can continue to operate without interference during these activities.

Examples of Criteria

1. Provides the ability to update the test environment without impacting the live system.
2. Provides a training environment that is separate from the live and test environments.

- *Response time.* **Response time** is the amount of time between a user action and the response from the information system. For example, after the user selects a lab test from a menu, the system requires a certain amount of processing time before that result can be viewed.

Examples of Criteria

1. Ensures instantaneous response time for all on-line transactions (one second or less).
2. Able to continuously track and monitor response time and provide reports containing this information.

- *Support of electronic technologies.* The information system should support other technologies that will enhance client care and business operations.

Examples of Criteria

1. Supports various methods of data entry by the user, including touch-screen entry and voice recognition.
2. Allows the use of bar-coding and scanning.

Administrative/General Administrative criteria describe how the system may be administratively controlled for appropriate and effective use of the information.

- *Security levels to comply with regulatory and legal requirements.* The Joint Commission for Accreditation of Hospital Organizations (JCAHO), for example, regulates the confidentiality, security, and integrity of hospital systems. The Health Insurance Portability and Accountability Act (HIPAA) imposes requirements for the protection of patient data and penalties for noncompliance.

Examples of Criteria

1. Allows various levels of security to be defined for different user groups. Each group should have access to only the information required for its client care or job duties.
2. Provides a mechanism to track and report what information has been accessed by which users.

- *On-line Help screens.* On-line Help screens display instructions to assist the user with completing a specific function.

Examples of Criteria

1. Help screens must be available and easily accessed by the user.
2. Help screens must be concise and easy to understand.

- *Purging and restoring data.* It is important to determine how long it is necessary to maintain on-line access to client data before purging it to other storage devices. Sometimes it becomes essential to restore these files for the purposes of audits, and the ease of performing these procedures must be considered. Advances such as the use of imaging technology to store diagnostic images and forms must be considered when purge criteria are defined.

Examples of Criteria

1. Includes a flexible client purge process, allowing both automatic and manual purge capabilities.

2. The process for restoring data that has been purged to storage must be convenient and readily accessible.

- *Report capabilities*. The system should provide a report-writing software component that allows specific types of information to be extracted from the database and presented in a report.

Examples of Criteria

1. Predefined reports should be produced automatically on a set schedule.
2. Users should be able to generate ad hoc reports on demand, with the capability to format them as desired.
3. Reports should be available on-line, eliminating concerns related to printing costs, labor, distribution, storage, and disposal of confidential materials.

Registration Criteria The registration criteria are essential for ensuring that the client is properly identified for all aspects of information management.

Examples of Criteria

1. Assigns each client a unique identifier across the organization.
2. Supports multiple registration sites. Clients may enter the health system at a number of points of service, including the physician's office, clinics, the emergency department, or the admissions office.
3. Provides the ability to change or update registration information.
4. Demonstrates the ability to track a client's location within the institution, as well as to track the use of system services.
5. Prevents the user from omitting required data before completing a function.

Order Entry/Results Reporting Criteria These criteria ensure that accurate entry of physician orders is accomplished in a timely and efficient manner, resulting in improved client care.

Examples of Criteria

1. Able to indicate details of orders such as frequency (for example, q6h or qd) and priority (stat, routine, and so on).
2. Notifies the user when a duplicate order is entered, and requests verification prior to accepting the new order. For example, the client may have a previously ordered daily chest x-ray. If a new order for a chest x-ray is now entered, the system should alert the user and request verification that this additional test is necessary.

3. Through order entry and results reporting, produces an audit trail that identifies the person who entered the order, the date/time of order entry and execution, and the status of the order (such as pending or completed).

4. Supports documentation of medications and treatments, and relates this documentation to the appropriate order.

5. Automatically generates client charges for specific orders or treatments as a result of entry or completion.

Medical Records Criteria The medical records criteria should support the storage of all pertinent client data obtained from various information systems, allowing the user to access a longitudinal record of all client activities and events or visits. The system should allow inquiry about clients, using various identifiers, including social security number, name, medical record, or account number.

Examples of Criteria

1. Provides support for automatic coding, including verification of codes entered with narrative description (for example, ICD-9-CM and CPT-4 codes).

2. Translates diagnosis and procedure terminology into numeric codes.

3. Produces deficiency lists on demand for individual records and individual physicians.

Accounting Criteria These criteria facilitate reimbursement for services rendered and help to ensure the financial stability of the enterprise.

Examples of Criteria

1. Generates summaries or detailed bills on demand.

2. Allows the user to enter the client's insurance verification data, insurance plan, and charges at any time during the stay, and to change the client's financial class.

3. Supports physician billing and captures data for linkage to physician billing services.

SYSTEM SELECTION

If the decision is made to purchase a new information system, the life cycle proceeds to Phase 2: system selection. This phase is critical to the success of the project. The extremely high purchase, installation, and maintenance costs associated with new or upgraded technology mean that the decision must be made carefully. The information gathered during the needs assessment phase is the basis for the system selection process and decision. Since it has been determined that a new system must be purchased, further information must now be gathered. Box 7–2 identifies some system selection considerations.

Additional Sources of Information

Trade shows and conferences are beneficial sources of information. Attendance at these events provides the opportunity to examine systems from various vendors in an informal atmosphere, compare and contrast system capabilities, and see actual demonstrations.

Other potentially helpful sources of information include weekly publications, trade newspapers, and monthly journals that address information and technology and local user groups. Textbooks and reference books also discuss system options. Published conference proceedings may also provide insight into pertinent issues and solutions. Finally, communication via the Internet and World Wide Web can furnish additional information, including insights from other users of a given system. This avenue may provide the most current and candid responses to questions.

Request for Information

An information systems **vendor** is a company that designs, develops, sells, and supports systems. Consideration of vendor characteristics is

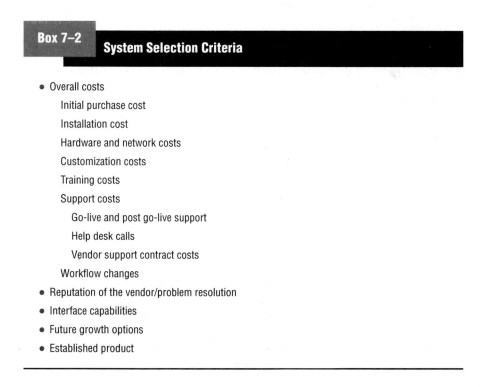

Box 7–2   System Selection Criteria

- Overall costs
    - Initial purchase cost
    - Installation cost
    - Hardware and network costs
    - Customization costs
    - Training costs
    - Support costs
        - Go-live and post go-live support
        - Help desk calls
        - Vendor support contract costs
    - Workflow changes
- Reputation of the vendor/problem resolution
- Interface capabilities
- Future growth options
- Established product

crucial in choosing a system that will be responsive to current needs and unanticipated changes. A great deal of information can be gleaned from vendors who are eager to make a sale. The **request for information (RFI)** is often the initial contact with vendors. An RFI is a letter or brief document sent to vendors that explains the institution's plans for purchasing and installing an information system. The purpose of the RFI is to obtain essential information about the vendor and its systems in order to eliminate those vendors that cannot meet the organization's basic requirements. One method for obtaining names of appropriate vendors is to complete reader response cards following advertisements in professional journals.

The RFI should ask the vendor to provide a description of the system and its capabilities. Often the vendor responds to the request by sending written literature. More information can be obtained by asking additional specific questions of the vendor. Some topics to consider for questioning include

1. The history and financial situation of the company, including the extent of its investment into research and development. This provides an indication of the company's commitment to enhancing and updating the product.
2. The number of installed sites, including a list of several organizations that already use the product you are considering.
3. System architecture, including the required hardware configuration.
4. Use of state-of-the-art technology.
5. Integration with other systems. Which other systems are currently integrated with the vendor's software in other hospital sites?
6. The methods of user support provided by the vendor during and following installation.
7. Future health care provider development plans.
8. Procedures for the distribution of software updates.

Request for Proposal

At this point, the steering committee will probably be overwhelmed with information. The next step is to evaluate this information and prepare a formal document called the **request for proposal (RFP)**. An RFP is a document sent to vendors that describes the requirements of a potential information system (Cross 1996). The RFP prioritizes or ranks these requirements in order of their importance to the organization. The purpose of this document is to solicit proposals from many vendors that describe their capabilities to meet the "wants" and "needs." The vendors' responses may then be used to narrow the number of competitors under consideration.

Strategies for a Successful RFP Because of the importance of the RFP, it must be structured to ensure successful system selection. All aspects of the document must be detailed and precise to facilitate an accurate response from the vendor. If questions are vague or poorly written, they could easily be misinterpreted by the vendor. For example, an ambiguous question might lead a vendor to indicate that the system meets a requirement when in fact it does not. It is advantageous to limit the number of requirements to those that are most important, and produce a simple and straightforward document. If an RFP is too lengthy, it will cost both the organization and the vendor a great deal of time and money to prepare and evaluate. It is difficult to evaluate a long document that is not focused on the important issues. Finally, a well-written RFP provides a framework that allows the steering committee to more accurately evaluate the vendor's proposal.

The format of RFP questions and answers may influence the authenticity of vendor responses. For example, for each question about a system feature, the RFP might offer four response choices, such as

1. *"Yes."* If the vendor indicates that this functionality is currently available, then the vendor must also provide a written explanation of how the system performs this function.
2. *"Available with customization."* The vendor must provide an estimated cost of customization and time frame for availability.
3. *"Available in the future."* The vendor must provide an estimated time frame for availability.
4. *"No."* No further information is required.

RFP Design Although the actual format of the RFP may vary from organization to organization, all RFPs must contain certain components that are essential for a complete and effective document. The RFP should include the following details:

- *Description of the organization.* The first objective of the RFP should be to familiarize the vendor with the organization. The RFP must describe the organization's overall environment, as well as the specific setting in which the system will function. The vendor needs to have enough information to facilitate proposal of appropriate systems and hardware configurations. The following information should be included:
  1. *Mission and goals.* The mission statement and any supporting documentation will provide the vendor with a view of the driving forces behind the selection process.
  2. *Structure of the organization.* The RFP should describe how the health care enterprise is structured, including all facilities and satellite areas that provide inpatient, outpatient, and home care services.

3. *Type of health care facility.* The RFP should specify whether the facility is a profit or nonprofit organization and contain descriptors appropriate to the organization, such as community, university, government, or teaching facility.

4. *Payer mix.* Additional information should quantify the proportion of clients for the various types of payers encountered. For example, the percentage of clients having private insurance, Medicare/Medicaid coverage, or HMO membership should be indicated.

5. *Volume statistics.* The RFP should provide volume statistics such as the following: number of inpatient beds, average occupancy, annual outpatient visits, emergency department visits, volume of lab tests performed, number of surgeries annually, and number of various categories of staff including physicians, nurses, and technicians.

- *System requirements.* Following the description of the organization, the RFP should include a comprehensive list of the system requirements previously developed by the committee. One point to consider when defining system requirements is to avoid limiting the vendor to specific configurations, such as the type and number of devices, because the vendor may be able to suggest better solutions.

- *Criteria for evaluation of responses.* Providing the vendor with an explanation of the RFP evaluation process may improve the quality of the vendor's response. If the vendors respond in the expected format, evaluating responses from multiple vendors can be more easily accomplished, and results more easily compared.

- *Deadline date.* Inform the vendor of the expected date of responses. Vendors who do not meet deadlines may be excluded.

Evaluation of RFP Responses

Once responses from various vendors have been received, the process of evaluation begins. Some initial considerations are related to how the vendor approached the RFP. For example, some questions to ask include:

- Was the response submitted by the deadline date?
- Was it the work of a professional team and company?
- Were the vendor representatives responsive and knowledgeable?
- Does the proposal address the requirements outlined in the RFP, or does it appear to be a standard bid?

Further evaluation is centered around the specific responses of the vendors to the requirements listed in the RFP. The prioritization and ranking of the requirements that were previously developed by the steering committee now are used to weight each item in the RFP. This produces an overall score for each vendor response. This score allows the vendors to be ranked objectively, based on their ability to meet the requirements. Vendors that are unable to meet all of the "musts" should be automatically eliminated.

The remaining vendors must now be evaluated in terms of benefits and costs. Examining the scores for the "wants" and discussing the vendor's proposed costs are components of the final decision-making process. It may be helpful to narrow the list to three finalists and then examine these more closely.

Site Visits The use of site visits is very helpful in selecting a system. Site visits allow the system to be seen in action at a location that is comparable in size and services provided. Comparison of site visit evaluations for the top three vendors may provide additional information that will facilitate decision making.

A successful site visit often begins with the preparation of a list of questions. Asking the same questions at each site visit helps the committee draw meaningful comparisons. It is helpful to request a demonstration of the live system. This will allow observations regarding the response time. It is also beneficial to examine reports and printed documentation produced by the system, and to interview people who are actually using the system. Often more candid information can be obtained if the vendors are not present during the interview process. Box 7–3 lists several questions that may be used during a site visit.

In addition, the vendor should provide a contact list of users from other organizations who are willing to be interviewed by phone (Cross 1996). Representatives from hospital departments may ask their counter-

---

Box 7–3 — Questions to Ask During a Site Visit

- How reliable is the system?
- How much downtime do you experience?
- How is the system backup accomplished, and how frequently is this done?
- Does the system use interface standards?
- How do customizations or enhancements get made to the system (in-house or by vendor)?
- How much training was required for users to learn the system?
- What do you like most about the system?
- What things would you like to change about the system?
- What features would you like to see added to the system?
- How is information access restricted, and how is security maintained?
- What have your experiences been with vendor support?

SOURCE: Adapted from *Choosing a Clinical Information System* by Hewlett-Packard Company, 1990, courtesy Hewlett-Packard Company.

parts in other organizations about the performance of the information system. This will provide insight into how the systems actually operate, as well as the support that the vendor provides.

Contract Negotiations

Once the decision has been made by the steering committee, the contract negotiations may be carried out by the enterprise's legal and purchasing representatives. They may request the names of the three highest ranked vendors, as well as their RFP responses. In this way, the contract negotiations will be able to address issues not specifically included in the RFP responses, such as cost justification and expected implementation schedules. The end result will be the selection of one vendor and a system that will be implemented in the enterprise. Following the signing of the contract, the implementation phase begins.

CASE STUDY EXERCISES

You are a member of the committee that will select a clinical documentation system for nurses. Prepare a timeline for the needs assessment and system selection phases. These processes should be accomplished over a 6-month period.

•　　•　　•

Develop a list of "musts" and "wants" and assign a weight to each item. Define what your weighting scale will be.

•　　•　　•

Create a list of questions related to this system selection process that you will ask at site visits.

SUMMARY

- The selection and implementation of an information system occurs through a well-defined process called the life cycle of an information system.
- The four phases of the life cycle of an information system are: needs assessment, system selection, implementation, and maintenance.
- The needs assessment process is often initiated when a deficit in the current method of manual or automated information handling is recognized.
- The system selection steering committee is an essential component of the assessment and selection processes, and leadership as well as membership of this group may impact the success or failure of the project.

- The needs assessment process should include an examination of the vision and mission statements of the organization, since these should guide the committee in looking to the future and determining the organization's information needs.

- A thorough understanding of how information is currently collected and processed is the starting point in performing a needs assessment.

- Determination of the system requirements should address criteria related to all aspects of system performance, including technical, administrative, registration, order entry, results reporting, medical records, and accounting criteria.

- The request for information is a letter or brief document sent to vendors that explains the institution's plans for purchasing and installing an information system. The purpose of the RFI is to obtain essential information about the vendor and its system capabilities in order to eliminate those vendors that cannot meet the organization's basic requirements.

- The request for proposal is a document sent to vendors that describes the requirements of a potential information system. The purpose of this document is to solicit from many vendors proposals that describe the capabilities of their information systems and support services.

- A weighted scoring strategy will facilitate the evaluation of complicated request for proposal responses from vendors, and will improve the ability of the steering committee to make an informed decision.

REFERENCES

Center of Healthcare Information Management. (1991). *Guide to Making Effective H.I.S. Purchase Decisions.* Ann Arbor, MI: Author.

Consulting Services. (1996). *Contingency Planning and Management, 1*(7), 20.

Cross, M. A. (1996). RFP: Simplifying the task of selecting a system. *Health Data Management, 4*(3), 99–105.

Hewlett-Packard Company. (1990). *Choosing a Clinical Information System.* Andover, MA: Author.

Oberst, B. (1991). Computerized doctor office systems: The benefit to the hospital, physician and patient. In M. J. Ball, J. V. Douglas, R. I. O'Desky, and J. W. Albright, (Eds.). *Healthcare information management systems* (pp. 51–61). New York: Springer.

Saba, V. K., and McCormick, K. A. (1996). *Essentials of computers for nurses.* Philadelphia: Lippincott.

Zielstorff, R. D., McHugh, M. L., and Clinton, J. (1988). *Computer design criteria for systems that support the nursing process.* Kansas City, MO: American Nurses Association.

System Implementation and Maintenance

After completing this chapter, you should be able to:

- Describe how implementation committee members are selected.
- Discuss the importance of establishing a project timeline or schedule.
- Explain the difference between the test, training, and production environments.
- List the decisions that must be addressed when performing an analysis of hardware requirements.
- Review the issues that must be addressed when developing procedures and documentation for users.
- Discuss the factors that contribute to effective training.
- Identify the components involved in go-live planning.
- Recognize several common implementation pitfalls.
- Name several common forms of user feedback and support.
- Explain the significance of providing ongoing system and technical maintenance.
- Recognize that the life cycle of an information system is an ongoing cyclical process.

T he previous chapter discussed the first two phases of the life cycle of an information system. This chapter explores system implementation and maintenance, which make up the third and fourth phases.

SYSTEM IMPLEMENTATION

Develop an Implementation Committee

Once the organization has purchased the information system, the implementation phase begins. A project leader is identified and a team of hospital staff is selected to support the project as a working committee. The steering committee chairperson or another member of the steering committee may serve as the implementation project leader. It is important, however, that the project leader be involved in the entire selection and implementation process (Saba and McCormick 1996). This ensures that the project leader has a firm understanding of the vision, goals, and expectations for the system.

The committee membership should include technical staff from the information services department as well as clinical representatives who are knowledgeable regarding current manual or automated procedures. Each group should be represented both by managers who have the authority to make the decisions and by department staff who have knowledge and experience of day-to-day operations. Recruiting efforts should be focused on people who display the characteristics that support effective group dynamics. In addition, the project leader should facilitate the development of effective group dynamics. Some of the characteristics of a successful implementation committee are listed in Box 8–1.

Install the System

The initial work of the implementation committee is to develop a comprehensive project plan or timeline, scheduling all of the critical elements

Box 8–1

Characteristics of a Successful Implementation Committee

Characteristics of Individual Members

- Communicates openly
- Efficiently uses time and talents
- Performs effectively and produces results
- Welcomes challenges
- Cooperates rather than competes

Group Characteristics

- Works toward a common goal
- Encourages members to teach and learn from one another
- Develops its members' skills
- Builds morale internally
- Resolves conflicts effectively
- Shows pride in its accomplishments
- Enhances diversity of its members

for implementation (Hewlett-Packard 1990). This plan should address who is responsible for accomplishing each element and when it must be completed (Figure 8–1). Project planning software may be helpful in developing the project timeline or schedule.

The committee members should first become familiar with the information system they will be implementing. This can be accomplished in several ways. The vendor can provide on-site training, hospital staff can receive training at the vendor's corporate centers, or third-party consultants may be hired. Once committee members have acquired an understanding of how the system functions, they will have the knowledge needed to analyze the base system as it has been delivered from the vendor. The next step is to decide whether this system should be used as is or customized to meet the specific needs of the organization. This decision will act as the implementation strategy that will guide the committee through the implementation process.

Regardless of which implementation strategy is followed, the committee must next gather information about the data that must be collected and processed. Consideration must be given to the data that is pertinent to each function and available to the user for entry into the system. A function refers to a task that may be performed manually or automated. Some examples include order entry, results reporting, and documentation. The output of the system should also be examined. For example, the format and content of printed requisitions, result reports, worklists, and managerial re-

Milestone	Person Responsible	Estimated Start Date	Completion Date
PHASE 3: SYSTEM IMPLEMENTATION			
Develop implementation committee			
Analyze customization requirements			
Perform system modifications and customizations			
Analyze hardware requirements			
Develop procedures and user guides			
System and integrated testing			
Provide user training			
Go-live conversion preparation and backloading			
Go-live event			

FIGURE 8–1 • Sample Template for a System Implementation Timeline

ports must be evaluated. A detailed analysis of the current work and paper flow will provide this information. Once decisions have been made regarding system design and modification, the appropriate department head should approve these specifications before the actual changes are made. Numerous changes delay implementation of the system and drive costs up.

At this point, the identified changes should be made to the system in the test environment. The **test environment** is one copy of the software where programming changes are initially made. After any changes are made, they must be tested to ensure that they display and process data accurately. Testing is best accomplished by following a transaction through the system for all associated functions. An example of this testing procedure might be to enter a physician's order for a chest x-ray into the system for a particular client. The correct printing of the requisition should be verified. Next, the results of the x-ray should be entered for this client. Both on-line results retrieval and printed report content should be verified. Finally, the system should be checked to make certain that the appropriate charges have been generated and passed to the financial system. It is important to realize that the test environment is not exactly the same as the live environment, since the live environment is much larger and more complex. As a result, the findings of the system test may not always indicate how well the system will perform in the live environment.

Analyze Hardware Requirements

A separate group of tasks related to the analysis of hardware requirements must also be addressed during the implementation phase. These tasks should be initiated early in the implementation phase, and continue simultaneously while system design and modifications are being completed. Some of these items include the following:

- *Network Infrastructure.* The determination of network requirements, cable installation, and wiring should be initiated early in the implementation phase. The processing power and memory capacity of network components must be addressed by the technical members of the implementation committee or other IS staff (Zeilstorff, McHugh, and Clinton 1988). Extensive rewiring and cabling may be needed, particularly if additional users are added. This can be an expensive process. Wireless technology may or may not be an alternative. Some functions that place a heavy demand on the network include digital imaging and archival or telemedicine.

- *Type of workstation device.* The system may be accessed via a number of different devices. These may include a networked personal computer (PC), thin client, wireless or handheld device, or mobile laptop PC that uses radio-frequency technology. Even a dumb terminal may provide access. The committee must investigate the advantages of each option and make recommendations regarding the type of hardware for purchase and installation. Once a decision has been made regarding the type of workstation, the appropriate number of devices per area or department must be determined.

- *Workstation location strategy.* A related workstation decision is the strategy for locating and using the hardware. Several options are available. **Point-of-care** devices are located at the site of client care, which is often at the client's bedside. Another strategy involves a centralized approach, where workstations are located at the unit station. A third option is to use hand-held or mobile devices that may be accessed wherever the staff finds it most convenient.

- *Hardware location requirements.* The area where the equipment is to be placed must be evaluated as to adequate electrical receptacles. In addition, the work area may require modifications to accommodate the selected hardware.

- *Printer decisions.* The various printer options should be examined. A choice must be made between laser printer technology, ink jet, and dot matrix, as well as specific features such as the number of paper trays and fonts.

Develop Procedures and Documentation

Comprehensive procedures for how the system will be used to support client care and associated administrative activities should be developed before the training process is begun. In this way, training may include procedures as well as hands-on use of the system. One approach is to examine the current nursing policy and procedure manuals and incorporate new policies and procedures related to automation. Information regarding downtime procedures should be included, so that staff are aware of what to do in the case of planned or unexpected system downtime. It may be beneficial to develop separate documentation that includes the downtime procedures and manual requisition forms, and have this in an easily identifiable and accessible location.

System user guides should also be developed at this point. These documents explain how to use the system and the printouts that the system produces (Saba and McCormick 1996). User guides provided by the vendor may be adequate if a limited number of modifications were made to the base system. However, if significant modifications have been made, it may be necessary to customize this documentation to reflect the system as the users will see it. In this case user guides cannot be completed until all modifications have been completed, tested, and approved for the live system.

Another important aspect of documentation is the development of a dictionary of terms and mapping terms from one system to another (Abbott 1996). This ensures everyone has a clear definition of terms and uses them in the same way.

Testing

The process of testing includes the development of a test plan, the creation of test scripts, system testing, and integrated testing. An effective test plan cannot be created until screens and pathways have been finalized and policies and procedures determined. Otherwise the plan must be revised one or more times. The test plan prescribes what will be examined within the new system as well as all systems that it shares data with. Successful testing requires the involvement of staff who perform day-to-day work because they know the current process and expected outcomes. The test plan should include patient types and functions seen in the facility. A review is then done to identify whether functions are completed without error. Problem areas should be tested again before the person responsible for that area indicates approval and signoff. After system testing, integrated testing can start. Integrated testing looks at the exchange of data between the test system and other systems to ensure that it passes in the fashion desired.

Provide Training

Once all modifications have been completed in the test environment, a training environment should be established. A **training environment** is a separate copy of the software that mimics the actual system that will be used. Many organizations populate the training database with fictitious clients, and make this database available for formal training classes during the implementation process and for ongoing education.

Training is most effective if the training session is a scheduled time independent from the learners' other work responsibilities, and at a site separate from the work environment. This allows the learner to concentrate on comprehending the system without interruptions. Planning should address providing adequate resources to allow for the scheduling of training sessions as close as possible to the go-live date. In addition, learners should have a place to practice following the formal classroom instruction.

Go-Live Planning

The committee should determine the **go-live** date, which is when the system will be operational and used to collect and process actual client data. At this point, the **production environment** is in effect. The production environment is another term that refers to the time when the new system is in operation. Some of the necessary planning surrounding this event includes the following:

- *Implementation strategy.* It must be determined whether implementation will be staggered, be modular, or occur all at once. An example of a staggered implementation strategy may be to go-live in a limited number of client units but in all ancillary departments. The remaining client units would be scheduled to go-live in groups staggered over a specified time frame.

- *Conversion to the new system.* Decisions must be made regarding what information will be **backloaded,** or preloaded into the system before the go-live date. This includes identification of who will perform this task and the methodology used to accomplish it. Plans for how orders will be backloaded must be developed. For example, a "daily × 4" order for a complete blood count should be analyzed to determine how many days will be remaining on the go-live date. This number should be entered when the backload is performed. Backloading may be needed to create accurate worklists, charges, or medication administration sheets. Plans for verification of the accuracy of preloaded data should be considered.

- *Developing the support schedule.* It often is necessary to provide on-site support around the clock during the initial go-live or conversion phase. Support personnel may include vendor representatives, information system staff, and other members of the implementation committee.

- *Developing evaluation procedures.* Satisfaction questionnaires and a method for communicating and answering questions during the go-live conversion should be provided.

- *Developing a procedure to request post go-live changes.* Priority must be given to changes required to make the system work as it should. Additional changes should go before the implementation committee or hospital steering committee to determine necessity. This process helps keep costs manageable.

Common Implementation Pitfalls

There are several common pitfalls with system implementation. Perhaps the most common is an inadequate understanding of how much work is required to implement the system, resulting in underestimation of necessary time and resources. If the initial timeline is not based on a realistic estimate of the required activities and their scope, the implementation process may fall behind schedule. Therefore, it is necessary to fully investigate the impact of the system and control the scope of the project in the early stages of planning.

Another serious problem that may occur during implementation is that of numerous revisions during design activities, creating a constantly moving target. As needed customizations and modifications are identified, it is imperative that the appropriate user department head approve and sign off on them before programming changes are made. Frequent changes can become very frustrating for the technical staff and result in missed deadlines. Ultimately, this can be very expensive and emotionally draining for the implementation team.

The amount and type of customization that is done to the information systems can also result in problems. To guide the implementation team, the implementation strategy must address the degree of customization that will be done. One strategy is using the system as it is delivered by the vendor, with minimal changes. The advantage of this strategy, which is often called the "vanilla" system, is an easier and quicker implementation. In addition, future software upgrades may also be implemented with greater ease and speed. The disadvantage of using the "vanilla" system is that user workflow may not match the system design.

The opposite implementation strategy is to fully customize the information system so that it reflects the current workflow. Although this may seem appealing, the disadvantages include a complicated, lengthy, and expensive implementation process. A further disadvantage is seen when system software upgrades are attempted. Many of the customizations may prohibit the upgrades from being installed without extensive programming effort. As a result, the present trend in the hospital information systems industry is to recommend use of the "vanilla" systems as they are delivered by the vendors.

Another common pitfall is providing insufficient dedicated resources to the implementation committee (Simpson 1996). Clinical representatives of this group cannot be expected to manage a full-time clinical position while contributing significant time to the implementation project. Since the end result of effective implementation is improved client care, it may be cost-effective to temporarily reassign clinical staff to the project.

There may also be problems with testing. These can include poorly developed test scripts, inadequate time to retest problem areas, and the inability to get other systems to exchange data with the test system. Inadequate testing can lead to unpleasant surprises at go-live.

All too often training suffers from inadequate allocation of time and resources. The training environment should mirror the testing environment and later the production environment. Design may not be completed when training starts. This creates a negative impression of the system among end users as well as confusion.

Finally, it is important to continually reinforce the concept that the implementation and the information system are owned by the users. If the users feel no ownership of the system, then they may not accept the system or use it appropriately, nor will they provide feedback regarding potential system improvements.

MAINTENANCE

Following implementation of the system, ongoing maintenance must be provided.

User Feedback and Support

One important aspect of maintenance is communication. Soon after the go-live event, feedback from the implementation evaluation should be acted on in a timely manner. This is usually the first aspect of system maintenance to be addressed. The results should be compiled, analyzed, and communicated to the users and IS staff. Any suggested changes that are appropriate may then be implemented.

Continued communication is imperative for sharing information and informing users of changes. Communication can be accomplished in a variety of ways. For example, a newsletter or printed announcement can be sent to the users, on either a regular or an as-needed basis. System messages can be displayed on the screen or printed at the user location. Focus groups or in-house user groups can be formed for discussion and problem solving.

Another form of user support is the help desk. The **help desk** provides round-the-clock support that is usually available by phone. Most organizations designate one phone number as the access point for all users who need help or support related to information systems. The help desk is usually staffed by personnel from the information systems area who have had special training and are familiar with all of the systems in use. Often they are able to help the user during the initial phone call. If this is not possible, the help desk may refer more complex problems or questions to other staff who have specialized knowledge. The help desk should follow up with the user and provide information as soon as it is available. The biggest problems during go-live are with sign-on and passwords. Users may have missed training or may not remember how to sign on to the system.

Visibility of the support staff in the user areas is another important form of support. By making regular visits to all areas, the support staff is able to gather information related to how the system is performing and impacting the work of the users. In addition, users have the opportunity to ask questions and describe problems without having to call the help desk.

System Maintenance

Ongoing system maintenance must be provided in all three environments: test, training, and production. This enables programming and development to continue in the test region without adverse effect on the training or production systems. Therefore, training can continue without interruption and the training environment can be upgraded to reflect programming changes at the appropriate time. Actual client data and workflow will not be impacted in the production system until the scheduled upgrade has been thoroughly tested in the test environment.

Requests submitted by users can provide input for upgrading or making necessary changes to the system. For example, a user might request changes to standard physician orders, such as a request to delete some lab tests to contain costs, or nursing documentation related to regulatory issues or Joint Commission on Accreditation of Healthcare Organizations (JCAHO) recommendations, such as adding advanced directives documentation. Advanced directives are used to convey whether the client wishes to be intubated, ventilated, or receive CPR or other life-saving or sustaining measures in the event of a medical emergency. The requesters must provide a thorough explanation of the desired changes, as well as the reason for the request. One method of facilitating this communication is to develop a request form, to be completed by the requesting users and submitted to the information services (IS) department. Upon receiving this form, the IS staff should determine if the change is feasible and should also consider whether any alternative solutions exist. Figure 8–2 provides an example of a request for services form.

Technical Maintenance

A large portion of ongoing maintenance is related to technical and equipment issues. This maintenance is the responsibility of the Information Services Department. Some examples of technical maintenance include:

- Performing problem solving and debugging
- Maintaining a back-up supply of hardware such as monitors, printers, cables, trackballs and mice for replacement of faulty equipment in user areas
- Performing file backup procedures

INFORMATION SERVICES REQUEST FOR SERVICES

Requested by: _____ Date: _____

Department: _____

Department Head (print) _____ Phone #: _____

Department Head (signature) _____

Priority: _____ Routine _____ Urgent Date Request Needed: _____

Requirement: _____

_____

_____

_____

_____

Reason for Request: _____ Cost Reduction   _____ Service Improvement

_____ Client Care Improvement   _____ Organizational Requirement

_____ Regulatory Requirement   _____ Other (explain) _____

Please provide other supporting details related to the reason for the request:

FIGURE 8–2 • Request for Information Services Form

- Monitoring the system for adequate file space
- Building and maintaining interfaces with other systems
- Configuring, testing, and installing system upgrades
- Maintaining and updating the disaster recovery plan

The Information System's Life Cycle

As users and technical support staff work with the system, they may come to identify problems and deficiencies. Eventually, these faults may become significant enough that the need to upgrade or replace the system becomes evident, illustrating the cyclical nature of the information system's life cycle. Phase 1, the needs assessment phase, is initiated once more and the life cycle continues. In other words, the life cycle is an ongoing process that never ends.

CASE STUDY EXERCISES

You are the project director responsible for creating an implementation timeline that addresses the training and go-live activities for a nursing documentation system that will be implemented on 20 units and involves

350 users. Determine whether the implementation will be staggered or occur simultaneously on all units, and provide your rationale.

• • •

Create the timeline for the training and go-live schedule for this implementation.

• • •

Your present manual Medication Administration Record is being replaced by an automated information system. Discuss the specifications you would recommend for reports that the system will generate to notify the nurse when medications are due. Determine how often the reports should print and what information they should contain.

You have been selected to develop test scripts for interface testing for a new patient care system. Develop a test script with multiple interfaces. Define the output that you should see for each system.

SUMMARY

- One important aspect of system implementation is the development of an effective implementation committee comprising clinical and technical representatives.
- The first task for the committee is the development of a timeline for system implementation activities.
- The implementation strategy must be determined by the committee. This strategy may call for using the system as it is delivered by the vendor or significantly customizing the system to match the current work needs.
- Identified modifications are made to the software in the test environment, so that actual client data and workflow are not affected.
- The following hardware considerations must be addressed during the implementation phase: type of workstation device, hardware location, printer options, and network requirements.
- User procedures and documentation are developed during the implementation phase, and provide support to personnel during training and actual use of the system.
- Training is a key element for a successful system implementation.
- Careful consideration must be given to planning the go-live conversion activities to minimize disruptions to client care.
- The implementation committee must be aware of the common pitfalls and problems that may negatively affect the implementation process.

- Maintenance, an ongoing part of the implementation process, includes user support and system maintenance.
- The information systems life cycle is a continuous cyclical process.

REFERENCES

Abbott, P. A. (1996). The nursing manager's role in successful system implementation. In M. C. Mills, C. A. Romano, and B. R. Heller, (Eds.). *Information management in nursing and health care* (pp. 116–127). Springhouse, PA: Springhouse Corporation.

Hewlett-Packard Company. (1990). *Choosing a clinical information system*. Andover, MA: Author.

Saba, V. K., and McCormick, K. A. (1996). *Essentials of computers for nurses*. New York: McGraw–Hill.

Simpson, R. L. (1996). Overcoming unrealistic expectations for IS implementation. *Nursing Management, 27*(3), 12–13.

Zielstorff, R. D., McHugh, M. L., and Clinton, J. (1988). *Computer design criteria for systems that support the nursing process*. Washington, DC: American Nurses Association.

9

Information Systems Training

After completing this chapter, you should be able to:

- Outline how learning objectives are determined for each group of users.

- Identify human factors that may negatively affect training.

- Compare and contrast the merits of various teaching approaches for system training.

- Recognize factors that affect learning and retention.

- Cite advantages and disadvantages associated with hospital-based trainers, vendor supplied trainers, and superusers.

- List content areas needed for all information system users.

- Describe methods to evaluate competence in system use.

- Review issues associated with training, including cost, staffing, computer requirements, confidentiality, realism, and teaching students.

As information systems become more prevalent in health care settings, nurses, allied health care professionals, and support staff are forced to master computer skills as a tool for the delivery and documentation of care. Some welcome the change, while others fear or resent what they perceive as the forced use of computers and possible job loss following the introduction of more technology. Computer skills are acquired through study and practice. Education is key to the successful use of any information system. Effective instruction may be costly and time-consuming, but the end result is greater efficiency in information handling, increased marketability of job skills, and improved quality of care. The organized approach to provide large numbers of hospital staff and health care students with the skills needed to use information systems is commonly called **training.** Some educators dislike this term because of its association with behavioral psychology, which focuses on changing the way that an animal or person acts by rewarding desired behavior or punishing undesirable behavior. This contrasts with cognitive psychology, which concentrates on restructuring the way that a person thinks through learning in order to change behavior.

Instructional success may be ensured through the development and implementation of a **training plan** that addresses the following areas:

- *A training philosophy*. Training is most effective when instruction occurs at a dedicated time independent of other work responsibilities and in an environment free from interruption.
- *Identification of training needs*. Prior to the initiation of training, it is necessary to determine who needs to be trained, what needs to be taught, the amount of instruction needed to master the prescribed tasks, what equipment is required, and when and where training will occur.
- *Training approaches*. Instructional decisions include whether to develop or purchase class materials and how the course will be taught:

for example, instructor-led discussion, self-paced modules, technology delivered training, or on-the-job training.

- *Identification of the group or persons who will coordinate or conduct training of hospital staff.* Administration may opt to use outside trainers or their own employees.

- *A timetable.* Those who draft the schedule must consider the number of users who need training prior to the planned date for system implementation, time required to complete training, and how soon trainees' new knowledge can be applied.

- *The budget.* Because it is time- and labor-intensive, training should be considered an investment in successful information system implementation that requires wise allocation of resources.

- *Evaluation strategies.* The ultimate success of training is measured by the ability of individuals to perform expected computer tasks. Tests and class evaluation comments may also be used. Technology delivered learning often provides a mechanism for evaluation (Newbold 1996).

A well-conceived and carefully executed training plan provides a comprehensive approach that ensures proper system use. The training plan should be in alignment with the strategic objectives of the organization (Boisvert 2000). The best plan can still fail if it lacks user acceptance.

IDENTIFICATION OF TRAINING NEEDS

Preparation begins with identifying user needs, followed by determining training class content, class schedules, hardware and software requirements, training costs, a location for training activity, approaches used in training, and evaluation strategies.

User Needs

Needs cannot be determined until the users have been identified. This is done through administrative decisions and analysis of job responsibilities. For example, administrators decide what functions will be automated first. These may include admission, discharge, and transfers; physician order entry; and documentation. Users are the persons who perform or document automated functions or who need to access automated information. See Box 9–1 for a list of personnel who may need information system training.

Despite the fact that different types of personnel often perform some of the same functions, individual job responsibilities differ, as do laws governing professional practice. Representatives from clinical areas can help identify user classes based on job descriptions. A **user class** is a level of personnel who perform similar functions. Not all user classes perform all information system functions, nor do they need training to use

---

Box 9–1 **Who Might Need Training?**

Clinicians

- Physicians
- Dentists
- Registered nurses
- Practical nurses
- Nurse practitioners
- Physician assistants
- Pharmacists
- Nutritionists
- Respiratory therapists
- Occupational therapists
- Speech therapists
- Physical therapists
- X-ray technicians
- Patient care and medical assistants

Students

- Students from all professional and technical health care programs

Support Personnel

- Admission clerks
- Dietary personnel
- Social service staff
- Home health care personnel
- Pastoral care staff
- Housekeeping personnel
- Central supply staff
- Case managers
- Infection control and quality assurance personnel
- Third-party payer certification and verification staff

---

all system functions. For example, licensed practical nurses (LPNs) comprise a user class. LPNs need to see and document client information, but they do not perform order entry. Registered nurses (RNs) have a larger scope of practice and a separate user class. Higher-level user classes include functions assigned to lower classes. This allows RNs to perform functions assigned to support personnel when these personnel are unavailable.

Supplemental staff and students who rotate through institutions with information systems are potential users. The level of automation in a given setting determines whether these groups require computer training. For example, if order entry is the only automated function, then neither students nor supplemental staff require training. When system access is required for the retrieval of data or documentation, training is necessary for supplemental staff to perform their jobs and for students to acquire educational information.

Learning objectives should be based on expected user functions. For example, if the trainee must document vital signs, the trainee must access the system, record vital signs, process the vital signs, and later retrieve them for view.

Training Class Content

Once identification of users and functions slated for automation is complete, class content and learning objectives can be determined. Training classes should address the following areas:

- *Computer-related policies*. Training is an excellent time to discuss client confidentiality, ethical computing, and sanctions for inappropriate system access. Upon completion of training, most institutions require employees to sign a document stating that system misuse may result in termination of employment. It is at this time that employees receive their access code. The **access code** is a unique identifier provided by the user's sign-on name and a password that limits computer use to authorized persons. Nonemployees sign a document stating that misused IS privileges may result in loss of clinical privileges and possible legal action. An example of misuse might include failure to properly handle and dispose of confidential computer printouts.

- *Human factors*. The implementation of an information system is a major change to the work setting. Many people are uncomfortable with change and computers, and fear job loss if they cannot adapt. These fears should be assuaged at the start of training to put users at ease. A review of how automation may benefit employees provides incentive to learn.

- *Basic computer literacy*. Many people lack fundamental computer skills and knowledge. An introduction to the primary parts and function of computers lays a foundation for system training.

- *Workflow*. Automation of manual processes changes the way that work is done. Classes must outline the new process in detail to help users understand how the system works and to make the transition to information systems.

- *The steps to perform specific functions*. For example, the demonstration of order entry must show all steps required to allow trainees to enter orders.

- *Help screens or on-line tutorials.* Help screens and on-line tutorials are beneficial to users, provided that users are aware of their existence and can use them. **Help screens** list specific actions to complete a particular task. **On-line tutorials** provide step-by-step instructions for how to use the software or one of its features. On-line tutorials are available on the computer for referral at any time. Training classes should introduce these features and demonstrate their access and use.

- *Error messages.* **Error messages** are text communications produced by the computer to warn the user that information is missing or improperly constructed. Error messages provide an opportunity to supply missing information or supply it in a format recognized by the information system. For example, a medication order must identify drug, dosage, route, and schedule. Failure to list any of these generates an error message. Class content should address how error messages are produced, avoided, and corrected.

- *Error correction.* Input errors result from typographical or spelling problems or incorrect choices. Errors may be corrected at the time of entry or at a later date. For example, some clinical documentation systems provide an opportunity to review and correct information prior to processing. Corrections are noted as made after data entry. Original entries remain as part of the record.

- *What to do when the system "freezes."* **Freezing** refers to a situation when the computer will no longer accept input or process what has been entered. Users need to know how the system should work and what to do in the event of malfunction, whether that involves referral to troubleshooting guidelines or a call to the information system help desk.

- *System idiosyncrasies.* What information systems can and cannot do is a function of programming and technical limitations. Computer programs often work differently than clinicians who perform a task manually. Major programming changes to accommodate clinicians are not always possible. For this reason, health care workers need to understand the limitations of their information system.

- *Basic equipment care and troubleshooting.* Some problems are as simple as a loose cable or cord or an empty paper tray or toner cartridge. In other cases lost icons, changes made to computer settings such as mouse speed or screen colors, or failure to properly log off of the system can cause difficulties. Users must learn how to deal with these problems.

- *Backup.* **Backup procedures** are alternative ways to accomplish functions normally done via the information system during downtime—times when the system is not operational or available for use. Downtime may be scheduled to perform tasks on a nightly basis or for system updates. Unscheduled downtime occurs as a result of problems. Backup may not be implemented unless downtime is lengthy. Manual requisitions and paper reports of lab results exemplify backup procedures. Backup procedures should be introduced during training and reviewed annually.

- *Alternative means to achieve a task*. It is often possible to accomplish a function in more than one way. Table 9–1 displays sample screen options that permit review of a client's lab results using any one of a variety of menu selections.

Class Schedules

Planning and scheduling class times can be challenging. Learner availability, needs, and attentiveness must be considered. Sessions of 1, 2, or 4 hours look good on paper, but it is difficult for employees to leave the clinical units and then they may feel rushed to return. It is also difficult for staff to arrive on time for sessions scheduled at the end of their shifts. Another problem occurs when workers are too tired or tense to benefit from instruction. For these reasons, dedicated training days often work best.

Class schedules must consider the available training days and the number of personnel who need instruction prior to go-live. When large numbers of people must be taught in a short period, around-the-clock training may be used. Extended class hours provide classes at times when off-shift employees are most attentive. Extra instructors may be needed to cover the additional hours. Preparation time for each class must be factored into the schedule as well. Training should also occur as close to scheduled system implementation time as possible to facilitate recall and application of new knowledge.

Table 9–1 Sample Screen Options for Reviewing Lab Results	
Screen Option	**Information Retrieved**
For the most recent tests	Provides results of the most recently completed tests
For today	Lists all lab findings for the current date
For the previous 2 days	Shows lab findings from the previous 2 days
From the time of admission	Displays all lab findings from admission to the present time, in either chronological or reverse chronological order
From previous admissions	Lists lab findings by dates of previous admissions
By department, e.g., chemistry, hematology, or microbiology	Allows practitioners to quickly find a particular result, such as a wound culture

Hardware and Software Requirements

The best way to learn how to use an information system is to train under conditions similar to working conditions. For example, learners should have the same equipment that is found in the clinical setting with a computer or terminal for their exclusive use. One workstation per individual ensures adequate practice opportunities for each person. Operation of printers and fax machines must be included in class content when these are an integral part of unit function. No training should occur on the actual system to protect client data from inadvertent view, change, or deletion. Client data is sometimes referred to as **live data.** For this reason, many hospital information system vendors offer the capacity to support separate databases for training and for actual system use. This feature allows learners to experience how the software works with simulated client information without jeopardizing confidentiality or interfering with treatment. Different sets of simulated data may be reserved for specific user groups or functions.

Training Costs

Training is expensive primarily because of the personnel hours required to develop, present, receive, and support educational activities (Filipczak 1996). For this reason, salary costs for the following staff must be considered:

- *Trainers.* Trainers spend many hours reviewing and developing materials for the class in addition to the time spent in instruction.
- *Employees undergoing training.* Compensation for time spent in training may be at the regular hourly rate or as overtime compensation if it is scheduled in addition to 40-hour work weeks.
- *Replacement staff.* Clinical units must be staffed while regular employees undergo training.
- *Support staff.* These employees perform jobs such as typing, copying, and collating instructional materials; preparing class audiovisuals; taking reservations for classes; and documenting attendance.

Even when vendors supply training materials, time must be spent to review the suitability of these materials prior to use. Other expenses are the purchase of hardware and software and preparation of a training area. Effective training limits instruction to personnel who need system access and to the functions they need to know.

A Training Center

Because client care is the top priority, no instruction should occur on the clinical units. The only permissible exceptions occur when inservices of 15 minutes or less are needed to address system updates. A dedicated training environment allows staff to focus on learning the system. A hospital site is convenient because employees are already there, travel time between clinical units and the center is nominal, and parking arrangements already exist. Unfortunately, space may not be available. Convenience of location, travel time, and parking or shuttle service are considerations with off-site facilities. Box 9–2 lists some factors to consider when selecting a training site.

No matter what site is selected, the training environment should facilitate learning through good lighting, a comfortable temperature, and good ergonomics. Chair and equipment position should minimize fatigue and repetitive stress injuries. Instructors must make an effort to create a comfortable atmosphere with frequent breaks and variations in teaching methods as a means to maintain student interest.

The training site may later serve a dual purpose because designated terminals or computers can be set up for either training or live system modes. This flexibility permits review of live data from the training area for a variety of purposes such as case management. Trainees cannot access the live system without their own unique access codes. This ability to set terminals or computers for either the training or live modes may also be used to provide additional practice opportunities for staff on the units as time permits.

Training Approaches

The overall training approach should be consistent with the institution's philosophy and reflect the fact that individuals learn at their own rate

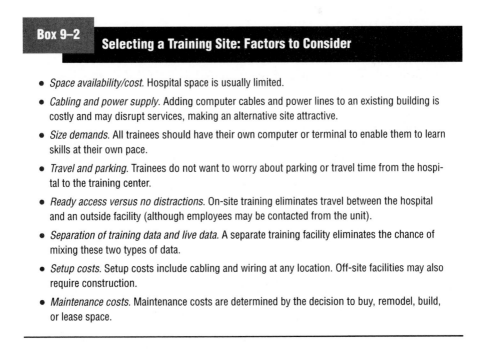

Box 9–2   Selecting a Training Site: Factors to Consider

- *Space availability/cost.* Hospital space is usually limited.

- *Cabling and power supply.* Adding computer cables and power lines to an existing building is costly and may disrupt services, making an alternative site attractive.

- *Size demands.* All trainees should have their own computer or terminal to enable them to learn skills at their own pace.

- *Travel and parking.* Trainees do not want to worry about parking or travel time from the hospital to the training center.

- *Ready access versus no distractions.* On-site training eliminates travel between the hospital and an outside facility (although employees may be contacted from the unit).

- *Separation of training data and live data.* A separate training facility eliminates the chance of mixing these two types of data.

- *Setup costs.* Setup costs include cabling and wiring at any location. Off-site facilities may also require construction.

- *Maintenance costs.* Maintenance costs are determined by the decision to buy, remodel, build, or lease space.

and in their own way (Abla 1995, Fender and Jennerich 1997, Glydura, Michelman, and Wilson 1995). A combination of instructional approaches improves overall retention for individuals with different learning styles. This strategy recognizes individual needs and values, and attempts to provide something for everybody. An example of a combination training approach may be seen with the instructor who uses a data projector to display the terminal to the class and provides written materials such as manuals, printouts of sample screens, exercises, self tests, and a training hospital. The **training hospital** is a collection of simulated client data assembled and stored for instructional purposes in a database separate from live client data. The training hospital offers all the automated functions found in the actual system but with no access to live client information. This use of multiple media in conjunction with hands-on practice enhances learning over any single approach. See Box 9–3 for factors to consider when choosing training methods.

Many options exist for training: traditional classroom instruction, computer-based training, on-line multimedia, on-line tutorials, on-the-job training, peer training, video, job aids, and self-directed text-based courses (Filipczak 1996, Mascara, Bartos, Nelson, and Rafferty 1994). Table 9–2 outlines advantages, disadvantages, and organizational tips for each instructional approach. Although traditional classroom training is heavily used, it is resource intensive (Zielstorff 1996). For this reason the popularity of alternative approaches is growing. A combination of self-paced and instructor-led approaches provides variety and offers the advantages associated with both methods. Case studies also help learners to work through ethical issues and apply new knowledge.

Training Materials Well-designed instructional materials are critical to successful information system training (Abla 1995, Filipczak 1996, Henry and Swartz 1995). **Learning aids** are materials intended to supplement or

---

Box 9–3 | **Selecting a Training Method: Factors to Consider**

- *Time.* Instructional approaches vary in the time required for development and presentation. For example, lectures can be written and revised quickly and provide content to large numbers of people at one time.

- *Cost.* Training methods vary in the number of personnel hours and money required for development and revision.

- *Learning styles.* People learn differently. For example, some people prefer to hear material, while others are visual learners. A combination of instructional methods aids overall learning.

- *Learning retention.* Repetition and the ability to apply learning via practice opportunities and application in the work setting help people to remember content.

Table 9–2 Advantages and Disadvantages Associated with Various Training Approaches and Tips for Effective Organizational Use

Training Approach	Advantages	Disadvantages	Tips for Effective Organizational Use
Instructor-led Class	Flexible Easily updated Can include demonstrations Allows for individual help Can test proficiency	Often relies on lecture ↑ class size ↓ demonstration effectiveness Consistency varies with trainer Difficult to maintain pace good for all	For each user group: • Keep a file with objectives and exercises. • Use the same presentation order. • Use generic examples unlikely to change over time. Never rely on just one trainer—leaves no paper trail for others to follow
Computer-based training (CBT)	Self-paced Interactive ↑ retention-uses technology to teach technology 24-hour availability Can be offered on-line or off-line Can be done in increments Facilitates mastery learning Emulates "real" system without threat of harm	Time- and labor-intensive to develop and revise Requires great attention to accompanying materials Limited usefulness of vendor supplied materials without customization	Trainer serves as a facilitator Needs specific, well-prepared learning aids
On-line multimedia	Interactive Stimulates multiple senses for ↑ retention Can test proficiency	Requires intense planning, resources for design, and revision Less flexible to revise	Use and revise carefully
On-line tutorials	24-hour availability Allows immediate application of learning Can test proficiency	Design and revision more involved than instructor-led training	Must have access from all locations and availability must be known
E-mail	Provides individual feedback on entry errors	All users must have e-mail Too slow for actual training	Must know how to use e-mail and have access

Table 9–2	Advantages and Disadvantages Associated with Various Training Approaches and Tips for Effective Organizational Use (Continued)		
Training Approach	**Advantages**	**Disadvantages**	**Tips for Effective Organizational Use**
Video	24-hour availability Easily revised/updated Extends resources	Not interactive Use for select content such as ethical dilemmas—not actual training	Use carefully
On-the-job training	Individualized Permits immediate application Can test proficiency	Trainer often does not know educational principles May lose productivity of two workers Seasoned employees may pass on poor habits Difficult to achieve with many interruptions	Trainer must know basic adult education principles May work well for unit clerks or working in pairs or to learn PC applications
Peer training	Training specific to function Can test proficiency	Trainer often does not know educational principles Seasoned employees may pass on poor habits	Trainer must know basic adult education principles May work well for unit clerks or working in pairs or to learn PC applications.
Superuser	Acquainted with clinical area and the information system May come from any user class Serves as communication link between user class and IS constraints	Spends time away from clinical responsibilities for additional information system training and meetings	May serve as resource persons particularly during off-shifts May assist with training other users
Job aids	↓ need to memorize ↓ training time ↓ help requests	Not effective if access is limited	Requires careful planning and structure Make accessible and user friendly
Self-directed text-based courses	Self-paced Can test proficiency Lacks interaction with training hospital/ system	Requires high level of motivation	Need highly structured materials

Source: Adapted with permission from Bush, A.M.P. (1993). "Computer-based training: Training approach of choice," *Computers in Nursing, 11*(4), 163–164; Sitting et al. (1995). "Evaluating a computer-based experiential learning simulation: A case study using criterion-referenced testing," *Computers in Nursing 13*(1), 17–24; the May 1996 issue of *Training Magazine.* Copyright © 1996. Lakewood Publications, Minneapolis, MN. All rights reserved.

reinforce lecture or computer-based training. Learning aids may include outlines, diagrams, charts, or conceptual maps. **Job aids** are written instructions designed for reference use in both the training and work settings. When vendor-supplied materials are available, they must be evaluated for quality of documentation and consistency with the current system. Vendor-prepared manuals do not usually reflect customization efforts. No training materials should be developed until system development is complete and the system works properly. User class representatives should review handouts and training materials for quality, clarity, and content prior to widespread training to guarantee that materials are accurate and easily understood.

Proficiency Testing

Proficiency tests are routinely included in IS training as a means to assure that learners can perform required functions. Any instructional approach can accommodate proficiency testing (Sittig, Jiang, Manfre, et al. 1995). Exams may be criterion- or norm-referenced. Criterion-referenced measures evaluate predetermined competencies, while norm-referenced tools assess performance relative to other persons. Norm-referenced testing is useful in competitive hiring situations where there are more applicants than positions available. However, this type of testing is not typically used with IS training. The tasks of administering, scoring, and storage and retrieval of individual exam scores are facilitated by technology delivered learning (Vaillancourt 2000).

IS Trainers Hospital administration decides who will conduct system training, based on cost factors and feedback from the IS department and representatives from the system selection committee. Instruction may be done by vendor-supplied personnel, consultants, or hospital employees. There are pros and cons for each approach. Vendor-supplied personnel and consultants typically know the information system well but lack knowledge of the institution's culture. Vendor-supplied trainers leave after the initial training is complete, forcing the hospital to find another means to train new employees as they are hired. Box 9–4 lists some factors to consider when selecting trainers.

Often hospitals develop and use a core set of instructors from their own personnel ranks. These individuals receive their initial system training from the vendor and then teach staff to use the system. They often come from the following groups:

- *Hospital-wide or staff development educators*. Educators know basic principles of adult education but may lack familiarity with specific day-to-day unit routines.
- *Clinicians*. Clinicians have expertise in their practice areas.
- *Department supervisors*. These individuals know their areas well but may not be able to leave their other responsibilities.

Box 9–4	Selecting a Trainer: Factors to Consider

- *Teaching skills and experience.* Previous experience is helpful.
- *Ability to work well with groups.* Interaction with a group differs from one-on-one communication. Most training occurs in a group setting, so this ability is an asset for system trainers.
- *Understanding user groups and their responsibilities.* Trainers may not represent every user group, but they must understand what every group does and the information they need to know to perform their jobs.
- *Training approach.* Trainers should be comfortable with the chosen approach. For example, if computer-based training is used, instructors must be acquainted with its features and help learners through it as needed.
- *Centralized versus departmental training.* Centralized hospital training presents general principles, while departmental training provides specific information related to individual responsibilities in a given area.

- *Information services personnel.* These individuals understand how the system works but lack a clinical perspective and may be unfamiliar with instructional theory.

A dedicated core of trainers helps to provide consistent instruction. Training does not end after initial system implementation; it continues as new employees are hired and additional functions are automated over the passage of time.

Superuser Another resource person is the **superuser,** a staff person who has become proficient in the use of the system and mentors others. Superusers may come from any of the user classes. Their specialized knowledge of both the system and clinical areas enables superusers to assist with training or help staff on other units. Superusers may be available on all shifts and can answer questions when IS staff are not available.

ADDITIONAL TRAINING CONSIDERATIONS

There are several issues related to training that should be addressed in every setting. These include but are not limited to the following:

- *Responsibility for training costs.* Institutions handle training costs differently. Some hospitals may charge each department a fee for training their personnel.
- *Responsibility for trainers.* Trainers frequently come from several departments. This may create confusion as to who their supervisors are or the length of their assignments. They may be temporarily assigned to the IS department.

- *Realistic training.* To be effective, training should incorporate examples seen in day-to-day practice.
- *Confidentiality.* Occasionally, simulated clients resemble actual cases or use celebrity names. This may raise concerns over confidentiality.
- *System updates.* Seasoned employees must be inserviced as additional functions are added, such as documentation of medication administration, nursing care plans, or critical pathway management.
- *The employee who fails to demonstrate system competence.* These situations should be handled individually. Learning time varies, and some people do not value the acquisition of computer skills. Inability to develop in this area may result in job loss.
- *Training personnel from other institutions.* As more hospitals merge, IS trainers must also teach staff from other hospitals that are at different stages of implementation.
- *Training students.* Responsibility for training and quality of clinical experiences are concerns.

Training Students

Training for students must be reevaluated periodically to keep abreast of needs and to ensure currency of information (Mascara et al. 1994). Students must be able to assess their clients, and review test results, document findings, and care on automated systems. Consideration must be given to the best ways to educate students because it is a costly undertaking in terms of time and resources. In fact, individual institutions derive few direct gains from training students unless the students seek employment within the enterprise after graduation. One IS strategy to minimize training efforts may be seen with the use of existing user classes for student use. This eliminates the need to create additional user classes and instructional materials. An example of this tactic is seen with the application of the vocational nurse user class for student professional nurses. Both of these populations demand access to client information and the ability to document assessment and care, but neither group requires order entry. Nursing assistant user functions may work well for medical assistant students.

Other options include making computer-based training available at affiliating schools, or utilizing faculty to instruct students on system use. IS training may also be incorporated into an elective course, enhancing marketability of graduates and possibly shortening their orientation period. The least satisfactory approach occurs when students receive no training or access, and faculty must enter all documentation for their students.

CASE STUDY EXERCISES

Kevin Gallagher, RN, has access to all client records on his medical–surgical unit. Consider each of the following situations:

- Kevin's mother is admitted to the unit. Is it appropriate for him to peruse his mother's electronic medical record? Why or why not?
- Kevin's unit clerk also has access to Mrs. Gallagher's record. Is it appropriate for her to view Mrs. Gallagher's record? Why or why not?
- Kevin's co-worker, Kaneesha, is a client on the unit assigned to another staff nurse's care. Is it appropriate for Kevin to review her chart or lab results? Why or why not?

· · ·

Nancy Whitehorse, RN, routinely accesses client records on her medical unit. Does she violate her confidentiality statement if she performs the following actions?

1. She reviews the information and doesn't discuss it with anyone else.
2. She discusses information obtained from client records with other health care workers on the unit.
3. She discusses clinical cases, omitting names, in social situations.

· · ·

Grace Elizaga has been given the charge of training the RNs and unit clerks from the first three client care units slated to start automated order entry at Potter's Medical Center (PMC). The target implementation date is in 2 months. A total of 93 RNs and 11 unit clerks must receive training prior to that time. Based on information from other agencies that have the same information system as PMC, 8 hours of training time is projected for each individual. As the nurse manager responsible for those units, you have been asked to work with Grace to develop a detailed plan to accomplish this task and submit this plan to your vice presidents of Client Care Services. Include the following in your plan and provide your rationale:

- Staffing
- Costs for your personnel
- Training start and completion dates
- Length and number of training sessions

SUMMARY

- Education is a key factor in the proper use of an information system. Education should be guided by a teaching plan that identifies user needs and includes a teaching philosophy, desired types of educators, and a timetable for training.

- Before user needs can be identified, it is necessary to identify the users. For IS purposes personnel levels are grouped into user classes by job description. Each class performs similar functions. For example, RNs, LPNs, physicians, and unit clerks each comprise separate user classes with different access privileges needed to do their work.

- IS training may be negatively impacted by discomfort with change or computers, the training environment, the class schedule, or instructional approach.

- The need for training must be evaluated for all potential IS users, not just staff. This group may include supplemental staff and students.

- No training should occur on client units or with live client information except for short updates. This protects the integrity of live information and provides an environment where learners can focus their attention on learning how to use the system.

- Training is a costly endeavor because it is labor- and time-intensive.

- IS training may be supplied by vendors or consultants, or drawn from any one of the following personnel groups: hospital educators, clinicians, or IS staff.

- Superusers are personnel with additional IS training or an above-average mastery of the system or both. They serve as resource persons in their departments, answering questions and helping others to work through IS problems. Superusers may come from any user class.

- Criterion-based competence tests may be included as part of training as a means to ensure that all learners demonstrate expected computer skills.

- Some training issues include determining responsibility for costs, staffing, trainer selection and chain of command, realism in training, confidentiality, how to handle system updates, what to do with the employee who fails to develop computer skills, and how to best meet the training needs of students.

REFERENCES

Abla, S. (1995). The who, what, where, when, and how of computer education. *Computers in Nursing, 13*(3), 114–117.

Boisvert, L. (2000). Web-based learning. *Information Systems Management, 17*(1), 35, 6 p.

Bush, A. M. P. (1993). Computer-based training: Training approach of choice. *Computers in Nursing, 11*(4), 163–164.

Fender, M., and Jennerich, B. (1997). The real key to success with new technology: Understanding people. *Enterprise Systems Journal, 12*(4), 38, 40, 42, 44, 46.

Filipczak, B. (1996). Training on the cheap. *Training, 33*(5), 28–34.

Glydura, A. J., Michelman, J. E., and Wilson, C. N. (1995). Multimedia training in nursing education. *Computers in Nursing, 13*(4), 169–175.

Henry, S. A., and Swartz, R. G. (1995). Enhancing healthcare education with accelerated learning techniques. *Journal of Nursing Staff Development, 11*(1), 21–24.

Mascara, C. M., Bartos., C. E., Nelson, R., and Rafferty, D. (1994). An effective approach for providing nursing students with HIS access. In S. J. Grobe and E. S. P. Pluyter-Wenting (Eds.), *Nursing informatics: An international overview for nursing in a technological era* (pp. 563–566). The proceedings of the Fifth IMIA International Conference on Nursing Use of Computers and Information Science. New York: Elsevier Science.

Newbold, S.K. (1996). Maximizing technology for cost-effective staff education and training. In M. C. Mills, C. A. Romano, and B. R. Heller, (Eds.). *Information management in nursing and health care* (pp. 216–221). Springhouse, PA: Springhouse Corporation.

Sittig, D. F., Jiang, Z., Manfre, S., Sinkfeld, K., Ginn, R., Smith, L., Olsen, A., and Borden, R. (1995). Evaluating a computer-based experiential learning simulation: A case study using criterion-referenced testing. *Computers in Nursing, 13*(1), 17–24.

Vaillancourt, S. (4 May 2000). Technology delivered learning. Presented at Tri-State Nursing Computer Network, Pittsburgh, PA.

Zielstorff, R. (1996). Training issues in system implementation. In M. C. Mills, C. A. Romano, and B. R. Heller, (Eds.). *Information management in nursing and health care* (pp. 128–138). Springhouse, PA: Springhouse Corporation.

10

Information Security and Confidentiality

After completing this chapter, you should be able to:

- Differentiate between privacy, confidentiality, information privacy, and information security.

- Discuss how information systems impact privacy, confidentiality, and security.

- Relate the significance of security for information integrity.

- Review several security measures designed to protect information and discuss how they work.

- Distinguish between appropriate and inappropriate password selection and handling.

- State examples of confidential forms and communication that are commonly seen in health care settings and identify proper disposal techniques for each.

- Discuss the impact that Internet technology has on health information security.

H ealth care information systems must provide rapid access to accurate and complete client information to legitimate users, while safeguarding client privacy and confidentiality. Health care administrators must demonstrate measures that protect information in order to comply with Health Insurance Portability and Accountability Act (HIPAA) requirements and meet accreditation criteria set forth by the Joint Commission on Accreditation of Healthcare Organizations (JCAHO) (Joint Commission 1996). Protection of client privacy and confidentiality requires an understanding of the concepts of privacy, confidentiality, information privacy, and security.

PRIVACY, CONFIDENTIALITY, AND SECURITY

While the terms *privacy* and *confidentiality* are often used interchangeably, they are not the same. **Privacy** is a state of mind, a specific place, freedom from intrusion, or control over the exposure of self or of personal information (Kmentt 1987, Windslade 1982). **Confidentiality** refers to a situation in which a relationship has been established and private information is shared (Romano 1987). Confidentiality is essential for the accurate assessment, diagnosis, and treatment of health problems. Once a client discloses confidential information, control over its redisclosure lies with the persons who access it (Curtin and Simpson 1999). Inappropriate redisclosure may be extremely damaging. For example, insurance companies may deny coverage based on information revealed to them without the client's knowledge or consent. Inappropriate disclosure can also damage reputations and personal relationships or result in loss of employment.

Information privacy is the right to choose the conditions and extent to which information and beliefs are shared (Murdock 1980). Informed consent for the release of specific information illustrates information privacy in practice. Information privacy includes the right to ensure accuracy of information collected by an organization (Murdock 1980). **Information security,** on the other hand, is the protection of information against threats to its integrity or inadvertent disclosure. Information systems can improve protection for client information in some ways and endanger it in others. Unlike the paper record that can be read by anyone, the automated record cannot easily be viewed without an access code. Poorly secured information systems threaten record confidentiality because they may be accessed from multiple sites with immediate dissemination of information. This makes clients highly vulnerable to the redisclosure of sensitive information.

INFORMATION SYSTEM SECURITY

Information system security is the protection of both information housed on the system and the system itself from threats or disruption (Brandt 1995, Eager 1995, Ettinger 1993, Liebmann 1995, Mitchell 1993). The primary goals of health care information system security are the protection of client confidentiality and information integrity. These goals are best met when security is planned rather than applied to an existing system after problems occur. Planning for security saves time and money and should be regarded as a form of insurance against downtime, breeches in confidentiality, and lost productivity. In addition to being secure, the system must still be easily accessible for legitimate users (Layland 1995, Schnaidt 1995).

Security Risks

Potential threats to information and system security come from a variety of sources (Baldwin 2000, Hoffman 1995, Kabay 1995, "PC Week executive" 1995). These threats may result in violations to confidentiality, interruptions in information integrity, and possible disruption in the delivery of services. A thorough risk analysis of the environment should be done when the system is implemented, with change, and whenever a problem occurs. Professionals may also be hired to test the system for vulnerabilities.

System Penetration Even the best-secured systems can be penetrated (Garner 1995, Robinson 1994). While no penetrations of health information systems have yet been reported, a survey conducted in the business sector found that more than half of its respondents claimed financial loss caused by inadequate security (Panettieri 1994). These respondents identified the greatest obstacles to better information security as a lack of personnel, insufficient funding and tools, and management apathy.

The main types of people who become involved in system penetration and computer crime include (Eager 1995, Slade 1994) the following:

- *Opportunists.* Opportunists take advantage of the situation and their access to information for uses not associated with their jobs.

- *Hackers.* Hackers are individuals who have an average, or above average, knowledge of computer technology and who dislike rules and restrictions. Hackers penetrate systems as a challenge, and many do not regard their acts as criminal. Others, however, break into systems with the intent of obtaining information.

- *Computer or information specialists.* These individuals are knowledgeable about how computers work and are in the best position to commit computer crime and disable systems while avoiding detection.

Unauthorized Users Although the most common fear is that of system penetration from outsiders, the greatest threat actually comes from employees who view information inappropriately, disrupt information availability, or corrupt data integrity. Such access constitutes unauthorized use and may occur at any level within an organization. Consideration must be given to the access rights accorded to all employees, including system administrators.

Even though health care professionals have codes of ethics to maintain client confidentiality, not all professionals act ethically. This is the reason that system safeguards are needed as well. As health care alliances grow and client records become more accessible, the likelihood of unauthorized system access will increase. Legal protection has been limited until recently, although the enactment of HIPAA will change this situation. Consumer groups and health care professionals need to serve as advocates for health care consumers in the protection of privacy and confidentiality.

Concern for client confidentiality is not limited to the period of active treatment. Record access may occur later through loopholes that exist in automated systems (Eager 1995, Hebda, Sakerka, and Czar 1994, Meranda 1995, Safran, Rind, Citroen et al. 1995). These loopholes will be found by curious users and must be corrected as soon as information system (IS) personnel and administrators become aware of them. One example may be illustrated with the automated system that restricts access to client records during treatment but allows retrieval of any record or lab value after client discharge. Health care alliance physicians and office staff often need to see test results after the client's admission but should be able to view the results only for their clients. This type of problem represents an oversight in the design process that must be revised.

Sabotage The destruction of computer equipment or records or the disruption of normal system operation is known as **sabotage.** This may be a problem with IS staff, but the majority of health care users are not accorded system privileges that would permit this type of destruction. Employees who are satisfied and well informed and feel a vested interest in maintaining information and system security are less likely to wreak havoc on the system. A positive environment, a well-defined institutional ethics policy, and intact security mechanisms help to deter intentional information, or system, misuse or destruction.

Errors and Disasters Errors may result from poor design or system changes that permit users more access than they require. This may be seen when information is restricted during the client's period of treatment but is available after discharge to any user. Errors may also arise from incorrect user entries such as inadvertent selection of the wrong client for data retrieval or documentation.

During disasters, manual backup procedures may compromise information because the primary focus is on maintaining services. One example of this is seen when paper reports of lab findings are not enclosed in envelopes for delivery to client care units.

Viruses, Worms, and Other Malicious Programs **Viruses** are deliberately written programs that use a host computer to spread and reproduce themselves without the knowledge of the person(s) operating the computer (Slade 1994). Viruses need normal computer operations to spread. Originally viruses attached themselves to other computer programs. They may, or may not, damage data or disrupt system operation. Some viruses are likened to electronic graffiti in that the writer leaves his mark by displaying a message. Infected boot sectors of diskettes and e-mail attachments are the most common methods of infection. The boot sector of a diskette contains start-up instructions for computers. When the computer is booted, or started, from the infected diskette, the virus is spread to the computer, which then infects the hard drive and diskettes used in that machine. Another type of virus requires execution of the infected file for spread. Viruses may use a combination of these approaches and are frequently widespread at the time of detection.

Viral infection may be spread through public access electronic bulletin boards; the Internet; e-mail attachment files, shareware, and commercial software; and infected diskettes taken from one computer or network to another. The infectious period for viruses is contingent upon viral type. Infection may occur with each run of the infected program or during any time that the infected program is run, or the virus may remain active in the computer memory until the computer is turned off.

Viruses are not the only program types that can damage data or disrupt computing (Slade 1994). Other malicious programs include worms, Trojan horses, logic bombs, and bacteria. See Table 10–1 for characteristics associated with each program type.

Occasionally peripherals, such as terminals and printers, may serve as **vectors** (Slade 1994). Vectors are devices that house viruses or other malicious programs until they can be spread to other computers. While antivirus software can locate and eradicate viruses and other destructive

Table 10–1	Characteristics of Malicious Programs

Program Type	Characteristics
Viruses	Require normal computer operations to spread May or may not disrupt operation or damage data
Worms	Named for pattern of damage left behind Often use LAN and WAN communication as a means to spread and reproduce
Trojan horses	Appear to do (or actually do) one function while performing another, undesired action One common example resembles a regular system log-in but records user names and passwords to another program for illicit use Do not self-replicate Are easily confined once discovered
Logic bombs	Are triggered by a specific piece of data such as a date, user name, account name, or identification May be part of a regular program or contained in a separate program May not activate upon the first program run May be included in virus-infected programs and with Trojan horses
Bacteria	Are a class of viral programs Do not affix themselves to existing programs

programs, the best defense against malicious programs is knowledge obtained from talking with computer users and experts about problems experienced. Some people are experts in viral detection and eradication. Box 10–1 provides tips for how to avoid malicious programs.

If a virus is contained on one machine, all diskettes used on it must be isolated (Phillips 1995, Slade 1994). Antivirus software must be used to disinfect diskettes and computers. Suspect files should be deleted. All backup diskettes should be considered suspect. It should not be necessary to reformat the hard drive to eliminate the virus(es).

Additional threats to information and system security come from poor password management, sharing passwords, and leaving logged-on terminals unattended (Gordon 1993, Miller 1993). Improper disposal of printed reports, and denial of receipt or authorship of documents also threaten information and systems.

SECURITY MECHANISMS

Security mechanisms use a combination of logical and physical restrictions to provide a greater level of protection than is possible with either approach alone ("PC Week executive" 1995, Safran et al. 1995). An example of a logical restriction is automatic sign-off. **Automatic sign-off** is

Box 10–1

How to Avoid Malicious Programs

- Use only licensed software.
- Use the latest version of virus detection software routinely. Upload updates on a regular basis.
- Never open any file attachment from an unfamiliar source.
- Use designated machines to check all new diskettes and software for viruses prior to use.
- Keep copies of computer start-up instructions, including CONFIG.SYS and AUTOEXEC.BAT files.
- Maintain a list of all program files, their size, and date of creation, and review these periodically for change.
- Retain backup copies of original software, work files, and directory structure for each PC. Backup can quickly restore system setup and work. However, since most software is now available on CD-ROM and can be reinstalled quickly, backup may not be necessary.
- Have lists of vendor, purchase date, and serial number for all hardware and software items to facilitate virus tracking.
- If a virus is found, send a copy to an expert for tracking purposes.

a mechanism that logs a user off the system after a specified period of inactivity on their terminal or computer. This procedure is recommended in all client care areas, as well as any other area where sensitive data exists.

Physical Security

Physical security measures include placement of computers, file servers, or terminals in restricted areas. When this is not possible, equipment may be removed or locked. Physical security is a challenge for remote access. **Remote access** is the ability to use the health enterprise's information system from outside locations such as a physician's office. This ability makes it difficult to determine whether the user is authorized or whether someone else is using the user's access code and password. Secure modems and encryption are particularly useful in conjunction with remote access.

Physical security is also challenged with the growing popularity of mobile wireless devices (Tabar 2000). This unique threat is seen with mobile devices such as personal digital assistants (PDAs) and laptops, which can fall into unauthorized hands. A future technology may involve radio tracking devices.

Passwords and Other Means of Authentication

Access codes and passwords are the most effective means for restricting automated record access (Houser 1995, Levin 1995, Liebmann 1995,

McCarthy 1996, Phillips 1995). A **password** is a collection of alphanumeric characters that the user types into the computer. This may be required after the entry and acceptance of an access code, sometimes referred to as the user name. IS administrators sometimes require this information to problem-solve or reissue passwords. The password does not appear on the screen when it is typed, nor should it be known to anyone but the user and IS administrators. Recommendations for password selection and use are given in Box 10–2. Obvious passwords are easily compromised. Software is available to test and eliminate easily compromised passwords prior to use.

Individuals should not share passwords or leave terminals logged in and unattended. System administrators must keep files that contain password lists safe from view or copying by unauthorized individuals. One compromised password can jeopardize information and the system that contains it. System administrators need to allow legitimate users the opportunity to access the system while refusing entry to others. One means to accomplish this is to shut a terminal down after a random number of unsuccessful access attempts and send security to check that area. Although passwords provide considerable system protection, other defenses are still necessary. These include measures to verify user identity. Figure 10–1 shows a screen shot of a log-in screen.

Sign-on access codes and passwords are generally assigned upon successful completion of system training (Liebmann 1995, Safran et al. 1995). Passwords may be difficult for the user to recall. This leads some people to write password(s) down and post them in conspicuous places. This practice should be prohibited. Passwords must be regarded as an electronic signature.

Frequent and random password change is recommended as a routine security mechanism (Brandt 1995). In truth, this can be an arduous, un-

Box 10–2   **Recommendations for Password Selection and Use**

- Choose passwords that are at least six characters long.
- Use combinations of upper- and lowercase letters, numbers, punctuation marks, and symbols.
- Do not use proper names, initials, words taken from the dictionary, or account names.
- Do not use words that are spelled backwards or with reversed syllables.
- Do not use dates or telephone, license plate, or social security numbers.
- Do not store or automate passwords in the computer.
- Avoid repeated numbers or letters.
- Keep passwords private.
- Change passwords frequently, with no reuse of passwords for a specified period.

FIGURE 10–1 • Screen Shot of a Logon Screen

pleasant task. There are, however, situations that mandate immediate change or deletion of access codes and passwords, including suspicion of unauthorized access and termination of employees. Codes and passwords should also be deleted with status changes such as resignations, leaves of absence, and the completion of rotations for students, faculty, and residents. Because IS staff can view any information in the system, all members of the department should receive new passwords when IS personnel leave. In the event that an IS employee is terminated, department door locks should be changed as well.

Firewalls

A **firewall** is a combination of hardware and software that forms a barrier between systems, or different parts of a single system, to protect those systems from unauthorized access ("Ensuring security" 1995, McCarthy 1996, Riley 1996, Semeria 1996). Firewalls screen traffic and allow only approved transactions to pass through them and restrict access to other systems or sensitive areas such as client information, payroll, or personnel data. Multiple firewalls can increase protection. Strong security policies and practices strengthen firewall protection. Once a user has passed through the firewall, controlling access to individual applications takes place elsewhere.

Application Security

Another area of concern is **application security,** which refers to protecting from harm a set of programs and the information that they store or create. Application security should be used with the client information system and other systems such as payroll records. Employees should sign off when they leave a terminal or computer or are finished using a particular software application, because failure to do so may allow others to use their code to access information. Automatic sign-off has been designed as a security measure when employees fail to properly exit a program or step away from the computer.

Antivirus Software

Antivirus software is a set of computer programs that can locate and eradicate viruses and other malicious programs from scanned diskettes, individual computers, and networks. The constant creation of new viruses makes it necessary to update antivirus software often. Antivirus software may come preloaded on new computers or be obtained in computer stores or over the Internet. Figure 10–2 shows a screen shot from an antivirus program indicating the presence of a virus.

ADMINISTRATIVE AND PERSONNEL ISSUES

Ultimately, the responsibility for protecting client privacy and confidentiality lies with health care administrators (Emery 1995, Faaoso 1992, Fried 1995, Kabay 1995, Smith and Kallman 1995). Upper management must have security awareness training and set a positive example. Next, administration must work with IS personnel to establish the following centralized security functions:

```
                                    Print Virus Information


****************************************************************
                    Virus Information
****************************************************************


Virus Name:   _1000
Aliases:
Infects:      .COM Files
Likelihood:   Rare
Length:       1000 bytes

Characteristics

Memory Resident   Yes   Triggered Event No
Size Stealth      No    Encrypting       Yes
Full Stealth      No    Polymorphic      No

Comments
No additional information.
```

FIGURE 10–2 • Screen Shot from an Antivirus Software Program

- *Correct, complete information security policies, procedures, and standards.* These should be published on-line for easy access, with e-mail notification of employees as new policies come out.

- *Information asset ownership and sensitivity classifications.* Ownership in this context refers to who is responsible for the information, including its security. Sensitivity classification is a determination of how damaging that information might be if it were disclosed inappropriately. The level of sensitivity may be used to determine what information should be encrypted.

- *Identification of security issues for managers.* Managers cannot properly safeguard information or information systems if they are unaware of actual or potential threats to either.

- *Identification of a comprehensive security program.* A well-defined security plan can avert or minimize threats. A key part of the plan is the identification of responsibility for information integrity and confidentiality.

- *Information security training and user support.* Education is an important component in fostering proper system use.

- *An institution-wide information security awareness program.* Formal IS training and frequent suggestions serve to remind users of the need to protect information. In reality, responsibility for system and information security is shared by health care administrators, IS and health care professionals, and all system users. Involving users in system development fosters ownership of this responsibility. This involvement can occur on an individual level or through an institutional security committee. Security committees should consider routine maintenance, third-party payer needs, legal issues inclusive of monitoring, ongoing security needs as the institution and system evolve, and disaster planning. The IS department should address these functions when there is no security committee. Individual users are responsible for protecting their passwords, saving and backing up work files on a regular basis, securing removable diskettes, and not leaving confidential information unattended on the computer screen (Smith and Kallman 1995). They should also be responsible for reporting any observed unauthorized access.

Levels of Access

Access should be strictly limited to a need-to-know basis. This means no personnel, including IS staff, should have routine access to confidential information unless it is required by a particular event, at which time an audit trail is established. IS personnel must be held to the same confidentiality statement that applies to other personnel.

Limits Access is determined by who needs the medical record and under what conditions and locations. Direct care providers require information on their clients. Access levels are decided by defining roles for every level of personnel. This process can be referred to as "user classes." Each user class has different privileges. Initial system access is contingent on successful completion of system training and demonstration of competence. User training should address appropriate uses of information and the consequences of information misuse.

User Authentication

Access by authorized individuals can be verified through user authentication (Hoffman 1995, Meranda 1995, Robinson 1994). One common form of authentication is the appearance of the user's name on the screen. In the event that other staff observe a discrepancy, they have the responsibility to report it immediately. More sophisticated means of authentication include passwords used along with either a "pass key" type of device or scanned employee identification (Tabar 2000). Encrypted key-based authentication is an emerging technology. An example is **public key infrastructure** (PKI). PKI utilizes an encrypted "pass key" that can be provided to the user in various formats, including a smartcard, port token, or wireless transmitter. The pass key provides a secret number that is verified against a registered digital certificate. The user submits the pass key information during the sign-on process, and the PKI system compares it against the registered digital certificate ID to verify a match. Security tokens that resemble key chain fobs are an example of this technology.

Scanned employee identification may include a name badge but generally refers to biometric authentication, which is based on a unique biological trait, such as a fingerprint, voice or iris pattern, retinal scan, hand geometry, or face recognition (Tabar 2000, Kearns 2000). This technology is now feasible and accurate. Unlike passwords or devices that can be forgotten or stolen, biometric measures are always with the individual. Many experts recommend a combination approach that requires a password plus either key-based authentication or a biometric measure.

Personnel Issues

Personnel issues for information handling include education and policy and procedure development and implementation (Eager 1995, Faaoso 1992). Staff education is a key element for information and system security. Education for information handling and system use includes an orientation, system training, and a discussion of what is acceptable behavior. Staff should also be informed of the consequences for unauthorized access and information misuse, the use of audit trails, and ongoing measures to heighten security awareness. Ongoing measures include periodic reminders that client information belongs to them and reminders about what comprises professional, legal, and ethical behavior. Yearly review of the ethical computing statement signed upon its receipt is one way to emphasize the importance of ethical behavior. Figure 10–3 displays an example of this statement. Education and monitoring activities show administrative commitment to ethical information use.

Explicit policies and procedures provide the discipline to achieve information and system security (Brandt 1995, Eager 1995, Ettinger 1993, Levin 1995, Liebmann 1995, Lindsay 1993, McCarthy 1996, Phillips 1995, Software Publishers Association 1995, Temin 1995). Policies and

---

ST. FRANCIS HEALTH SYSTEM
INFORMATION SYSTEM
USER SIGN-ON CODE RECEIPT

[] St. Francis Medical Center
[] St. Francis Hospital of New Castle
[] St. Francis Central Hospital
[] _____

ST.
FRANCIS
HEALTH
SYSTEM

Hospital Personnel or Hospital Based Physician Sign-On codes are confidential. Disclosure of your Sign-On code, attempts to discover another person's Sign-On code, or unauthorized use of a Sign-On code are grounds for immediate dismissal.

I, the undersigned, acknowledge receipt of my User Sign-On Code and understand that:

1. My User Sign-On Code is equivalent of my signature; (Please note that the electronic signature is recognized by the Health Care Finance Administration (HCFA) and the Commonwealth of Pennsylvania).

2. Accessing the system via my Sign-On Code, is recorded permanently;

3. If assigned a User Sign-On Code, I will not disclose this code to anyone;

4. I will not attempt to learn another user's User Sign-On Code;

5. I will not attempt to access information in the system by using a User Sign-On Code other than my own;

6. I will access only that information which is necessary to perform my authorized functions;

7. If I have reason to believe that the confidentiality of my User Sign-On Code has been broken, I will contact Information Services immediately so that the suspect code can be deleted and a new code assigned to me; and

I understand that if I violate any of the above statements, it will be referred to the appropriate authority.

I further understand that my User Sign-On Code will be deleted from the system when I no longer hold an appointment or am no longer employed at St. Francis or authorization is otherwise revoked.

I have read the above statements and understand the implications if confidentiality of Sign-On code is violated.

_____ Social Security #_____-_____-_____
Name (Please print)

Dept:_____Supervisor:_____ Position:_____

System: MIS:_____   MEDIPAC:_____   G/L:_____   A/P:_____   CYBORG:_____   OTHER:_____

Signature of Code Recipient_____ Date:___/___/___

* Trainer Signature:_____ Date:___/___/___

* Dept. Head Authorization:_____ Date:___/___/___

Issuer Signature:_____ Date:___/___/___
        Information Services

Code will not be issued without proper identification and signature in presence of issuer.
* Signature <u>must</u> be present prior to issuance of code.   MIS User Class:_____

FORM H-1280 Date of Origin: 2/85
        Revised: 10/95

File: Personnel Department
Physicians: Medical Staff Office

FIGURE 10–3 • Sample Ethical Computing Statement (reprinted by permission of St. Francis Health System, Pittsburgh, PA) procedures should address information ethics, training, access control, system monitoring, data entry, backup procedures, and exchange of client information with other health care providers. Information ethics policies should do the following:

- *Plan for audit trails.* **Audit trails** are a record of IS activity. Users should know that their system access is monitored.
- *Establish acceptable computer uses.* This includes authorized access and using only legal software copies. One example of how this might be enforced is requiring licenses for all software used within the institution.
- *Collect only required data.* Limiting collection of information to what is needed, but no more, eliminates the danger of inappropriate disclosure of unneeded information and may lighten the workload.
- *Encourage client review of files for accuracy and error correction.* Client inspection of records ensures information integrity.

Information ethics policies are most credible when practiced by top administrators and IS personnel (Smith and Kallman 1995).

System Security Management

System security involves protection against deliberate attacks, errors, omissions, and disasters. Good system management is a key component of a strong framework for security because it encompasses the following tasks (Fried 1995):

- Monitoring
- Maintenance
- Operations
- Traffic management
- Supervision

Monitoring entails observing all system activity and alerting managers to problems such as intruders or the introduction of a virus. Maintenance encompasses all activity needed for proper operation of hardware, including preventive measures such as testing and periodic replacement of select components to ensure that data is available when it is needed. Operations management includes all activities needed to provide, sustain, modify, or cease telecommunications. Traffic management permits rerouting transmissions for better system performance. Supervision requires monitoring traffic and taking measures to prevent system overload and crashes (Arpege Group 1994).

While software is available to facilitate system management tasks, few commercial packages exist for comprehensive systems and network management (Wilkerson 1996). This situation forced institutions to develop in-house solutions or use outsourcing agents for customized applications.

Many organizations have different staff members for network and systems management. Network staff traditionally focus on hardware and connections, while IS personnel track information and software use. The security officer plays a pivotal role in tracking personnel information relative to system use. It is the security officer who may assign access codes and passwords to authorized users and deletes codes for staff no longer with the organization. Increased computing needs and limited budgets require greater staff efficiency. Wise use of system and network management tools will help to provide that efficiency, minimize the number of required support staff, reduce support costs, and improve information security.

Audit Trails

Auditing software helps to maintain security by recording unauthorized browsing (Baldasserini 1995, Brandt 1995, Phillips 1995). The Computer Security Institute of San Francisco estimates that more than half of unauthorized data access occurs in-house (Tabar 2000). Audits can show access of records by user or by password, and all access by an individual or level of employee. Frequent review of audit trails for unusual activity quickly identifies inappropriate use. Audit trail records should be kept for at least several months. Department managers must be advised when audit trails indicate that their staff have accessed records without a need.

In the event that an audit trail identifies unauthorized access, it is important to enforce written policy. At the very least this is a verbal reprimand or possibly a notation on the employee's performance evaluation. In many institutions, however, employees are held to the statement they signed upon receipt of their access code and password acknowledging termination of employment as a possible consequence of inappropriate system use. When employees are terminated for this reason, they may be escorted off the premises by the security department. This prevents any further opportunity for unauthorized access.

Audit trails may also reveal unauthorized access from outside sources, although little legal recourse has been available to punish the guilty parties until recently (Meranda 1995, Miller 1993). The best protection is offered through improved security mechanisms.

HANDLING AND DISPOSAL
OF CONFIDENTIAL INFORMATION

While most people recognize the need to keep medical records confidential, many are less attentive to safeguarding information printed from the record or extracted from it electronically for report purposes. All client record information should be treated as confidential and not left lying out for view by unauthorized persons.

Computer Printouts

The primary sources of unauthorized release of information are printing and faxing (Meranda 1995). For tracking purposes, each page of output should have a serial number or other means of identification. Control must be established over the materials that users print or fax. Some institutions include on printouts such as lab results a header that displays the word, "Confidential," in large letters. This reminds staff to dispose of materials appropriately. Paper shredders should be accessible and employed for immediate disposal of unneeded copies. When shredders are not available, there should be designated waste cans in secure areas.

Faxes

Sound institutional and departmental policies are needed for the use of fax machines that consider what types of information can be sent, who should receive the transmissions, the location to which transmissions are sent, and verification of receipt ("Faxes reduce errors" 1996, Phillips 1995). Information should not exceed that requested or required for immediate clinical needs. Legal counsel should review policies for consistency with federal and state law. Clients should sign a release form prior to faxing information. The following measures enhance fax security:

- *The use of a cover sheet.* This is a particularly important practice when the fax machine serves a number of different users. A cover sheet eliminates the need for the recipient to read the fax transmission to determine who gets it. The cover sheet may also contain a statement to remind recipients of the presence of confidential information. Figure 10–4 displays an example of a fax cover sheet.

- *Authentication at both ends of the transmission prior to data transmission.* This action verifies that the source and destination are correct.

- *Programmed speed-dial keys.* Programmed keys eliminate the chance of dialing errors and misdirected fax transmissions.

- *Encryption.* Encoding transmissions makes it impossible to read confidential information without the encryption key. This safeguards fax transmissions that might be sent to a wrong number.

- *Sealed envelopes for delivery.* The enclosure of confidential information in sealed envelopes provides a barrier to discourage casual viewing.

- *Fax machine placement in secure areas.* Secure areas have limited traffic and few, if any, strangers.

- *Limited machine access by designated individuals.* Restricting access to a few people makes it easier to enforce accountability for actions and identify any transgressions.

- *Inclusion of a request to return documents by mail.* Inadvertent entry of a wrong phone number can jeopardize sensitive information. In the event that information is faxed to a wrong number, a request to return documents may limit further disclosure.
- *A log of all fax transmissions.* A roster of all faxes sent and received provides a means to keep track of what information is sent and to help ensure that only appropriate information is sent.

ST. FRANCIS MEDICAL CENTER
FAX TRANSMITTAL FORM

ST.
FRANCIS
HEALTH
SYSTEM

DATE: _____   NO. OF PAGES: _____
(including cover sheet)

FROM: _____

FACILITY: _____

DEPARTMENT: _____

TELEPHONE: _____   FAX:_____

TO: _____

FACILITY: _____

DEPARTMENT: _____

TELEPHONE: _____   FAX:_____

COMMENTS: _____

_____

_____

_____

_____

_____

This fax contains privileged and confidential information intended only for the use of the recipient named above. If you are not the intended recipient of this fax or the employee or agent responsible for delivering it to the intended recipient, you are hereby notified that any dissemination or copying of this fax is strictly prohibited. If you have received this fax in error, please notify sender listed above; and return the original to the above address via U.S. mail.

This information has been disclosed to you from records whose confidentiality is protected by state and federal law. Any further disclosure of this information without the prior written consent of the person to whom it pertains may be prohibited.

FIGURE 10–4 • Sample Fax Cover Sheet (reprinted by permission of St. Francis Health System, Pittsburgh, PA)

E-mail and the Internet

E-mail is discussed at length in the chapter on electronic communication and the Internet. Policy should dictate what types of information may be sent via e-mail. E-mail is a great means of disseminating information, such as announcements, to large numbers of people quickly and inexpensively. However, information that is potentially sensitive should not be sent via e-mail unless it is encrypted. Nonencrypted messages can be read and public e-mail password protection of mailboxes can be cracked. When looking at encryption, ask whether your e-mail software encrypts all messages between users, whether messages are encrypted both in transit and when stored in the mailbox, and whether messages remain encrypted when sent between different e-mail packages. Unauthorized, or dormant, mail accounts should be destroyed and firewalls used for additional protection (Baldasserini 1995).

Web-Based Applications for Health Care

There is a high level of concern over the security of health information transmitted via the World Wide Web. The debate over whether the Web is safe enough to use for health information is likely to continue for some time. Technology and know-how can provide adequate security (Baldwin 2000). Economic concerns may diminish safeguards. Internet use for health care information over the Web continues to grow. Protection of health information can be ensured by spelling out liability for its compromise and insurance.

Electronic Storage

Confidential information may also be copied from the system in the form of electronic records. Administrators may download these records for report purposes. Once the records are no longer needed, electronic copies of sensitive data should receive the same treatment as any other data that has met its purpose. In this case, a software shredder can be employed. A **software shredder** overwrites files with meaningless information so that sensitive information cannot be accessed (Phillips 1995).

CASE STUDY EXERCISES

In the course of conversation your nurse manager tells you that she loaded a copy of the spreadsheet program she uses on her home office PC onto one of the unit PCs so that she can work on projects at both locations. Your institution has a well-publicized policy against the use of unauthorized, unlicensed software copies. As a staff nurse, what should you do? Explain your response.

•   •   •

You notice several of the new residents playing computer games on the nursing unit. You had not been aware of these games previously. What, if any, action should you take? Explain your rationale.

• • •

To remember her computer system password, university nursing instructor Pat Pawakawicz taped her password to the back of her name pin. When Ms. Pawakawicz lost her name pin recently, it was turned into hospital security and subsequently the IS department with her password still attached. When Ms. Pawakawicz picked up her name pin, she expressed intent to use the same password. Is this an appropriate way to treat a password? Should she use the same password again? Provide your rationale. What, if any, legal ramifications might there be for Ms. Pawakawicz regarding use of her password by unauthorized users?

• • •

The administration at St. John's Hospital takes pride in their strong policies and procedures for the protection of confidential client information. In fact, St. John's serves as a model for other institutions in this area. However, printouts discarded in the restricted access IS department are not shredded. On numerous occasions, personnel working late observed the cleaning staff reading discarded printouts. What action, if any, should these personnel take relative to the actions of the cleaning staff? What action, if any, should be taken by IS administration? Provide your rationale. If current practices are maintained, are there any additional potential risks for unauthorized disclosure of client information? If you answer yes, identify what these risks might be.

• • •

The secretary on 7 Tower Oncology receives a fax transmission about a client consult. The fax was intended for a physician's office in the adjacent building. She places the fax in the out bin of her desk to be delivered later by volunteers. No in-house mailer was used. Is this action appropriate? Explain why or why not.

SUMMARY

- The primary goals of health care information system security are the protection of client confidentiality and information integrity.
- Privacy and confidentiality are important terms in health care information management. Privacy is a choice to disclose personal information, while confidentiality assumes a relationship in which private information has been shared for the purpose of health treatment.
- Information privacy is the right to choose the conditions under which information is shared and to ensure the accuracy of collected information.

- Threats to information and system security and confidentiality come from a variety of sources, including system penetration by hackers, unauthorized use, errors and disasters, sabotage, and viruses.

- Planning for security saves time and money and is a form of insurance against downtime, breaches in confidentiality, and lost productivity.

- Security mechanisms combine physical and logical restrictions. Examples include automatic sign-off, physical restriction of computer equipment, strong password protection, and firewalls.

- Ultimately, health care administrators are responsible for protecting client privacy and confidentiality through education, policy, and creating an ongoing awareness of security.

- One aspect of system security management includes monitoring the system for unusual record access patterns, as might be seen when a celebrity receives treatment.

- Health information on the Internet requires the same types of safeguards provided for information found in private offices and information systems.

- All chart printouts and forms containing client information should be given the same consideration as the client record itself in order to safeguard confidentiality.

REFERENCES

Arpege Group (Ed.). (1994). *Network management: Concepts and tools.* New York: Chapman & Hall.

Baldasserini, M. (1995). Playing with fire. *Computer Shopper, 15*(6), 606+.

Baldwin, F. D. (2000). In Web we trust? *Healthcare Informatics, 17*(5), 56–58, 60, 62, 64, 66.

Brandt, M. (1995). CPR alert: Ten steps to end the great paper chase. *Healthcare Informatics, 12*(2),105–108.

Curtin, L., and Simpson, R. (1999). Privacy in the information age. *Health Management Technology, 20*(7), 32–33.

Eager, W. (1995). *The information payoff: The manager's concise guide to making PC communications work.* Englewood Cliffs, NJ: Prentice Hall.

Emery, K. H. (1995). *How to be a successful systems manager in a PC environment.* New York: McGraw-Hill.

Ensuring security in an online world. (1995). *The Workgroup Computing Report, 18*(4), 10+.

Ettinger, J. E. (1993). Introduction: Key issues in information security. In J. E. Ettinger (Ed.). *Information security: Applied information technology* (pp. 1–10). London: Chapman & Hall.

Faaoso, N. (1992). Automated patient care systems: The ethical impact. *Nursing Management, 23*(4), 46–48.

Faxes reduce errors, but threaten confidentiality. (1996). *The American Nurse, 28*(6), 2.

Fried, L. (1995). *Managing information technology in turbulent times*. New York: Wiley.

Garner, R. (1995). The growing professional menace. *Open Computing, 12*(7), 32+.

Gordon, J. (1993). Data encryption and its applications to computer security. In J. E. Ettinger (Ed.). *Information security: Applied information technology* (pp. 115–128). London: Chapman & Hall.

Hebda, T., Sakerka, L., and Czar, P. (1994). Educating nurses to maintain patient confidentiality on automated information systems. In S. J. Grobe and E. S. P. Pluyter-Wenting (Eds.). *Nursing informatics: An international overview for nursing in a technological era, The Proceedings of the Fifth IMIA International Conference on Nursing Use of Computers and Information Science*. New York: Elsevier Science.

Hoffman, L. (1995). How safe is your system? *Beyond Computing, 4*(5), 42–44.

Houser, W. R. (1995). It's high time to tighten security and penalize lapses. *Government Computer News, 14*(12), 33.

Joint Commission on Accreditation of Healthcare Organizations. (1996). *Medical records process*. Chicago: Accreditation Manual for Hospitals.

Kabay, M. (28 September 1995). No more excuses: Protect the Net now. *Communications Week*, 54+.

Kearns, D. (2000). Biometrics not an invasion of privacy. *NetworkWorld*. Available online at http://www.nwfusion.com/columnists/2000/0522kearns.html.

Kmentt, K. A. (Winter 1987). Private medical records: Are they public property? *Medical Trial Technique Quarterly, 33*, 274–307.

Layland, R. (1995). A plan of attack for network security. *Data Communications, 24*(7), 19+.

Lee, J., and Hudspeth, L. (1995). Crash-proof your PC. *Home Office Computing, 13*(9), 71+.

Levin, C. (1995). Net security reawakening. *PC Magazine, 14*(11), 31.

Liebmann, L. (28 September 1995). How to protect distributed data. *Communications Week*, 54+.

Lindsay, D. (1993). An overview of leading security issues. In J. E. Ettinger (Ed.). *Information security: Applied information technology* (pp. 11–19). London: Chapman & Hall.

McCarthy, B. (1996). Building a firewall. *Datamation, 42*(10), 74–76.

Meranda, D. (1995). Administrative and security challenges with electronic patient record systems. *Journal of AHIMA, 66*(3), 58–60.

Miller, D. (1993). Preserving the privacy of computerized patient records. *Healthcare Informatics, 10*(10), 72–74.

Mitchell, C. J. (1993). Management of secure systems and security within OSI. In J. E. Ettinger (Ed.). *Information security: Applied information technology* (pp. 47–60). London: Chapman & Hall.

Murdock, L. E. (1980). The use and abuse of computerized information: Striking a balance between personal privacy interests and organizational information needs. *Albany Law Review, 44*(3), 589–619.

Panettieri, J. C. (28 November 1994). Are your computers safe? *InformationWeek*, 34–48.

PC Week executive: Guide to data security. (1995). *PC Week, 12*(14), E7+.

Phillips, K. (1995). Securing the enterprise: Without adequate safeguards, corporate data lies exposed to outside and inside threats. *PC Week, 14*(12), N1+.

Riley, W. D. (1996). Behind the wall. *Datamation, 42*(10), 33.

Robinson, E. N. (1994). The computerized patient record: Privacy and security. *M.D. Computing, 11*(2), 69–73.

Romano, C. (1987). Confidentiality, and security of computerized systems: The nursing responsibility. *Computers in Nursing, 5*(3), 99–104.

Safran, C., Rind, D., Citroen, M., Bakker, A. R., Slack, W. V., and Bleich, H. L. (1995). Protection of confidentiality in the computer-based patient record. *M.D. Computing, 12*(3),187–192.

Schnaidt, P. (1995). Less inconvenience, more security. *Network Computing, 6*(10), 31+.

Semeria, C. (1996). Internet firewalls and security. *Enterprise Systems Journal, 11*(7), 32–38.

Slade, R. (1994). *Guide to computer viruses*. New York: Springer.

Smith, H. J., and Kallman, E. A. (October 1995). Ethical growth: The sequel. *Beyond Computing, 4*(10),16–17.

Software Publishers Association. (1995). *Software use and the law: A guide for individuals, businesses, educational institutions, and user groups.* Washington, DC: Software Publishers Association.

Tabar, P. (2000). Data security: Healthcare faces a tricky conundrum of confidentiality, data integrity and timeliness. *Healthcare Informatics, 17*(2), 50–52.

Temin, T. R. (1995). Security alert. *Government Computer News, 14*(6), 32.

Wilkerson, R. (1996). Still to come: Melding of systems and network management. *PC Week, 13*(3), N3+.

Windslade, W. J. (1982). Confidentiality of medical records: An overview of concepts and legal policies. *Journal of Legal Medicine, 3*(4), 497–533.

11

System Integration

After completing this chapter, you should be able to:

- Discuss the importance of network integration for health care delivery.

- Explain what an *interface engine* is and how it works.

- Identify several integration issues, including factors that impede the process.

- Discuss the relevance to system integration efforts of the data dictionary, master patient index, uniform language efforts, and clinical data repository.

- Consider how standards for the exchange of clinical data impact integration efforts.

- Review the benefits of successful information system integration for health care providers and health care professionals.

- Define the role of the nurse in system integration efforts.

- Understand how emerging Web-based tools can provide an alternative method for obtaining patient information from diverse information systems.

M ost hospitals and health care providers have automated information systems in some, if not all, of their major departments. Historically, financial systems were implemented by an organization first, followed by registration, laboratory systems, order entry, pharmacy, radiology and monitoring systems (not necessarily in that order). Some of these systems may have been implemented as stand-alone systems. Most departments select the information system that best meets their needs or that hospital administration approves for reasons of cost, vendor promises, or the preexistence of other products by the same vendor in the institution. It is rare for all departments in a given health care institution to agree that one vendor's product meets their information system needs. As a consequence, most institutions have several different systems that do not readily communicate or share data. Often each of these systems is highly customized to meet individual department and institutional specifications. This customization, however, complicates integration. Integration needs have increased dramatically as single institutions and providers use more systems internally, and as they join with other institutions to form enterprises, alliances, and networks. In addition, integration must be achieved before the computer-based patient record (CPR) can be realized.

Integration is the process by which different information systems are able to exchange data in a fashion that is seamless to the end user. The physical aspects of joining networks together are not nearly as complicated as getting unlike systems to exchange information in a seamless manner. Traditionally, communication between and among most disparate systems has been the result of costly, time-consuming efforts to build interfaces (Kooh 2000). In other words, interfaces are the tools used to achieve integration. An **interface** is a computer program that tells two different systems how to exchange data.

Without integration, providers cannot realize the full advantages of automation, since sharing data across systems is limited and redundant data entry by various personnel takes place. When this occurs, the likelihood of errors is increased. This situation is unacceptable in a time when managed care forces institutions to realize the benefits of automation in order to compete in today's health care delivery system. Box 11–1 lists some benefits associated with integration.

INTERFACE ENGINES

Interfaces between different information systems should be invisible to the user. Many vendors claim their products are based on **open systems technology,** the ability to communicate with other systems. The reality is that there is little incentive for vendors to market products that readily work with their competitors' products. Another problem is that the customization of vendor products by individual providers precludes off-the-shelf interface solutions. This necessitates costly and time-consuming design of custom interfaces. Another problem with customized interfaces is pinpointing the responsibility for problems. Each vendor responsible for developing an interface tends to blame the other for any difficulties encountered. Without a determination of responsibility, problem resolution is delayed and no one can be held accountable for the cost of solving the problem. All too often the institution must absorb the costs for this process; yet competition in a managed care environment does not permit this luxury. In addition, the timely flow of information is critical to cost-cutting measures and institutional survival. An alternative solution to this dilemma is now available via the interface engine.

An **interface engine** is a software application designed to allow users of different computer systems to access and exchange information both in real-time and batch processing. **Real-time processing** occurs immediately, while **batch processing** typically occurs once daily. In this situation, data is often not processed until the end of the day, and therefore is not available to users until that time. Although batch processing

---

| Box 11–1 | The Benefits of Integration |

- Allows instant access to applications and data
- Improves data integrity with single entry of data
- Decreases labor costs with single entry of data
- Facilitates the formulation of a more accurate, complete client record
- Facilitates information tracking for accurate cost determinations

was very common in the past, the current trend is toward real-time processing.

The interface engine provides seamless integration and presentation of information results. Interface engines work in the background and are not seen by the user. This technology allows applications to interact with hardware and other applications. Interface engines allow different systems that use unlike terminology to exchange information. This is done through the use of translation tables to move data from each system to the **clinical data repository,** a database where collective data from all information systems is stored and managed. The clinical data repository provides data definition consistency through mapping. **Mapping** is the process where terms defined in one system are associated with comparable terms in another system. Box 11–2 discusses some of the benefits associated with the use of interface engines.

Interface engines require new skills in the information services department. Staff may now include an integration analyst who will identify initial and ongoing interface specifications, coordinate any changes that will impact interfaces, and maintain a database for translation tables. This analyst must ascertain that data integrity is intact for all data to be sent correctly through the interface engine.

Interfacing of laboratory orders and results provides an example of how the interface engine is used in a hospital setting. On admission, the client's demographic information is entered in the hospital registration system, and portions of this data are transmitted to the clinical data repository via the interface engine. When a laboratory order is entered into the order entry system, the appropriate client demographic information is retrieved from the clinical data repository and used by the order entry system. After the order is entered, the order information may be

---

Box 11–2 **Interface Engine Benefits**

- Improves timeliness and availability of critical administrative and clinical data
- Decreases integration costs by providing an alternative to customized point-to-point interface application programming
- Improves data quality because of data mapping and consistent use of terms
- Allows clients to select the best system for their needs
- Preserves institutional investment in existing systems
- Simplifies the administration of health care data processing
- Simplifies systems integration efforts
- Shortens the time required for integration
- Improves management of care, the financial tracking of care rendered, and efficacy of treatment

transmitted via the interface engine to the clinical data repository and the laboratory system. When testing is complete, the results are transferred via the interface engine from the laboratory system to the clinical data repository. At this point, they are available for retrieval using the order entry system or another clinical information system.

INTEGRATION ISSUES

Integration is a massive project within institutions and enterprises. It generally requires more time and effort than originally projected. Several factors contribute to this situation. First, vendors frequently make promises about their products to make a sale; often these promises cannot be delivered. Second, merged institutions may prefer to keep their own systems rather than accept a uniform standard that would be easier to implement. The strategy adopted in this situation may require further negotiation and additional programming. Third, as each department and institution tries to retain its own identity and political power, it is difficult to come to an agreement on a common data dictionary, data mapping, and clinical data repository issues. Another issue is that integration brings a number of concerns for individuals, including changes in job description, learning new skills, the fear of job loss, and the general fear of change. Box 11–3 identifies several factors that may impede the integration process.

Box 11–3 **Factors That Slow Integration**

- *Unrealistic vendor promises.* Vendors may promise that their information system easily interfaces with other systems. Many customers find they face difficult, lengthy, and costly integration efforts after they have already purchased the system.

- *Unrealistic institutional timetable.* This is often based on a lack of understanding of the complexity of the integration process.

- *Changing user specifications.* As the integration process proceeds, users frequently request additional capabilities or change their minds regarding initial specifications.

- *Lack of vendor support.* Vendors may not provide enough support and assistance to facilitate the integration efforts.

- *Insufficient documentation.* Information regarding existing systems and related programming is imperative for achieving successful integration.

- *Lack of agreement among merged institutions.* Individual facilities within a merged enterprise may wish to continue use of their existing systems. This means there are more systems to integrate.

- *All components of a vendor's products may not work together.* Although difficulties are expected in attempts to integrate competing vendors' products, there may also be problems in integrating products developed by the same vendor.

THE NEED FOR INTEGRATION STANDARDS

The need to exchange client data is rapidly increasing in response to the demands placed by managed care as well as consumer demands for improved levels of health care. To derive the utmost benefit from data, it must have a consistent or standard meaning across institution, enterprise, and alliance boundaries, facilitating the exchange of client data. This is the basis for developing a data dictionary within an enterprise and a uniform language for use on a national and global scale.

Data Dictionary

The **data dictionary** defines terminology to ensure consistent understanding and use across the enterprise. Terms defined in the data dictionary should include synonyms found in the various systems used within the enterprise. This may be achieved, in some cases, through the use of the interface engine. For example, a term or data element may be a diagnosis or a lab test such as potassium. Potassium may be known in the nursing order entry system as "potassium," but be called "K" in the lab system. The use of the data dictionary and interface engine facilitates integration and also allows for the collection of aggregate data.

Master Patient Index

The integration process may require enhancements to the data dictionary, the clinical data repository, and the master patient index. The **master patient index** (**MPI**) is a database that lists all identifiers assigned to one patient in all the information systems used within an enterprise (Bazzoli 1996). It assigns a global identification number for each patient and allows patients to be identified by demographic information provided at the point of care. The MPI may use first and last names, birthdates, social security numbers, and driver's license numbers. It cannot rely on a single type of number such as the social security number, because of duplicates and the fact that some people, such as noncitizens, may not have one. When the MPI can't match records based on demographic data, all possible matches are provided for the user to view and select. The MPI is a critical component in supporting successful integration. Not all health care enterprises have a data dictionary, a clinical data repository, or MPI, or these components may be in various stages of development. The move toward creating a lifetime patient record creates the need to access patient encounters across time. This is particularly important in a multi-institutional enterprise. The MPI, data dictionary, and clinical data repository are tools that support this effort.

The MPI saves work because key information can be obtained from the database instead of needing to be rekeyed for each patient visit. This decreases the possibility of making a mistake and eliminates the inadvertent creation of duplicate records. As a result, the admission clerk now plays a greater role in the maintenance of data integrity.

Some of the key features of an effective MPI include the following:

- It locates records in real time for timely retrieval of information.
- It is flexible enough to allow inclusion of additional identification.
- It is easily reconfigured to accommodate network changes.
- It can grow to fit an organization of any size.

Uniform Language

One step in the integration process is the development of a uniform definition of terms, or language. This is essential for the easy location and manipulation of data. Many efforts to develop uniform languages are underway in the health care arena. For example, the National Library of Medicine has developed the Unified Medical Language System, which includes the Uniform Nursing Language. In addition, the American Nurses Association sponsors the Congress of Nursing Practice Steering Committee on Databases ("ANA revises criteria" 1996). This group addresses issues including nursing classification schemes, uniform data sets, data elements, and national databases. One of its primary goals is to develop a mapping system to link various classification schemes. This would allow the development of national data sets for use by nursing.

Data Exchange Standards

In addition to the uniform definition of terms, integration standards also facilitate the exchange of patient data by providing a set of rules and structure for formatting the data. A major standard for the exchange of clinical data for integration is Health Level 7 (HL7). **HL7** refers to both an organization and its standards for the exchange of clinical data. In particular, these standards address definitions of data to be exchanged, the timing of the exchanges, and communication of certain errors between applications (Hammond 1996). HL7 provides a structure that defines data and elements and specifies how the data is coded. The structure of the data element must follow HL7 rules, such as those specifying the length of the fields and the code nomenclature. Use of HL7 standards in individual applications will improve the integration of these applications with other applications or systems. Benefits include easier and less costly integration within an organization, and more accurate and useful data integration nationally and globally. Integration efforts and the development and use of integration standards, including HL7, are taking place at many levels. For example, integration is seen beyond the hospital setting in the form of **integrated delivery systems** (IDS). Although efforts are underway to develop both national and international health data networks, competition does not encourage this type of sharing of information. Standards may be in place, but not necessarily be used. Another factor is that HL7 standards may be somewhat modified by information system vendors to support various applications. These variations must be addressed during the integration process.

HL7 standards are not the only standards that have been evolving to fit the changing health care model. Other organizations have also been instrumental in supporting the development of standards and in helping to define data exchange. These organizations include the Computer-Based Patient Record Institute, the MEDIX International Standards Organization, the American Society for Testing and Materials, and the Institute of Medicine.

BENEFITS OF INTEGRATION

One major benefit of integration and the ability to exchange client data is the development of the computer-based patient record (Marrs and Kahn 1997). In this case, integration allows data from many disparate information systems to be accessed from one point by the user, providing a complete record for each client. The **clinical data repository** is a key element of the computerized patient record. It provides a storage facility for clinical data over time. The data in the clinical data repository may be generated from various systems and locations. For example, lab data may be generated by a laboratory system and may be collected in an acute, ambulatory, or long-term care setting. Other data may be included from clinical systems such as radiology, pharmacy, and order entry. Decision support applications that use clinical repository data can be used at other facilities if data from all facilities can be mapped to the data dictionary. One of the stumbling blocks to the creation and maintenance of the clinical data repository may be poor documentation regarding term definitions in the individual systems collecting the data. Figure 11–1 depicts an example of mapping with laboratory test terms.

Hospitals and health care enterprises also benefit from integration. Using integration strategies will permit data exchange within each hospi-

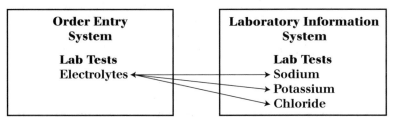

The order entry system lists a test called Electrolytes. The laboratory information system does not list a test called Electrolytes but lists its individual component tests. Before the interface engine can allow exchange of data, the relationships between the tests listed in both systems must be established by mapping.

FIGURE 11–1 • Mapping of Laboratory Test Terms

tal and across health care networks or enterprises, allowing them to find trends in financial and clinical data. Integration can open up a realm of possibilities for new ways to chart data trends, for example, by provider, by diagnosis, or by cost. In this way, health care providers can obtain improved information, making them better able to react to market changes and maintain a competitive edge.

The lack of data integration is a barrier to effective data reporting and analysis (Merlo and Freundl 1999). For example, executive information needs may require data regarding all aspects of an obstetric patient's care, including prenatal care, risk factors, complications before admission, length of hospital stay, and cost of the entire episode of care. Some of this information may be stored in an independent information system in the physician's office. Other data may be found in the hospital clinical information system, and in the financial system. Without effective integration of clinical, financial, and administrative data, it is difficult to provide a complete system information base for management and decision support (Mills and O'Keefe 1991).

Another benefit of integration is that it facilitates data collection for accreditation processes. For example, JCAHO (Joint Commission on Accreditation of Health Care Organizations) requirements call for the ability to provide aggregate data (Joint Commission 1996). These requirements include the following:

- A uniform definition of data
- Uniform methods for data capture
- The ability to provide client-specific as well as aggregate data

These information standards allow JCAHO to compare data within and among health care enterprises.

INTEGRATION IMPLICATIONS FOR NURSING

There are also particular concerns for nursing in relation to system integration. A primary consideration is that nursing involvement is essential in the interface design phase. Nurses must be involved in identifying and defining data elements that an interface may be able to supply. One way to ensure this is to recruit staff nurses to provide input during the interface design.

Another concern is ensuring that data will be collected in only one system and shared via the interface engine and clinical data repository with all other systems requiring it (Merlo and Freundl 1999). This eliminates redundant effort while ensuring data integrity. For example, a client's allergies should be collected by a nurse and entered into a clinical information system. This data is then transmitted to the clinical data repository via the interface engine, where it is available for retrieval by other systems that may require it, such as a pharmacy system.

Nursing can also benefit from integration and data exchange. For example, trends in client care data and cost analysis can be used to justify nursing staffing levels in the hospital setting. In addition, integration provides a tool to build nursing knowledge.

EMERGING INTEGRATION SOLUTIONS

The traditional integration process is an enormous project that is costly and may require many years to complete. An emerging solution for providing interim access to data from disparate systems involves the use of Web-based tools and a hospital's intranet or the Internet (Turisco 1999). These tools often require a Web browser, security clearance, and an intranet or Internet connection. Most of these tools allow view-only access to various diverse applications used within the enterprise. Some may provide a minimal level of update capability. Access to patient data from many systems is managed by the use of a common patient identifier, or MPI, which will allow the user to identify the patient only once, then view that patient's information from a number of separate information systems. Although this Web-based approach provides immediate data access, it is not a replacement for integration between information systems. Its value is that it requires minimal maintenance effort, while remaining a low-cost interim solution.

CASE STUDY EXERCISES

You have been selected as a member of the Integration Project Team, which is charged with identifying ways that system integration could improve information flow. You work on an inpatient unit that uses a stand-alone nursing documentation system that is not interfaced or integrated with any other hospital information system. Identify the implications of this situation, and suggest integration options that could improve information flow.

• • •

You are working to identify elements in your health care enterprise that could be used for a master patient index (MPI). List five basic elements and describe how each could be used for an MPI.

SUMMARY

- An interface is a computer program that tells two different systems how to exchange data.
- Most health care providers have a variety of automated information systems that do not readily share data unless major efforts are made to build interfaces.

- Integration is the process by which different information systems are able to exchange data without any special effort on the part of the end user.

- The creation of networks to exchange data between systems and the process of integration are essential in today's health care information world, where an institution or enterprise may have multiple disparate clinical information systems.

- The interface engine is a software application designed to allow users of different information systems to exchange information without the need to build direct customized interfaces between systems.

- Other processes that facilitate the move toward integration and the exchange of client information include the clinical data repository, mapping, the data dictionary, the master patient index, uniform language efforts, and data exchange standards.

- The clinical data repository is a database that collects and stores data from all information systems.

- Mapping of terms establishes the relationship between terms defined in one system and those used in another.

- The data dictionary defines terms used within an enterprise to ensure consistent use.

- The master patient index (MPI) lists all identifiers assigned to one client in all information systems and assigns a global identification code as a means to locate all records for a given client.

- Standardization of clinical terms through a uniform language is one means to facilitate the exchange of information across health care enterprises. The Congress of Nursing Practice Steering Committee on Databases and the National Library of Medicine (through its Unified Medical Language System) is working on uniform language issues.

- HL7 is a standard for the exchange of clinical data that provides rules and structure for how data is formatted.

- Integration improves data integrity and access for caregivers, eliminates redundant data collection, and improves data collection for staffing, for finding financial trends and client outcome trends, and for meeting requirements of regulatory and accrediting organizations.

- Integration is a necessary component for the development of the computerized patient record and for integrated delivery systems.

- An interim solution to the costly and time-consuming process of integration is the use of Web-based tools to access patient data from various systems using the hospital's intranet or the Internet.

REFERENCES

ANA revises criteria for evaluating nursing vocabularies, classification systems. (November/December 1996). *The American Nurse*, 9.

Bazzoli, F. (1996). Providers point to index software as key element of integration plans. *Health Data Management*, *4*(9), 61–65.

Hammond, W. E. (June 1996). Politics and standards. *HL7 News*, 1, 13.

Joint Commission on Accreditation of Health Care Organizations. (1996). *Medical records process*. Chicago: Accreditation Manual for Hospitals.

Kooh, L. (2000). Integrating data is key to enhancing information systems. *Ophthalmology Times*, *25*(1), 13–14.

Marrs, K. A., and Kahn, M. G. (13 February 1997). Extending a clinical repository to include multiple sites. On the Web at: *http://osler.wustl.edu/~mars/test.html*.

Merlo, J., and Freundl, M. (1999). Overcoming the barriers to cross-continuum information integration. *Healthcare Financial Management*, *53*(6), 35–38.

Mills, M. E., and O'Keefe, S. (1991). Computerization: A challenge to nursing administration. In M. J. Ball, J. V. Douglas, R. I. O'Desky, and J. W. Albright (Eds.). *Healthcare Information Management Systems* (pp. 103–113). New York: Springer.

Turisco, F. (1999). Using internet technology to extend access to legacy systems. *Healthcare Financial Management*, *53*(5), 86.

12

The Computer-Based Patient Record

After completing this chapter, you should be able to:

- Discuss the similarities and differences between the electronic medical record (EMR) and the computer-based patient record (CPR).

- Define the term *computer-based patient record.*

- Understand the twelve characteristics of the computer-based patient record, as defined by the Institutes of Medicine.

- Discuss the benefits associated with the computer-based patient record.

- Review the current status of the CPR, including impediments.

- List several concerns that must be resolved prior to the implementation of the CPR.

T he current environment in the health care arena is one of confusion. The move toward managed care is causing rapid and uncontrolled changes in all aspects of health care. In particular, the requirements for management of client information are expanding, resulting in the transformation of the way health care providers access information. The traditional paper medical record, which simply records client status and results in one place, no longer meets the needs of the health care industry. The drawbacks of the paper record include the fact that it is episode-oriented, with a completely separate record for each client visit. Therefore, no continuous or integrated client record is available. Another drawback is the limited accessibility to the actual record for physicians and other caregivers, who must obtain the record from the medical records department, meaning that only one person can access the record at any given time. The solution to this dilemma is the **computer-based patient record** (CPR). The CPR is not simply the computerization of the paper client record, but an information system developed to enhance and support client care (Stetson and Andrew 1996).

DEFINITIONS

It is evident that there is a great deal of confusion regarding terminology and definitions related to the CPR. Some of the terms frequently used include *electronic medical record, computer-based patient record,* and *computer-based patient record system,* as described below.

Electronic Medical Record The EMR is an electronic version of the client data found in the traditional paper medical record (Andrew and Dick 1996). The EMR includes **unstructured data,** which is data that does not follow any particular format and often is seen as a text report. Examples are reports produced by transcription services, including history and physical assessments, consultation findings, operative reports, and discharge summaries. The EMR also includes **structured data,** which is data that follows a predefined format and is often presented as discrete data elements. Structured data is often obtained from automated ancillary reporting systems. A primary example is laboratory results from an automated laboratory information system. Another type of data that may be included in the EMR is electronic imaging produced by diagnostic studies, including tomography, ultrasound, and magnetic resonance imaging. Although the EMR is often confused with the CPR, the EMR is generally defined as one component of the CPR. The CPR is a comprehensive lifetime record, while the EMR is the record for a single treatment episode. Figure 12–1 displays one example of an electronic medical record.

Computer-Based Patient Record According to the Institutes of Medicine (IOM) an electronic patient record resides in a system designed to support users through availability of complete and accurate data, bodies of medical knowledge, and other aids (Andrew and Dick 1997). The CPR consists of multiple components that include documentation by health care providers, test results, and related information.

Computer-Based Patient Record System (CPRS) The CPRS, as defined by the Institutes of Medicine, is the set of components that forms the mechanism by which patient records are created, used, stored, and retrieved. It includes people, data, rules and procedures, processing and storage devices, and communications and support facilities (Andrew and Dick 1996). This system is accessed at a clinical workstation and is used to collect and retrieve all clinical data for a client beginning with the client's first encounter with the health care system. The result is a longitudinal client record. In many settings, initial efforts toward a CPRS are directed at integrating the various information systems already in use across the enterprise, including nursing information systems, demographic and registration systems, and ancillary department systems.

CHARACTERISTICS OF THE CPR

The Institutes of Medicine identified the following 12 major components of the CPR, which they consider the "gold standard" attributes (Andrew and Dick 1996):

1. *Provides a problem list that indicates the client's current clinical problems for each encounter.* A problem list should also denote the number of occurrences associated with all past and current problems, as well as the current status of the problem (Dick and Gabler 1995).

2. *Evaluates and records health status and functional levels using accepted measures.* These outcome measures have not been effec-

```
MIS  -0010-01(R)    ST. FRANCIS HEALTH SYSTEM      (TEST #5)
06/02/00 10:27 AM    (QAT$$P)    PAGE 001

= = = = = = = = = = = = = = = = = = = =
CPR,CHARLES                      M  77 35031-
MR #: 320024            ADM: 06/02/00
PAT#: 320024370154                              PATIENT RECORD
= = = = = = = = = = = = = = = = = = = =          = = = = = = =

        DATA ENTERED DURING:   06/02/00 12:00 MN TO 10:27 AM
= = = = = = = = = = = = = = = = = = = = = = = = = = = = = = = = =

ALLERGIES:


 CODEINE, ALLERGY.
 PT./R.O. STATES REACTION TO CODEINE RASH                     PCAN
 SHELLFISH, ALLERGY                                           PCAN

VITAL SIGNS:

 DATE:  TIME:      T-A     T-O    T-R   P-R   P-A   R      RECORDER:
 06/02 08:00AM            099.8         90        24         PCAN

MISC VS-OBSV:

              114/86                                         PCAN
              UNABLE TO WEIGH PT                             PCAN


MEDICATIONS:

DIGOXIN TAB 0.125MG (LANOXIN)
 06/02 09:30AM #1,PO,GIV                 CZAR,PATRICIA   HSP5
FUROSEMIDE TAB 20MG ('LASIX')
 06/02 09:00AM #1,PO,GIV                 CZAR,PATRICIA   HSP5
MEPERIDINE INJ 25MG (DEMEROL),
 06/02 09:40AM IM,GIV,INJ SITE,LUOQ,PAIN RATING
             ,3,USING THE,0-10 SCALE     CZAR,PATRICIA   HSP5
POTASSIUM CHLORIDE 10MEQ TAB ('KDUR')
 06/02 09:30AM #1,PO,GIV                 CZAR,PATRICIA   HSP5

OTHER PATIENT DATA:

 06/02 09:15AM ADM ASSESSMENT                                PCAN
              PT HAS AN ADVANCE DIRECTIVE YES               PCAN
              PAIN ASSESSMENT: ARE YOU HAVING ANY
                    PAIN/DISCOMFORT NOW , YES.
                    LOCATION:--CHEST.
                    DURATION: INTERMITTENT.
                    TYPE: SHARP                              PCAN

                      CONTINUED
```

```
 CPR,CHARLES                                      PATIENT RECORD
```

FIGURE 12–1 • Example of an Electronic Medical Record

tively addressed by vendors in most cases. In the current competitive health care market, increased attention to measuring outcomes and quality of care are imperative, and must begin to be addressed by IS departments and vendors.

3. *Documents the clinical reasoning/rationale for diagnoses and conclusions.* Allows sharing of clinical reasoning with other caregivers, and automates and tracks decision making.

```
06/02/00 10:27 AM    (QAT$$P)    PAGE 002                \\\\        \\\\
                                                            \   \       \   \
                                                            \\\\  \\\\ \\\\
= = = = = = = = = = = = = = = = = = = = = =                  \           \  \
CPR,CHARLES                          M  77 35031-            \           \  \
MR #: 320024               ADM: 06/02/00                     = = = = = = = = =
PAT#: 320024370154                                          PATIENT  RECORD
= = = = = = = = = = = = = = = = = = = = =                   = = = = = = =
      DATA ENTERED DURING:    06/02/00 12:00 MN TO 10:27 AM
= = = = = = = = = = = = = = = = = = = = = = = = = = = = = = = = = = = = =

  06/02 10:24AM PT ENROLLED IN ORGAN DONOR PROGRAM- NO            PCAN
  06/02 10:27AM REINFORCE MED INSTRUCTION                         PCAN
                PROVIDE EMOTIONAL SUPPORT TO PT/FAM               PCAN
                I HAVE SEEN THE PT, VALIDATED/COLLECTED THE
                       DATA & I AM INITIATING THE PLAN OF
                       NSG CARE BASED ON MY EVAL OF THE
                       ASSESSMENT                                 PCAN
                PLAN OF CARE DEVELOPED WITH CONSIDERATION OF
                       AGE AND FUNCTIONAL STATUS                  PCAN
                FALL PRECAUTION INITIATED                         PCAN
                RED FALL PRECAUTION ARM BAND ON                   PCAN

                    ** END OF SECTION **

                       LAST PAGE
```

CPR,CHARLES   PATIENT RECORD

FIGURE 12–1 • Continued

4. *Provides a longitudinal or lifetime client record* by linking all of the client's data from previous encounters.

   5. *Supports confidentiality, privacy, and audit trails.* System developers must supply multiple levels of security to ensure appropriate access to confidential client information.

   6. *Provides continuous access to authorized users.* Users must be able to access the client record at any time.

7. *Allows simultaneous and customized views of the client data* for individuals, departments, or enterprises. This ability improves efficiency for the specific users by allowing the data to be presented in a format that is most useful to them. The flexibility to support multiple different and simultaneous views of client data is a feature that many vendors find difficult to achieve.

8. *Supports links to local or remote information resources,* such as various databases using electronic mail, CD-ROM, or hard disk. Access to pertinent information from various external sources will provide the caregiver with needed information in a timely and effective format that can be used to support client care. Examples include access to literature searches and drug information databases.

9. *Facilitates clinical problem solving by providing decision analysis tools.* Examples include simple support, such as timely reminders regarding health maintenance activities, and rules-based alerts that supply decision-making support for the physician.

10. *Supports direct entry of client data by physicians.* The question of how to provide a simple and acceptable mechanism for direct entry of data by physicians without relying on dictation continues to be a problem for vendors.

11. *Includes mechanisms for measuring the cost and quality of care.* This area has not yet been addressed by the majority of information system vendors, but is vitally important in providing a significant competitive edge in today's health care market.

12. *Supports existing and evolving clinical needs by being flexible and expandable.* Many information systems address specific areas of specialty such as emergency or ambulatory care. These systems may be difficult to customize and expand to meet the specific needs of the health care enterprise.

Most of the data included in the CPR is automated structured data. Other data formats may also be linked to the CPR, including dictation and transcription, images, video, and text. This data, and collective data from all systems, is stored and managed in the **clinical data repository.** This database allows retrieval of multiple elements of client data regardless of their system of origin. For example, the user may retrieve a lab result from the clinical data repository that was originally produced by the laboratory information system (LIS), along with a radiology report that was generated in the radiology information system (RIS) from a transcribed dictation. Collectively, these various systems and the clinical data repository make up the CPR.

The development of **data exchange standards** is instrumental for the implementation of the CPR. These standards will allow the uniform capture of data that is required to build a longitudinal record comprising in-

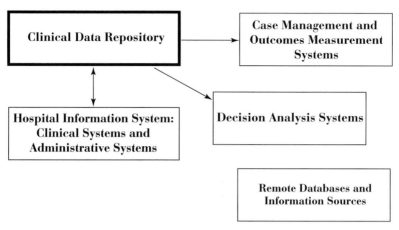

The CPR comprises the systems shown above. Client data flows between the systems as indicated by the arrows. External databases and information sources may also be accessed by the CPR, even though no client data flows to them.

FIGURE 12–2 • A Sample of CPR Components

tegrated information systems from multiple vendors. Figure 12–2 shows some sample components of the CPR.

BENEFITS OF THE CPR

The driving force for the development of the CPR is managed care. A well-developed CPR facilitates the management of both cost and quality of client care. The powerful framework of the CPR optimizes the collection, presentation, and communication of client data. This results in time and money savings for anyone who participates in the health care delivery process, including clients, physicians, and health care providers and payers.

The benefits of the CPR can be best understood when considering the needs of various groups of users. Some of the benefits are general, but others relate specifically to nurses, physicians, and the health care enterprise.

General Benefits

- Improved data integrity, since information is more readable, better organized, and more accurate and complete.
- Increased productivity. Caregivers are able to access client information whenever it is needed, and at multiple convenient locations. This can result in improved client care due to the ability to make timely decisions based on appropriate data.
- Improved quality of care. The CPR supports clinical decision-making processes for physicians and nurses.

- Increased satisfaction for caregivers. Caregivers are able to take advantage of easy access to client data as well as other services, including drug information sources, rules-based decision support, and literature searches (Amatayakul 1997).

Nursing Benefits

- Current data and data from previous events are easily compared.
- The nurse can maintain an ongoing record of the client's education and learning response across various encounters or visits.
- Baseline demographic and assessment data does not have to be repeated for each encounter.
- Data that has been entered is universally available to all who have access to the CPR.
- Data for research is more readily available and of better quality.
- It provides prompts to ensure administration and documentation of medications and treatments.
- It facilitates automation of critical and clinical pathways.

Physician Benefits

- Multiple users can access the client record simultaneously.
- Physician can easily access previous encounters.
- Chart access is faster. No need to wait for old records to be delivered from the medical records department.
- Better reporting tools. Trends and clinical graphics are available on demand.
- Physicians can save time and reduce liability through better documentation (Barrett 2000).

Health Care Enterprise Benefits

- Client record security is improved (McFall 1993).
- Less space is needed for record storage.
- The medical record department saves costs because of decreased need for pulling, filing, and copying of charts.
- Client eligibility for coverage in managed care settings is easily verified (Amatayakul 1997).
- Cost evaluation is improved based on clinical outcomes and resource utilization data (Barrett 2000).

CURRENT STATUS OF THE CPR

As of this writing in mid 2000, the perfect CPR system has not been widely implemented (Gaillour 1999). Although many health care systems have automated part or all of the paper client record, this alone does not fulfill the vision of a CPR. Box 12–1 lists six qualities of a successful CPR. While many organizations struggle with the slow piecemeal conversion to electronic medical records, unintended negative outcomes may be seen. These include increased workloads and delayed information retrieval as clinicians search multiple data sources for patient information (Barrett 2000).

Impediments to CPR Development

Information system vendors as well as health care providers are, for the most part, aware of the pressing need to develop the CPR, and are continuously working toward its evolvement. Development of an electronic infrastructure and cost are the two major impediments to the creation of a fully functioning CPR. The principal requirement is that the major participants in the health care arena, including health care facilities, payers, and physicians, must be linked electronically. This is a very costly undertaking in many cases. Other impediments include the lack of a common vocabulary, and resistance among caregivers.

Electronic Infrastructure The health care facilities, payers, and physicians must all have the ability to access and update the client's longitudinal record. In other words, the various information systems that support these stakeholders must be linked electronically by the network infrastructure (Anderson and Bunschoten 1996). Agreements must first be reached regarding the nature and format of client data to be stored, as well as the mechanisms for data exchange, storage, and retrieval. This

Box 12–1	Qualities of a Successful CPR
1. Fast	The user is able to quickly enter and retrieve data.
2. Familiar	The CPR follows familiar graphical user interface (GUI) conventions.
3. Flexible	The CPR allows personalization of documentation style, enabling it to meet the information needs of many types and categories of users.
4. Enhances Workflow	The CPR improves work efficiency and effectiveness.
5. Improves Documentation	The user sees the CPR as improving the process of documentation.
6. Meets Regulatory Requirements	The CPR supports the regulatory requirements related to data content and security measures.

SOURCE: "The CPR: Getting Physicians on Board," by D. S. Stetson and P. E. Andrew, 1996, *Healthcare Informatics, 13*(6), 20–24.

means that all participants must use common data communication standards. First and most important is the decision regarding the recognition of a universal client identifier, such as a Social Security Number, so that all client data can be associated with the correct client. Improvements in connectivity alone are not enough to support the CPR. It is also important to include components such as interoperability, comparability, decision support, and point of care data capture to achieve the true integration necessary for the CPR (Amatayakul 2000).

Cost Another impediment to the CPR is cost (Dick and Steen 1991, Gaillour 1999). The development of the electronic links forming the infrastructure is costly, and the allocation of fiscal responsibilities has not yet been addressed. Currently each health care enterprise or system is paying for its own electronic medical record development. Links to other facilities and agencies are rare and for the most part limited to provider–payer arrangements. Further progress in CPR development is likely to be minimal until decisions regarding cost allocation are reached.

Vocabulary Standardization There is little standardization in health care settings regarding the medical vocabulary or language used in client records. This lack of standards prevents the integrating of discrete and disparate data from multiple sources into one complete record (Anderson and Bunschoten 1996). Additional progress in the development of a universal medical and nursing language will support the development of the CPR. This effort is already underway with the development of the Nursing Minimum Data Set.

Caregiver Resistance Resistance on the part of caregivers such as physicians and nurses also acts as an impediment to the development and use of the CPR (Stetson and Andrew 1996). The fully developed CPR necessitates mandatory use of computers by caregivers as part of their daily routine. Some individuals are unable or unwilling to use computers. This may be related to various factors such as the complexity of software, the availability of PCs or terminals, and resistance to change in the work patterns. Some physicians feel that data entry is demeaning and a waste of time, and interferes with their ability to provide client care on a timely basis. Actual practice reveals that nearly all physicians will do some data entry, but only a few will do a lot (Gaillour 1999).

CONCERNS ASSOCIATED WITH THE CPR

Several concerns must also be addressed as the CPR is developed. These include data integrity, ownership of the electronic patient record, privacy and confidentiality, and electronic medical signature.

Data Integrity

Data integrity can be compromised in three ways: incorrect entry, data tampering, and system failure. In general, data integrity can be improved by implementing security measures, including the use of audit trails, as well as the development of detailed procedures and policies.

Incorrect Data Entry The client data found in the CPR is only as accurate as the person who enters it and the systems that transfer it. Therefore, critical information, such as allergies and code status, should be verified for accuracy at each encounter. This will allow the correction of data entry errors and also screen for changes that have occurred in client status. This is especially crucial since data may be entered or modified from many different encounters in the health care arena, such as hospitals, clinics, and home care visits.

Data Tampering In addition to accidental data entry errors, it is possible that an individual may make malicious data modifications. An effective audit trail procedure will permit the tracking of who entered or modified each data element, allowing appropriate follow-up measures.

System Failure Hardware and software malfunctions, such as a system crash, may result in incomplete or lost data. Once the problem has been resolved, it may be necessary to verify the client data that could have been affected.

Ownership of the Patient Record

Currently, paper medical records are the property of the institution at which they are created. This institution is responsible for ensuring the accuracy and completeness of the record. With the development of the CPR, however, ownership issues become more complex (Ellsasser, Nkobi, and Kohler 1995). Since many providers will be using the same data, it is unclear who actually owns it and is responsible for maintaining its accuracy. Because the data is shared and updated from many sites, decisions must be made regarding who can access the data and how it will be used. In addition, it must be determined where the data will actually be stored.

Privacy and Confidentiality

Preservation of the client's privacy is one of the most basic and important duties of the health care provider (Anderson and Bunschoten 1996). Since one of the key attributes of the CPR is the ease of data sharing, the client's privacy rights may not be guarded by all who have access to the record. Legislation must be initiated that will address electronic access to client records. In addition, health care providers must address client privacy rights when developing the electronic record.

Electronic Signature

The health care provider has always been required to authenticate entries into the paper medical record with a handwritten signature. This cannot be done with the CPR, since all entries are electronic. An **electronic signature** must be used to authenticate electronic data entries (Feste 1993). A user's computer access code and/or password recognizes that individual by name and credentials and allows access to the system. The user is required to sign a confidentiality statement before obtaining an access code, stating that no other person will be permitted to use the code. Other newer technologies, such as private encryption keys and biometric authentication, should be considered when developing an electronic signature mechanism (Tabar 2000).

Systems typically affix a date and time log to each entry, as well as the identity of the user in the form of an audit trail. The electronic signature is automatically and permanently attached to the document when it is created. This electronic signature cannot be forged or transferred to any other transaction, and provides authentication of the health care provider.

SMART CARDS

One of the evolving technologies associated with the CPR is the smart card (Broomberg 1995). The **smart card** is used to store client information such as demographics, allergies, blood type, current medications, current health problems, including recent findings, and payer or insurance provider. Some cards may also include the client's photograph. The smart card is similar in appearance to a plastic credit card. Those smart cards that contain a microprocessing chip are able to store thousands more bits than a magnetic strip card (Tabar 2000).

At the present time, smart cards are just beginning to be introduced in the United States; use is more widespread in Europe. A person carrying a smart card presents it to the health care provider at the time of treatment, and it is processed through an electronic card reader. The card provides detailed client information that is not part of an electronic network, thus ensuring accuracy and making information readily available. According to Broomberg (1995), "the success of a smart card system is based entirely on planning. If your planning is good, you can be assured of a worthwhile application."

CONSIDERATIONS FOR THE FUTURE

One of the stumbling blocks in the development of the CPR is the quest for the perfect system. Although many health care organizations have automated large portions of the patient's medical record, others hesitate to implement the CPR because they have not yet found the perfect system that meets the Institutes of Medicine's criteria. It is suggested that these organizations implement something useful, even though it may not be perfect (Gaillour 1999). This will provide the capability to automate workflow with the goal to reduce steps and improve accuracy. Connectivity will allow the sharing of core patient information across the organization. Finally, data will be available for reporting and analysis, providing the ability to benchmark patient types and individual patient progress and outcomes (Barrett 2000).

CASE STUDY EXERCISES

You are a member of the committee charged with designing the CPR at your facility. Identify which components of nursing documentation should be retained in the clinical data repository. For example, would you want to include all client vital signs from the current hospital admission? Explain why you would include or exclude the various components.

• • •

Identify several external sources of information that would be useful as part of the CPR for access by a home health nurse.

• • •

Discuss the implications of providing nurses in a hospital setting with access to all electronic client information. Identify which types of information are appropriate for access by nurses.

SUMMARY

- The computer-based patient record (CPR) is an electronic patient record that includes client data, medical knowledge, and other essential health care information.
- The Institutes of Medicine has identified 12 major components or characteristics of the CPR, which are designated as the "gold standard" attributes.
- The CPR offers benefits to nurses, physicians, and other health care providers, as well as to the health care enterprise.
- As of mid 2000, the perfect CPR has not been widely implemented.
- Infrastructure, cost, vocabulary standardization, and caregiver resistance are the major impediments to the development of a CPR.
- Issues that must be considered when developing the CPR include data integrity, ownership of the patient record, privacy, and electronic signature.
- An emerging technology related to CPR development is the use of smart cards to store client information.

REFERENCES

Amatayakul, M. (1997). Making the case for electronic records. *Health Data Management*, 5(5), 56–63.

Amatayakul, M. (2000). Critical success factors: Steps to achieve a truly integrated information system. *Health Management Technology*, 21(5), 14–18.

Anderson, H. J., and Bunschoten, B. (1996). Creating electronic records: A progress report. *Health Data Management*, 4(9), 36–44.

Andrew, W., and Dick, R. (1996). On the road to the CPR: Where are we now? *Healthcare Informatics*, 13(5), 48–52.

Andrew, W., and Dick, R. (1997). Where we've been and where we're headed. *Healthcare Informatics*, 14(2), 52–56.

Barrett, M. J. (2000). The evolving computerized medical record. *Healthcare Informatics*, 17(5), 85–93.

Broomberg, B. (1995). Hints on developing a smart health card system. *Toward an Electronic Patient Record '95—Proceedings*, Vol. 2, 502–512.

Dick, R. S., and Gabler, J. M. (1995). Still searching for the "Holy Grail." *Health Management Technology*, 16(3), 30–35.

Dick, R. S., and Steen, E. B. (1991). *The computer-based patient record: An essential technology for health care.* Washington, DC: National Academy Press.

Ellsasser, K. H., Nkobi, J., and Kohler, C. O. (1995). Distributing databases: A model for global, shared care. *Healthcare Informatics*, 12(1), 62–68.

Feste, L. K. (1993). Electronic signature as it is today. *Journal of AHIMA*, 64(4), 18–19.

Gaillour, F. R. (1999). Rethinking the CPR: Is perfect the enemy of good? *Health Management Technology*, 20(4), 22–25.

McFall, E. (1993). An electronic medical record—delivering benefits today. *Healthcare Informatics*, 10(10), 76, 78.

Stetson, D. S., and Andrew, P. E. (1996). The CPR: Getting physicians on board. *Healthcare Informatics*, 13(6), 20–24.

Tabar, P. (2000). The latest work: A glossary of healthcare information technology terms. *Healthcare Informatics*, 17(3), 75–133.

13

Regulatory and Accreditation Issues

After completing this chapter, you should be able to:

- Review important legislation for the protection of health care records, including HIPAA.

- Discuss the impact of major accrediting agencies and reimbursement issues on the design and use of information systems.

- Review some design and implementation considerations for automated documentation systems in specialized facilities.

PRIVACY AND CONFIDENTIALITY LEGISLATION

Until recently, legal protection of data confidentiality has been poor. The 1996 passage of the **Health Insurance Portability and Accountability Act (HIPAA),** also known as the Kennedy–Kassebaum Bill, represents the first federal legislation to protect automated client records. This legislation calls for the establishment of an electronic patient records system and privacy rules (Information Policy Committee 1997).

Previous attempts to legislate medical records privacy included the Individual Privacy Act, the Fair Health Information Practices Act of 1995, and the Medical Records Confidentiality Act of 1995 (Thomas 1997). However, none of these bills were passed. Table 13–1 provides a synopsis of each of these proposed bills.

The Medical Records Confidentiality Act, otherwise known as the **Bennett Bill,** was notable because it contained the following points (Braithwaite 1996):

- A definition of *health information trustee* as a person or entity that creates, receives, obtains, maintains, or transmits protected health information, and any employee, agent, or contractor of same

- Conditions for the inspection and copying of protected information

- Provisions for the correction or amendment of protected health information

- Time limits and additional constraints over disclosure of information

- Authorization and accountability for disclosure of information, including electronic disclosure

- Stiff sanctions for inappropriate access or use of health-related information

Although the Bennett Bill did propose safeguards for health care information, the American Civil Liberties Union (ACLU) and several con-

| Table 13–1 | Previous Attempts at Legislation to Protect the Privacy of Medical Records |

Title	Synopsis
Individual Privacy Protection Act of 1991	Designed to amend the Privacy Act of 1974, increasing the minimum amount of civil damages when records are not properly maintained Provided penalties for violations of privacy rights Established an individual privacy protection board
The Fair Health Information Practices Act of 1995	Required health care providers, information service organizations, benefit plan sponsors, and health researchers to allow individuals to examine their own records Set forth provisions concerning the use and disclosure of protected information Established penalties for violations of the act
Medical Records Confidentiality Act of 1995	Designed to ensure medical record privacy Defined *health information trustee* Established circumstances for disclosure Required trustees to establish safeguards and to maintain records of disclosures not related to treatment Established penalties for failure to comply with the act
Medical Privacy in the Age of New Technologies Act of 1997	Established safeguards for health information Restricted the use and disclosure of information Proposed civil and criminal sanctions for failure to comply with the act
Fair Health Information Practices Act of 1997	Required health care providers to allow individuals to examine their records Restricted the use of protected information to the purpose for which it was collected or for which disclosure authorization has been obtained Mandated the establishment of standards for electronic document transmission, receipt, and maintenance Established civil and criminal penalties for violations of the act Authorized research on protecting health information

SOURCE: Adapted from "Legislative information on the Internet," Thomas, 1997. On the Internet at: *http://thomas.loc.gov/home/thomas.html.*

sumer rights groups opposed the bill because they thought it did not adequately address client control over the use and dissemination of health information. Other critics felt its wording would prevent legitimate exchange of client information between institutions (Braithwaite 1996, Barrows and Clayton 1996). Box 13–1 lists some principles identified by the ACLU for the formulation of a health information privacy policy.

The **Privacy Act of 1974** protects federally managed records, such as those of Medicare and Medicaid, and mandates that federal agencies develop, implement, and disclose their plans for maintaining the security of stored data (Hebda, Sakerka, and Czar 1994, Frawley 1995, Robinson 1994, Rothfeder 1995). Veteran Affairs Administration Hospitals have

Box 13–1   American Civil Liberties Union (ACLU) Principles for Formulating a Health Information Privacy Policy

- Strict limits on access and disclosure of all personally identifiable health data
- Individual control of all personally identifiable health records, with no disclosure without informed consent
- Security measures that protect against unauthorized access or misuse by authorized persons
- No access to personally identifiable health information for employers or potential employers
- Individuals have the right to access, copy, and/or correct any information contained in their own medical records
- Full notification of clients of all uses of their health information
- The establishment of a private right of action and government enforcement to prevent or correct wrongful disclosures or information misuse
- The establishment of a federal system to ensure compliance with privacy laws and regulations

SOURCE: Adapted from "Privacy, confidentiality, and electronic medical records" by R. C. Barrows and P. D. Clayton, 1996, *Journal of the American Medical Informatics Association, 3*(2), 139–148; and *Toward a new health care system: The civil liberties issues*, an ACLU Public Policy Report, 1994. Extracts from the CINAHL® database reprinted by kind permission of Cinahl Information Systems, Glendale, California, telephone (818) 409-8005 ext. 4483.

published these plans. No similar federal mandate exists for private institutions and providers. European agencies refuse to transmit medical information to the United States for this reason.

It is important to note that the Privacy Act of 1974 was enacted prior to widespread computer use. As a result, protection of medical records varies from state to state. Practitioners must be familiar with the regulations of the states in which they practice. Some states have regulations, statutes, and case laws that recognize the confidentiality of medical records and limit access. Breach of confidence may lead to disciplinary action for health care professionals by their state boards for licensure. Some states have criminal sanctions against violations of client confidentiality, but enforcement and quantification of damage are difficult.

Several groups besides the ACLU express a strong interest in privacy issues for medical records. These include the Center for Democracy and Technology, the National Coalition of Patient Rights, and the Electronic Privacy Information Center. Each group maintains its own Web site.

The need for legislation regarding privacy and confidentiality continues to be addressed. Recently proposed bills include the Medical Records Privacy Act of 1997. This is a comprehensive bill that provides medical record privacy for patients. It allows a patient to access their own automated information and provides the capability to allow or deny the release of information and limit the extent of disclosure (Curtin and Simpson 1999). Another recent proposal is the Health Care Personal Information Nondisclosure Act of 1998. Unlike the Medical Records Privacy Act of 1997, this proposal denies patient access to their own medical record if it could cause mental harm (Curtin and Simpson 1999).

THE HEALTH INSURANCE PORTABILITY AND ACCOUNTABILITY ACT

Although other legislation has been proposed but not passed, the Health Insurance Portability and Accountability Act (Pubic Law 104-191) was passed into law by Congress in 1996 (Proposed standards 2000). Once the final rules and regulations are published in 2000, facilities must begin using the standards within two years. The impact of HIPAA will be at least as great as Y2K, if not greater. Some estimates suggest that HIPAA compliance will result in spending that is twice the amount spent in Y2K preparation.

HIPAA has the following objectives (Haramboure 1999, Hellerstein 2000):

- To assure the portability of health insurance
- To prevent health care fraud and abuse
- To assure the security and privacy of health information
- To enforce health information standards that will improve the efficiency of health care delivery, simplify the exchange of data between health care entities, and reduce cost
- To reduce the paperwork associated with processing health care transaction

HIPAA will impact all organizations and individuals involved in the delivery of health care. Organizations, including hospitals, physician offices, home health agencies, and nursing homes, must prepare for the provisions of this legislation. Also affected will be payers, employers, data services, regulatory agencies, as well as information system vendors, Medicare, and Medicaid. HIPAA will impact individual care providers, including physicians, nurses, other clinicians, instructors, students, and volunteers. Others who have direct or indirect access to patient information will also be impacted. Examples include utilization review staff as well as housekeeping and maintenance personnel.

HIPAA Standards

HIPAA includes specific standards that address the security and privacy of patient information. Health care organizations must ensure that information systems containing patient data require proof of user identity. In addition, policies and procedures related to information security should be reviewed and updated to support this legislation.

Authentication of user identity is an essential component of HIPAA. Authentication may include the following elements (LaRochelle 1999):

- *What the user has or possesses.* Examples are smart cards and encryption keys, or PKIs.
- *What the user knows.* Examples include sign-on ID and passwords.
- *Physical attributes.* This includes fingerprints, voice recognition, retinal scanning, and other biometric parameters.

HIPAA also includes requirements for electronic signature standards. Although electronic signatures are not required by HIPAA, specific standards are described if an organization chooses to use them. Electronic or digital signatures include an encrypted digital tag added to an electronic document (Tabar 2000). This technology has the following features:

- User authentication that guarantees the user's identity.
- Provides evidence that supports the validity of the signature.
- Ensures the integrity of the message.

HIPAA Compliance

One of the most effective measures in preparing for HIPAA compliance is the designation of a chief security officer or privacy official (Hellerstein 2000). The responsibility of overseeing efforts to meet HIPAA's security standards should be formally assigned to a specific person or organization. The security officer should do the following during preparation for HIPAA:

- Educate IS staff and administration regarding HIPAA.
- Perform a risk analysis that reviews current systems and procedures.
- Identify changes that must be made, including system changes.
- Develop a plan to carry out needed revisions.
- Communicate and educate all staff regarding system revisions and updates to policies and procedures.

Box 13–2 lists examples of current security measures that should be evaluated for HIPAA compliance.

The HIPAA legislation includes descriptions of the various penalties for noncompliance, which could be severe. For example, the penalty for violating transaction standards is up to $100 per person per violation, and up to $25,000 per person per violation of a single standard per calendar year. Penalties for wrongful disclosure of patient information include large fines as well as possible imprisonment.

ACCREDITATION AND REIMBURSEMENT ISSUES

Several agencies have a major impact on health care providers. Accreditation or approval determines whether providers receive funding, enhances the provider's image, instills confidence in the quality of services

Box 13–2	Evaluation of Current Security Measures for HIPAA Compliance

Examples of Security Measures That Should Be Evaluated

- *Determine what types of data are stored on PCs and storage media such as diskettes.* Do they hold patient data?

- *Secure workstations.* Do workstations require a unique sign-on for each user? Are workstations and point-of-care devices protected from theft?

- *System security.* Is there an auto–log-off procedure in place?

- *Evaluate network security.* Is your network protected from unauthorized access?

- *Update your hardware and software inventories.*

- *Examine physical features in accordance with security requirements.* Identify location of backup media and workstations in relation to public access.

- *Printout security.* How are paper reports containing patient information disposed of?

rendered, and attracts qualified professionals. This process has direct implications for how documentation and information systems are structured. These agencies may be subdivided into accrediting bodies and agencies that dictate reimbursement criteria. The Joint Commission for Accreditation of Healthcare Organizations (JCAHO) and the Commission on Accreditation of Rehabilitation Facilities (CARF) fall into the first group, with Medicare and Medicaid and other third-party payers in the second group, as well as Ambulatory Payment Classifications (APCs). Each is discussed below.

JCAHO

The mission of the **Joint Commission for Accreditation of Healthcare Organizations (JCAHO)** is to improve the quality of care delivered to the public, develop standards of quality in conjunction with health professionals, and encourage organizations to meet or exceed these standards through the accreditation process. Once limited to acute care facilities, JCAHO standards now exist for ambulatory, long-term, home health, mental health, and hospice care, as well as managed care. JCAHO accreditation benefits providers by helping them to meet all, or portions of, state and/or federal licensure and certification requirements. JCAHO accreditation also expedites third-party payment and provides guidelines for the improvement of care, services, and programs. Other benefits include community confidence in the organization and improved staff recruitment and retention.

JCAHO standards shape organization practice and documentation, thereby impacting information system documentation design (Joint Commission 1996). When accreditation standards change, documentation must reflect additional requirements. Furthermore, JCAHO now has information management standards for health care organizations. A brief description of current JCAHO information standards follows.

1. *Measures that protect information confidentiality, security, and integrity,* inclusive of
   - Determining user need for information access and level of security
   - Easy, timely retrieval of information without compromising security or confidentiality
   - Written and enforced policies restricting removal of client records for legal reasons
   - Guarding records and information against loss, destruction, tampering, and/or unauthorized use

2. *Uniform definitions and methods for data capture* as a means to facilitate data comparison within and among health care institutions.

3. *Education on the principles of information management and training for system use.* This may include education about the transformation of data into information for subsequent use in decision support and statistical analysis.

4. *Accurate, timely transmission of information* as evidenced by the following characteristics:
   - 24-hour availability in a form that meets user needs
   - Minimal delay of order implementation
   - Quick turnaround of test results
   - A pharmacy system designed to minimize errors
   - An efficient communication system

5. *Integration of clinical systems* (i.e., pharmacy, nursing, lab, and radiology systems) *and nonclinical systems* for ready availability of information.

6. *Client-specific data/information.* The system collects, analyzes, transmits, and reports individual client-specific data and information related to client outcomes that can be used to facilitate care, provide a financial and legal record, aid research, and support decision making.

7. *Aggregate data/information.* The system generates reports that support operations and research and improve performance and care. For example, information may be provided by practitioner, client outcomes, diagnosis, or drug effectiveness.

8. *Knowledge-based information.* Literature is available in print or electronic form.

9. *Comparative data.* The system can extract information useful to compare the institution against other agencies. Deviations from expected patterns, trends, length of stay, or numbers of procedures performed may be noted.

Information standards may be demonstrated through the presence of the following: planning documents; institutional and departmental policy and procedures; data element definitions and abbreviations; observations; continuing education outlines and records; interviews with administrators and staff; and meeting minutes. A scoring system notes the degree to which each standard is met. Scoring criteria can be found in the JCAHO's accreditation manual.

CARF

The **Commission on Accreditation of Rehabilitation Facilities (CARF)** is another health care accrediting body (McCourt 1993, CARF 1996). Its focus is the improvement of rehabilitative services to people with disabilities and others in need of rehabilitation. CARF provides a template for operations as well as a tool for evaluation. CARF is a private, nonprofit organization that uses input from consumers, rehabilitation professionals, state and national organizations, and third-party payers to develop standards for accreditation. Although similar in purpose and structure to JCAHO, CARF places a greater emphasis on the following factors:

- Accessible services
- Comprehensiveness and continuity in individual treatment plan
- Input from consumers about CARF and its decision making
- Safety of persons with disabilities and their evacuation in the event of an emergency
- Postdischarge outcomes

Like JCAHO standards, CARF standards shape institutional practices and documentation requirements. This may necessitate changes in automated documentation systems to comply with CARF standards.

Reimbursement Issues

Medicare, Medicaid, and other third-party payers dictate reimbursement criteria to health care organizations. Health maintenance organizations (HMOs) also have numerous criteria that must be met for reimbursement of services. Failure to demonstrate client need for a service may result in denial of that service or reimbursement for that service. For example, Medicare will pay for a client's care in a transitional or subacute care unit only if the client has a preceding hospital stay. It also requires a demonstrated daily need for skilled services. Documentation plays an essential role in this process. Automated documentation systems should support entry of information about client need through initial screen design and the use of prompts to elicit needed information. Automated systems can also remind providers of remaining days of coverage for each client, as well as services not covered by Medicare, Medicaid, or their third-party payers.

Ambulatory Payment Classification (APC) describes new reimbursement criteria for ambulatory procedures that became effective in August 2000 (Micheletti 2000). Specific coding guidelines have been developed for ambulatory reimbursement, as well as guidelines for managing APC compliance. Preparation for APC compliance requires several areas of concentration:

- Verify the integrity of the charge description master. Ensure that there is no duplicate payment for supplies and services.

- Address the charges of multiple departments, including overlap and duplication.

Box 13–3 **Minimum Data Set for Nursing Home Resident Assessment and Care**

- Identification and background information
- Cognitive patterns
- Communication/hearing
- Vision patterns
- Physical functioning and structural problems
- Continence in last 14 days
- Psychosocial well-being
- Mood and behavior patterns
- Activity pursuit patterns
- Disease diagnoses
- Health conditions
- Oral/nutritional status
- Oral/dental status
- Skin condition
- Medication use
- Special treatment and procedures
- Identification information
- Resident information
- Discharge information

- Develop appropriate management reports for reviewing APC reimbursement.

SPECIAL FACILITY ISSUES

Specialized facilities have unique needs with implications for automated documentation systems. Not all of these needs are covered by JCAHO accreditation. State regulations, including mental health legislation, play an important role in dictating standards for information systems. No attempt is made here to address each type of facility, but pertinent considerations are noted.

Section B. Cognitive Patterns

1 Comatose
- ❏ Yes (skip to Section E)
- ❏ No

2 Memory
Short-term—recall after 5 minutes
- ❏ OK
- ❏ Problem

Long-term
- ❏ OK
- ❏ Problem

3 Memory/recall ability
- ❏ Current season
- ❏ Location of own room
- ❏ Staff names/faces
- ❏ That he/she is in a nursing home
- ❏ None of the above

4 Cognitive skills for daily decision making
- ❏ Independent
- ❏ Modified independence—some difficulty in making new situations only
- ❏ Moderately impaired—poor decisions, requires supervision
- ❏ Severely impaired—never makes decisions

5 Indicators of delirium/disordered thinking
- ❏ Less alert, easily distracted
- ❏ Changing awareness of environment
- ❏ Episodes of incoherent speech
- ❏ Periods of motor restlessness or lethargy
- ❏ Cognitive ability varies over course of day
- ❏ None of the above

6 Change in cognitive status
- ❏ None
- ❏ Improved
- ❏ Deteriorated

FIGURE 13–1 • Sample Screen Shot from an Automated Summary for a Nursing Home Resident

Geriatric and Long-Term Facilities

Because of long stays and high client ratios for each nurse, documentation in nursing homes and long-term facilities must be concise, while addressing specific problems for this client population. Many institutions have developed their own forms to expedite this process and address required areas in accord with the mandated frequency of charting for reimbursement. For example, monthly comprehensive summaries on each resident are required. Box 13–3 identifies areas that a monthly summary might include. Figure 13–1 displays a sample documentation screen from an automated summary. When long-term or skilled beds (beds occupied by clients who require specialized nursing care) are located within an institution with automated documentation, additional screens are needed to meet the special needs of this population. Automation can speed updates, provide prompts to ensure appropriate response, decrease entry errors on ICD-9 reimbursement codes, and generate automated plans of care.

Documentation of Restraint Application/Assessment

Time applied: __:__ (Maximum time policy identifies for removal automatically shown)
Time scheduled for release: __:__
Reasons for use: (indicate all that apply)
❑ Behavior harmful to self/to others
❑ Necessary to prevent injury
❑ Assaultive behavior
❑ Increased agitation
❑ Impulsive behavior
❑ Other (Specify): _____

Type of restraint applied:
❑ Soft wrist
❑ Waist
❑ Jacket posey
❑ Geriatric chair
❑ Locked leather wrist
✓ One
✓ Two
❑ Locked leather ankle
✓ One
✓ Two
Time restraints removed: __:__
Neurovascular status distal to restraints:
-Pulses: may select from predetermined responses or indicate "other" and describe
-Color: may select from predetermined responses or indicate "other" and describe
-Sensation: may select from predetermined responses or indicate "other" and describe
Frequency of nursing assessments: __:__

FIGURE 13–2 • Suggested Screen Design for Restraint Use in an Automated Documentation System

Screen design of documentation requires an increased emphasis on psychosocial functioning and several other areas. JCAHO, Medicare, and Medicaid requirements are driving forces in documentation design.

Psychiatric Facilities

Each state has its own public health and mental health legislation and regulations that impact information system design. For example, regulations relative to the use of restraints vary from state to state. Documentation must comply with state law as well as JCAHO requirements. For example, important points for charting on the application of restraints include date and time applied, reason for use, type of restraint applied, length of time the client remains in restraints, neurovascular status distal to the restraint, and the frequency of assessments done on the client in restraints. Policy must be established that includes these areas and identifies a maximum length of time that a client may remain in restraints without a renewal order from a physician. This policy should be reflected in time limits on documentation screens. Seclusion policies should be basically the same. Figure 13–2 shows a suggested documentation screen for restraint use and seclusion.

There is also a greater tendency for interdisciplinary documentation in psychiatric care, due to the need to provide adequate system and record access to many different personnel. Nursing staff, psychiatrists, psychologists, social workers, and recreational therapists require access to psychiatric client records no matter what unit the client is admitted to.

CASE STUDY EXERCISES

You are teaching an undergraduate course titled Nursing Informatics. One class session is scheduled for a discussion on the protection of client record information. How would you summarize the current status of legislative safeguards in the United States? What, if anything, would you suggest that students might personally consider to improve this situation?

• • •

You have been appointed to the Clinical Information Systems Committee, which is charged with looking at ways that automation can facilitate data collection for the next JCAHO accreditation visit. List examples of how your community hospital demonstrates adherence to JCAHO information standards, and state your rationale for why you feel these examples display compliance.

• • •

You are the general nursing information systems (IS) liaison person at Wilson Rehabilitation Institute. CARF accreditation is coming up. What would you do to ensure that your automated documentation is in compliance with CARF standards? Explain your rationale.

SUMMARY

- Current legal protection for health record privacy and confidentiality is addressed by HIPAA legislation, which is currently expected to become effective in 2002.

- Accrediting agencies such as JCAHO and CARF, Medicare and Medicaid regulations, third-party payer demands, state and federal laws, and Ambulatory Payment Classifications dictate documentation requirements.

- Information systems and the design of automated documentation must incorporate safeguards for information privacy as well as standards for quality of care imposed by accrediting agencies.

- Automated documentation can facilitate the collection of data for accrediting bodies, third-party payers, and state and federal requirements.

- Special care facilities have documentation requirements that require additional automated screen design.

REFERENCES

American Civil Liberties Union. (1994). *Toward a new health care system: The civil liberties issues*. An ACLU Public Policy Report. New York: American Civil Liberties Union.

Barrows, R. C., and Clayton, P. D. (1996). Privacy, confidentiality, and electronic medical records. *Journal of the American Medical Informatics Association, 3*(2), 139–148.

Braithwaite, W. R. (1996). National health information privacy bill generates heat at SCAMC. *Journal of the American Medical Informatics Association, 3*(1), 95–96.

CARF. (30 September 1996). *CARF mission statement*. On the Web at: *http://www.carf.org*.

Curtin, L., and Simpson, R. (1999). Privacy in the information age. *Health Management Technology, 20*(8), 32–33.

Frawley, K. (1995). Achieving the CPR while keeping an ancient oath. *Healthcare Informatics, 12*(4), 28–30.

Haramboure, D. (1999). An industry unready for HIPAA's proposed privacy legislation. *Health Management Technology, 20*(8), 16–17.

Hebda, T., Sakerka, L., and Czar, P. (1994). Educating nurses to maintain patient confidentiality on automated information systems. In S. J. Grobe and E. S. P. Pluyter-Wenting (Eds.). *Nursing informatics: An international overview for nursing in a technological era*. The Proceedings of the Fifth IMIA International Conference on Nursing Use of Computers and Information Science. New York: Elsevier Science.

Hellerstein, D. (2000). HIPAA and health information privacy rules: Almost there. *Health Management Technology, 21*(4), 26–31.

Information Policy Committee National Information Infrastructure Task Force. (April 1997). *Options for promoting privacy on the National Information Infrastructure.* On the Web at: *http:/www.iitf.nist.gov/ipc/privacy.htm.*

Joint Commission on Accreditation of Healthcare Organizations. (1996). *Medical records process.* Chicago: Accreditation Manual for Hospitals.

LaRochelle, B. (1999). Fundamental and trade-offs of IT security. *Health Management Technology, 20*(8), 18–21.

McCourt, A. E. (1993). *The specialty practice of rehabilitation nursing: A core curriculum*, 3rd ed. Skokie, IL: The Rehabilitation Nursing Foundation of the Association of Rehabilitation Nurses.

Micheletti, J. A. (2000). APC environment poses new compliance risk. *Health Management Technology, 21*(6), 54–56.

Proposed standards for privacy of individually identifiable health information. (2000). U.S. Department of Health and Human Services. On the Web at: *http://aspe.os.dhhs.gov/admnsimp/pvcsumm.htm.*

Robinson, E. N. (1994). The computerized patient record: Privacy and security. *M.D. Computing, 11*(2), 69–73.

Rothfeder, J. (1995). Invasion of privacy. *PC World, 13*(11), 52+.

Tabar, P. (2000). The latest work: A glossary of healthcare information technology terms. *Healthcare Informatics, 17*(3), 75–133.

Thomas, Legislative information on the Internet. (16 June 1997). On the Internet at: *http://thomas.loc.gov/home/thomas.html.*

14

Community Health Information Networks

After completing this chapter, you should be able to:

- Define *community health information network (CHIN)*.
- List the four major components of a CHIN.
- Explain how connectivity is provided when developing a CHIN.
- Review the importance of data formats in CHIN development.
- Discuss client confidentiality and data security issues as they relate to CHINs.
- Identify the two major benefits associated with CHINs.
- List several limiting factors to the development of CHINs.
- Describe the current status of CHINs in the United States.

Community Health Information Networks (CHINs) are a rapidly emerging technology within progressive health care settings. A CHIN can be defined as an organization that offers electronic connections that enable all providers, payers, and purchasers of care to exchange financial, clinical, and administrative information in a defined geographic location, eliminating redundant data collection and reducing paperwork (Tabar 2000). In other words, a CHIN is a public wide-area network, linking various participants in a community of care (Gordon 1996). These networks are among the newest form of information sharing available to health care professionals, and are likely to be used by nearly all major health care providers in the near future. Physicians are major users of CHINs and often are the initial source of client data that is transmitted within the CHIN (Gilchrist 1994). Users of CHINs outside of the hospital include insurance providers, employers, regulatory agencies, and financial institutions (Bir and Zerrenner 1995). Figure 14–1 shows the relationship between the various CHIN participants within the community.

COMPONENTS OF A CHIN

Information sharing within a CHIN should be accomplished in a manner that conveys data in a seamless, standardized electronic format. A CHIN can be thought of as a network of networks, connecting the various networks of participating organizations into one large network. This allows for the retrieval of information without the user having to know where the information actually resides. According to Bir and Zerrenner (1995), the four primary features of a CHIN are

1. *Open communications.* Open communications, facilitated by an interface engine, are necessary for providing access to the data throughout the CHIN. This provides connectivity between the

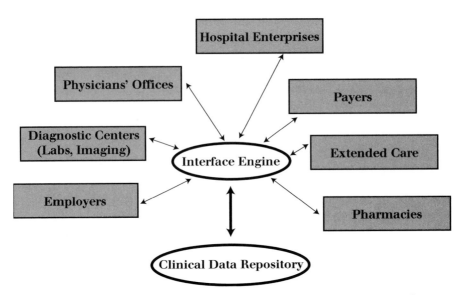

FIGURE 14–1 • Relationship Between CHIN Participants (Gordon 1996; copyright ©
Healthcare Technology Management magazine, HealthTech Publishing Company, East
Providence, RI)

computer-based patient record, various data repositories, and
payer information, so that all data is available to the various participants in the CHIN.

2. *The computer-based patient record (CPR).* Access should be provided to the CPRs from all participating CHIN members.

3. *Clinical data repository.* The CHIN clinical data repository is a
combination of all clinical data available from the various individual data repositories of each participating organization. Box 14–1
lists some specific types of information available in the CHIN clinical data repository.

4. *Mechanisms for cost, outcome, and utilization analysis.* This type
of analysis is based on information provided by the payers, as well
as the outcomes recorded by the health care providers. The data is
able to be manipulated and analyzed by decision support software,
including rules-based analysis. For example, a clinical information
system can suggest a treatment plan based on an analysis of the
collective data from many clients available within the CHIN data
repository.

In addition to providing access to client data, CHINs may also provide
members with other types of services that facilitate and improve the
management of client care. A list of the major services that may be available in a CHIN is seen in Box 14–2.

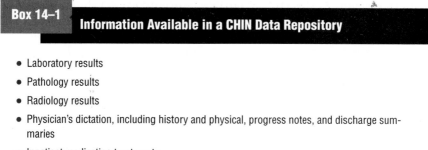

Box 14–1 **Information Available in a CHIN Data Repository**

- Laboratory results
- Pathology results
- Radiology results
- Physician's dictation, including history and physical, progress notes, and discharge summaries
- Inpatient medication treatments
- Nursing care documentation
- Client demographic information
- Client health care insurance information
- Names of primary and consulting physicians

DEVELOPMENT OF A CHIN

Connectivity

Interfaces are developed to connect existing networks belonging to the various providers, payers, and other facilities within the community. An **interface engine** is used to translate data that is generated within one organization into a standardized format that can be used throughout the CHIN and understood by users from any participating organization.

The interface engine must use industry standards for data formatting in order to promote effective sharing of information across systems. The most common standard for electronic data exchange in health care is **Health Level 7 (HL7).** This is a flexible protocol that permits the exchange of key sets of data among different application systems. Accord-

Box 14–2 **Services Provided by CHINs**

In addition to providing access to client data, CHINs may also provide the members with other types of services that facilitate and improve the management of client care. These may include the following:

- Voice mail, electronic mail, and faxing capability
- Clinical results reporting
- Access to client demographic information
- Ability to make physician consult and referral requests
- Ability to view claim status
- Access to enrollment and eligibility status for health care reimbursement

ing to Hammond (1996, p. 1), HL7 was originally developed to define standards for the interchange of clinical data, but "the focus has changed with the expansion of the health care model into enterprise systems and integrated delivery systems and community, geographic, and state-wide health care information systems."

The basic building blocks of a CHIN include hardware, software, and the infrastructure that is needed to facilitate connectivity. A master communications server is used to manage the integration of the many independent network systems from each organization participating in the CHIN. Connectivity can be accomplished using technologies such as routers and specialized cabling. The use of **integrated services digital network (ISDN)** cable allows the transfer of large volumes of data at high rates of speed. This is particularly important because client records have become more complex and exist in a variety of formats that may not be transmitted using standard cables. For example, some client record components such as history and physical notes, operative notes, and pathology and radiology reports are in the format of text documents. Other information is available in the format of diagnostic images, including MRI and CT scan results. Ultrasound and cardiac catheterization findings may be communicated using video technology. Finally, signal tracking may be used to store information obtained from fetal and cardiology monitoring. ISDN technology will provide the capability to transfer these varying types of client data.

Data Elements

An important consideration in developing a CHIN is the use of a **unique patient identifier.** The utilization of a single identifier, such as the social security number, will ensure that the correct data is associated with each client. Since data is transmitted into the CHIN repositories from multiple sources and organizations, it is imperative to design a system that will ensure data accuracy and integrity.

It is also important to develop a cross-reference of codes used throughout the CHIN. For example, different codes may be used by various organizations to identify the client as an outpatient. Users must be able to understand the codes entered by other organizations in order to effectively use the available data.

The CHIN must provide all of the pertinent basic identifying data related to each client visit or encounter. This includes the client name and identifiers, date of service, and location of the encounter. In addition, the purpose of the visit or inpatient stay should be available.

Centralized Data Repository

Another component of a CHIN is a centralized data repository that stores information obtained from the existing databases of various providers. Ideally, information stored in the data repository can then be queried and extracted by the participants of the CHIN. The users can extract information related to a single client, or may extract aggregate information related to a large number of clients. This ideal data repository does not actually exist in CHINs today, because of legal and data security reasons (Gordon 1996). Instead, users may be provided with an index identifying the location of a particular database storing the desired information. This information can then be requested from the specific organization owning the database, and transmitted electronically.

CHIN Developers

The major participants in the development of a CHIN include vendors that specialize in software application development, telecommunications, database management, and interface engines (Wakerly 1994). These vendors must work closely with the actual providers, payers, and other members of the CHIN to develop a network that meets the need of the subscribers as well as the clients for whom they care. The key to building an effective CHIN is the collaboration and cooperation of all involved parties.

BENEFITS ASSOCIATED WITH CHINs

Access to Client Information

The major benefit seen with the use of a CHIN is increased access to client care information. Since the information from various providers and payers is pooled, a large volume and variety of information is contained within the network. Access to this information by various CHIN members may lead to increased productivity and reduced costs. Productivity is improved because of the quicker responses to requests for client information. Improved communications may result in a reduced length of stay for inpatients (Bazzoli 1995), as well as improved medical decision making and quality of care. Smaller hospitals that are CHIN members may gain access to a larger repository of information and services. The quickly changing health care environment demands easy and swift access to information from many sources. Nursing may also benefit from access to the wide array of information available in the CHIN. Specific client-related data, such as past medical history and treatments, may now be available regardless of the fact that treatment was provided in different health care organizations or enterprises within the community. If these organizations are CHIN participants, the exchange of client data will support and improve client care. In addition, nurses may utilize aggregate client data obtained from the CHIN for research and to develop treatment protocols.

Cost Reduction

Cost reduction is another benefit associated with CHINs. The manual transmission of client data requires more staff involvement and is generally more expensive than the automated transmission of client information. Therefore, use of a CHIN by health care providers to transmit and access client information may result in cost savings. Significant savings may also be realized because of electronic communications between providers and payers using a CHIN. Information such as eligibility, verification, and preauthorization and approvals are exchanged frequently in relation to both inpatient stays and outpatient services.

LIMITING FACTORS

Although the anticipated rapid emergence of CHINs in the mid 1990s indicated their need and acceptance within the health care community, this development has not yet been realized. It is doubtful that any current networks actually meet the requirements of an ideal CHIN. Since the development of a CHIN database can be accomplished using technologies that are already in existence, one might wonder why the development of CHINs falls short of the vision that was first developed.

Client Confidentiality Issues

The major stumbling block is the issue of maintaining client confidentiality and privacy (Gordon 1996). Since client information is shared across a large number of organizations within the CHIN, it can be difficult to limit access to only those professionals who have a need to know. The problem is compounded by the fact that CHIN subscribers have access not only to the information they are seeking on one client, but also to information on many other individuals contained within the database. One way to ensure that an individual user sees only relevant data is to permit access to only pertinent categories of information. For example, a billing clerk should be given access only to diagnostic and procedure billing codes, and not have access to clinical knowledge (Frawley 1995).

Ownership of the CHIN

A related limiting factor to the development of a CHIN is the question of ownership. Since many providers and payers throughout the community are participants, ownership must be clearly established before the system is developed. Many of the participants will want to share and access information while retaining control of their own data (Rubin and Aukema 1995). The CHIN participants must develop policies and procedures that define data ownership while supporting and enforcing reciprocity in data sharing.

Initial Development Costs

Another limiting factor in the development of a CHIN may be cost. Start-up fees may be prohibitive, and may include building the infrastructure of cabling and wiring, purchasing computer hardware and software, and coordinating with other facilities. In addition, all of this planning and development takes a great deal of time, and hospital information services departments may have other priorities. Some may question whether the long-term advantages are worth this initial investment. It seems, however, that most progressive health care communities are proceeding with the development of CHINs, indicating they believe the advantages outweigh the disadvantages and risks.

CURRENT STATUS OF CHINs

The movement of health care providers and payers toward the development of CHINs saw steady progress in the early 1990s. The Wisconsin Health Information Network, developed in 1993, was the first CHIN in the United States. By November 1996, there were approximately eight functioning CHINs (Bazzoli 1996). The popularity of the CHIN concept seemed to diminish in the late 1990s, however. By 2000, the use of newer Internet technologies enabled the development of an Internet-based CHIN in Pittsburgh (Patrick 2000). The use of the Internet to wirelessly access information over a network may be a strategy for overcoming the limitations and difficulties in integration of disparate information systems. This new technology may rekindle the health care industry's interest in CHINs.

CASE STUDY EXERCISES

You are an administrator of a home health care agency in a community that has recently developed a CHIN. Explain how access to this network will improve the ability of your staff to provide appropriate client care.

•   •   •

Describe the types of information that your staff will be accessing from the CHIN, as well as the data that will be added to the CHIN from your agency.

SUMMARY

- Community health information networks (CHINs) are networks that allow the exchange of data among health care providers, payers, and purchasers of care within a defined geographic community.

- The four primary components of a CHIN are open communications, the computer-based patient record, a clinical data repository, and mechanisms for cost, outcomes, and utilization analysis.

- Connectivity between CHIN participants is a major factor in the development of the network, and utilizes technology such as interface engines, Health Level 7 (HL7) data standards, and integrated services digital network (ISDN) cable.

- Issues that must be addressed when developing a CHIN include patient identifiers, cross-references for codes, and the clinical data repository structure.

- The two major benefits associated with CHINs are increased access to client care information and cost reduction.

- The factors limiting the development of CHINs include client confidentiality issues and initial start-up costs.

- Steady progress was seen in the development of CHINs in the United States in the early 1990s, but little development in the later 1990s. Internet technology may provide a new strategy for the development of CHINs.

REFERENCES

Bazzoli, F. (1995). Will CHINs hit the jackpot or break the bank? *Health Data Management, 3*(10), 50–59.

Bazzoli, F. (1996). Restoring the image of networks. *Health Data Management, 4*(11), 39–47.

Bir, N., and Zerrenner, W. (1995). Network design and implementation of a CHIN from a hospital's perspective. *Toward an electronic patient record '95—Proceedings*, Vol. 2, 50–58.

Frawley, K. (1995). Achieving the CPR while keeping an ancient oath. *Healthcare Informatics, 12*(4), 28–30.

Gilchrist, G. (1994). Physicians as front-end users of CHINs. *Healthcare Informatics, 11*(8), 80.

Gordon, M. S. (1996). Get ready to take it on the CHIN. *Health Care Technology Management, 7*(5), 36–39.

Hammond, W. E. (June 1996). Politics and standards. *HL7 News*, 1.

Patrick, S. (2000). Medical record keeping is going high-tech. *Dallas Business Journal, 23*(31), 19.

Rubin, R., and Aukema, M. (Fall 1995). CHIN overview: When you've seen one, you've seen one. *Infocare*, 22–23.

Tabar, P. (2000). The latest work: A glossary of healthcare information technology terms. *Healthcare Informatics, 17*(3), 75–133.

Wakerly, R. T. (Ed.). (1994). *Community health information networks, creating the health care data highway*. Chicago, IL: American Hospital.

15

Disaster Planning and Recovery

After completing this chapter, you should be able to:

- Identify events that can threaten information system (IS) operation.
- Review the advantages associated with IS disaster planning.
- Outline the steps of the disaster planning process.
- Describe how to recover from a disaster.
- Discuss how information obtained from a mock or actual disaster can be used to improve disaster response.
- Discuss legal and accreditation requirements for contingency plans.

U ntil recently, disaster planning received little attention. However, as reliance upon timely access to data grows, so does the recognition of the importance of contingency planning for all organizations dependent on timely access to and processing of information for continued operation. This is no less true for health care agency information systems, networks, and freestanding PCs. Health care providers must determine how a disaster may impact delivery of services, and identify strategies to ensure continuity of care.

WHAT IS DISASTER PLANNING?

A disaster is an occurrence that disrupts or disables necessary business functions (Corrigan 1995, Fried 1995). Disasters strike without warning. For this reason, **disaster planning** is essential for every institution. Disaster planning is an organized approach that anticipates potential system problems, maintains the security of client information under adverse or unexpected conditions, and provides an alternative means to support the retrieval and processing of information in the event that the information system fails. Disaster recovery plans allow organizations to resume system operations. The importance of information to everyday work dictates the priority given to IS disaster planning. Plans should ensure uninterrupted operation or expedite resumption of operation after a disaster while maintaining data integrity and security. Potential risks, critical information, general policy and procedures, hardware and software options, troubleshooting, revisions as changes occur, data backup, training, testing, and overall costs must be considered. Disaster plans need to encompass the multiple vendor platforms found in most organizations and address the implications for other agencies of an inoperable system. For example, if a health care information system is down for a lengthy period of time, information will not be available to third-party payers and suppliers. A comprehensive **disaster** plan actually consists of separate plans for each of the following areas (Cerullo and Cerullo 1998):

- *The emergency plan.* Provides direction during and immediately after the incident.
- *The backup plan.* Maps out steps to ensure the availability of key employees, vital records, and alternative backup facilities for ongoing business and data processing operations.
- *The recovery plan.* Restores full operational capabilities.
- *The test plan.* Uncovers and corrects defects in the plan before a real disaster occurs.
- *The maintenance plan.* Provides guidelines ensuring that the entire plan is kept up-to-date.

Consideration of each of these areas as separate plans may provide for better division of responsibility and increased awareness of significance.

It is also important to consider the human factor when developing and implementing a disaster plan (Cerullo and Cerullo 1998, Simonelli 2000). At times of disaster the institution should be prepared to assist employees and their families, including providing such amenities as transportation to work and possibly temporary housing. Restoration of employees' peace of mind is just as important as recovering data from a computer. This includes reestablishing user confidence once the system is up and running as well as addressing the emotional impact that the disaster had on employees.

Agency personnel may develop a disaster plan, but consultant expertise on the team can develop a plan more quickly, objectively, and knowledgeably because no one individual can know everything needed to implement an effective disaster plan for a large, complex system (Corrigan 1995, Fried 1995, Mannion and Persson 1996, Piellucci 1996). Once developed the plan should be carefully reviewed for weak spots (Morrissey 1999). A successful plan requires commitment from top management down (Ivancevich, Hermanson, and Smith 1998).

The security officer should have a key role in disaster planning. This starts with a basic understanding of the plan development process to help direct the effort (Leary 1998). Part of the security role is the protection of information.

ADVANTAGES OF DISASTER PLANNING

It is not always possible to avoid a disaster, but a good plan can minimize losses incurred by damage, particularly from an internal disaster (Cerullo and Cerullo 1998, Corrigan 1995, Hussong 1996, Fisher 1996, Kutner 1996, McDaniel 1996, Reshaur and Luongo 2000). A good plan does the following:

- Identifies vulnerabilities within the organization and strategies for correction

- Provides a reasonable amount of protection against downtime and data loss
- Allows time for restoration of equipment, the facility, and services
- Ensures continuity of the client record and delivery of care
- Expedites reporting of diagnostic tests
- Captures charges and supports billing and processing of reimbursement claims in a timely fashion
- Ensures open communication with employees and assures customers of availability of services or interim arrangements
- Provides a mechanism to capture information need for regulatory and accrediting bodies
- Helps to ensure compliance with federal legislation and Joint Commission for Accreditation of Hospital Organizations (JCAHO) requirements
- Establishes backup and restoration procedures for systems, databases, and important files

In short, an effective disaster plan saves money up front and over time through limiting loss of data, equipment, and services. Any agency that requires information integrity and availability cannot afford to be without a disaster plan. A good plan can make the difference between institutional survival or demise when the likelihood of bankruptcy increases with each moment that data is unavailable.

Environmental Disaster Versus System Failure

Hazards come from a variety of sources, ranging from environmental disasters to equipment failure (Corrigan 1995, Hussong 1996). Table 15–1 lists some IS threats. A thorough appraisal by IS personnel can minimize the risk of damage from various situations. Environmental disasters may be natural or man-made. Plans must anticipate the predictable and the unpredictable, inclusive of climate, location, building features, internal hazards, such as fire or smoke damage, and utility service. Many hospitals lack the infrastructure to accommodate and support information systems. Often the system and data are housed in areas threatened by potential plumbing leaks or exposure to dangerous materials, such as oxygen, anesthetic agents, or other hazardous chemicals. Both the security of the IS power supply and availability of backup power to sustain uninterrupted computer operation must be considered. The hospital utility lines may be at risk because of their location, particularly if construction is underway and power or telephone lines have not been marked and protected from inadvertent damage.

Disaster may also result from human error, such as accidental file deletion, failure to follow proper backup procedures, the introduction of viruses or vandalism, theft, or loading incomplete programs (Corrigan

Table 15–1	Threats to Normal System Operation

Threat	Examples
Accidents	Loss of power
	File corruption
	Transportation accidents
	Chemical contamination
	Toxic fumes
Natural disasters	Avalanche
	Floods
	Earthquakes
	Hurricanes
	Tornadoes
	Blizzards
Internal disasters	Hardware or software errors
	Water line breaks
	Construction accidents
	Fire
	Sabotage
	Theft
	Ex-employee violence
Malicious or violent acts	Hackers
	Bombs
	Terrorism
	Civil unrest
	Armed conflict

1995). An example of the latter might include a vendor software update that was inadequately tested prior to distribution.

System or equipment failure may occur in the absence of any of the preceding environmental disasters (Corrigan 1995). System failure may result from the failure of a component part or parts. Central processing unit (CPU) crashes, cabling and software problems, and even loose plugs may cause difficulties. When feasible, spare parts such as hubs, patch cables, extra printers, PCs, and servers as well as trained support staff should be available to troubleshoot system problems, avert downtime, and initiate recovery. Redundancy in system design raises the initial system cost but increases IS reliability. A well-executed physical system prevents many problems or makes them easier to discover. A review of the facility, system, policies and procedures, and disaster plan conducted quarterly can identify vulnerable areas. A review should also be done whenever major changes are introduced. Box 15–1 lists areas for consideration.

Box 15–1 **Suggested Areas for Review to Avert System Disasters**

- Documentation
- Network access controls
- Physical security
- Archived data
- Vital records
- Backup procedures
- Recovery procedures
- Backup equipment
- Backup facility
- Test plan
- Network diversity

- Communications links
- Spare parts inventory
- Backup services
- LAN configurations
- Personnel availability
- Off-site storage
- Operations personnel
- Technical personnel
- Vendor service and maintenance agreements

SOURCE: Adapted from Jackson, R. (1996). "Quantifying a business impact analysis." *Disaster Recovery Journal, 9*(1), 21, 23, 25.

STEPS OF THE DISASTER PLANNING PROCESS

A disaster plan for information services does the following: identifies information essential to maintain daily operations; develops policies and procedures to establish how disasters and recovery will be handled; selects and tests backup strategies and storage provisions; and educates staff on the initiation of backup alternatives; and makes recovery arrangements.

Identification of Essential Information

Determining vital information for system operation requires IS staff to complete the following tasks:

- Ascertain what information is necessary for daily operations
- Identify applications and databases that support these critical functions
- Identify computer platforms and communications facilities needed to support these applications
- Distinguish between essential operations and support functions such as administration or billing

These tasks are best achieved by interviewing employees. At the conclusion of the interviews the disaster recovery team should identify the following for each critical mission process (Fried 1995, Nicolet 1996):

- Description, purpose, and origin of the information

- Information flows
- The recipients, or users, of the information
- Requirements for timeliness
- The implications of information unavailability

Once these points have been identified, the disaster recovery team should verify their findings with system users.

Even after information critical to system users has been identified, it is important to realize that critical information is more than the information required for direct client care (Corrigan 1995, Moore 1996). Individual areas within the institution have vendor contracts, personnel files, financial or claim documentation, permits, building blueprints, regulatory compliance documentation, equipment manuals, and reporting data in a variety of formats and places. Much of this information would be difficult or time-consuming to replace. For this reason each area should develop a disaster plan and complete a physical vital record inventory such as the one depicted in Figure 15–1. This inventory should specify:

- Volume and description of information
- Format; for example, whether it is maintained on paper, disk, or tapes
- When the information was created, its use, and how it relates to other records
- When the information is transferred to storage or destroyed
- Equipment used to store critical information
- Consequences for the loss of this information

IS Policy and Procedure Development

Well-documented backup systems and procedures are essential for disaster recovery (Corrigan 1995, Leary 1998, Moore 1996). While each institution and system is different, the disaster plan should identify:

- General system policies and procedures, including who can declare a disaster and the mechanism for calling a disaster
- The emergency telephone tree/call schedule (inclusive of telephone and beeper numbers) and the length of time required for each identified person to arrive, whether the person is an employee or any other individual key to the recovery process
- Alternative communication methods, such as cell phones and pagers
- Responsibilities for each administrator
- System configurations
- An outline of what users should do in the event of a disaster, including their responsibilities with manual systems
- A projected timeline for system restoration

Make one copy of this page for each record listed. When parentheses appear, select one response from within them.

Record name:
> Scheduled and Unscheduled Meds Due lists/Parenteral Therapy lists

Purpose of record:
> Used to administer medications to patients

Who is responsible for this record:
> HIS*-generated document based on MD orders

Media (paper, fiche, mainframe, etc.):
> HIS paper document

Where is the record stored:
> HIS system, on nursing units for 24 hours

Volume/frequency of change:
> Many times/day

Retention requirement:
> 24 hours

Originating office:
> Nursing units

Location of any copies:
> Nursing units/outdated copies

The record is: (irreplaceable, unique/difficult to replace/not hard to replace)

The record is: (essential for business/not essential but important/not important)

How would you obtain this record if your copy were destroyed?
> If HIS system available, reprint; if not, go through each patient's chart

How would you re-create the information on this record?
> Through patient's chart and current hard copy of Patient Care Plans

How long after a disaster could you work without this record?
> Few hours—would use documents available

How is this record protected from destruction? (not protected, sprinklered office area, fireproof cabinet, duplicates kept in other locations, sprinklered warehouse, mainframe computer files, easily re-created, etc.)
> HIS backups—paper documents not protected

Duplication and off-site storage is: (already being done/should be done/is not necessary)
> Already being done—HIS

Are you prepared to supply input data, or work in progress, to allow the rerun of your critical applications from the last off-site backup?

Who is in charge of removing/restoring this record if it is damaged? What provisions have been made to restore/remove damaged records? What is the relocation destination? Who will transport damaged records and what is this person's 24-hour phone number and security clearance?

* HIS, hospital or health care information service.

FIGURE 15–1 • Example of a Physical Vital Records Inventory Sheet

- Troubleshooting and problem resolution
- Data backup and restoration procedures
- Repair procedures
- A list of basic resources required to perform services
- A vital record inventory that includes, but is not limited to, vendor/service provider and warranty information
- Provisions for nonclinical vital record access, backup, and if needed, appropriate restoration techniques for each type of storage medium used
- Vendor service agreements along with identification numbers

Documentation must be explicit since support people come and go. For example, instructions should provide details on how to load tapes and the order in which to load them. Key information, such as people responsible for implementing the plan and the roles they play, must be updated as needed. An independent party should review documentation for clarity and completeness regularly and after a disaster. Documentation should include goals for the implementation of suggested and/or required changes.

Backup and Storage

Backup allows restoration of data if, or when, data is lost (Casey and Kohler 1996, Zeidman 1996). Data loss may occur with disk or CPU crashes, file deletion, file corruption secondary to power or application problems, or overwritten files. Traditional backup dumps data to a storage medium such as a tape for transfer to another site for storage and, if needed, system restoration. Storage media differ, but should permit permanent or semipermanent record keeping. Magnetic tape is a popular, and relatively inexpensive, storage medium. Optical disks are another storage option with a longer shelf life and a higher cost. Electronic transfer over high-speed telephone lines to another site is a faster, more reliable means of backup that eliminates transportation concerns. When electronic transmission is not an option, a second set of backup media should be made and transported separately to ensure against accidental loss or destruction.

Backup may fail because of faulty software, bad network connections, worn tapes, or poor storage conditions (Corrigan 1995, "Defusing the backup bomb" 1995). For this reason backup should be verified and periodically tested. Newer tape drives have well-developed error correction, eliminating the need to verify backup copies but not the need to test stored media. Storage conditions must be climate controlled and free from electromagnetic interference to avoid degradation of media. Agencies may opt to outsource storage to cold sites. A **cold site** is a commercial service that provides storage for backup materials or the capacity to handle the disaster-stricken facility's computer equipment (Amelyn 1996, Leary 1998). Often backup materials are found on a combination of different media. Materials are shipped from the institution to the cold site, where backups from multiple organizations are kept in protected vaults under controlled conditions. Agency personnel are responsible for backup, dating, and labeling materials for storage. Cold sites should be located in areas free from floods and tornadoes, and at least five miles away from the agency to avoid disaster conditions.

Electronic transfer of data for storage at another site may also be outsourced. **Remote backup services** (**RBSs**) are commercial enterprises that provide backup services for customers. They offer a simple, inexpensive option for customers in client–server environments (Zeidman 1996). RBSs provide customers with backup software that is installed at their site and at a central, remote file server. The customer dials to the remote server to back up data. Each customer has a separate account, and file access is limited to authorized persons. RBS staff protect both data and data integrity. Data retrieval, when needed, is limited only by the speed of the communication link. RBSs also provide reports to show which files have been backed up.

Personal Computers Although the primary focus for IS disaster plans is on the major systems, large amounts of information important for daily operations are also found on PCs. For this reason, IS disaster plans need to include PCs. Routine PC maintenance prevents many problems (Carlisle 1996, Lee and Hudspeth 1995, Hoffman 1995, Sands 1996). Box 15–2 lists tasks suggested for PC maintenance. Agencies cannot assume that PC users know how to perform these chores and should offer instruction and assistance. For example, computer support personnel should perform PC backup. This has the added benefit of standardizing PC backup procedures and media.

Manual Versus Automated Alternatives

The decision to use manual alternatives when the system is down has implications for the delivery of care, the cost of care given, record management, and employee system training. A backup alternative is a different means to accomplish a common task than what is ordinarily used. An example of a manual backup alternative is when staff must complete requests for laboratory tests via paper forms that must then be delivered to the lab instead of selecting the ordered test from a menu option on a computer screen. Implementation of a backup alternative may delay delivery of services for several reasons. First, personnel are less familiar with the alternative procedure and will take longer to accomplish their work. Results reporting and processing requests for services will be delayed. Manual forms may no longer exist or may not be current in listing available tests or test names. Because automation eliminated personnel

Box 15–2 Recommended PC Maintenance

- Create several DOS boot diskettes. Boot diskettes allow the PC to start even if the hard drive won't work. Keep at least one copy with backup tapes/diskettes.
- Keep original software handy in the event that it must be reinstalled.
- Print out copies of SYSTEM.INI, AUTOEXEC.BAT, CONFIG.SYS, and WIN.INI files, update them every time new software is added, and keep the printouts in an accessible area.
- Establish a secure place for backup diskettes or tapes away from the PC, preferably in a fire-proof safe or file cabinet. Backup diskettes stored under poor conditions or kept in the same area as the PC are vulnerable to the same threats.
- Do an incremental backup daily, a full backup weekly, and a full system backup monthly.
- Test backup tapes/diskettes to ensure that they are good. Establish a policy for routine replacement of backup media.
- Periodically delete files from the hard drive that are no longer needed.
- Defragment all hard drives monthly.
- Maintain air flow around the PC to allow cooling.
- Keep diskettes away from magnetic fields, including electronic devices.
- Periodically clean PCs.
- Run virus protection software regularly and obtain updated versions as available.

that supported the manual process there may be few people available that know the manual alternative. Automated backup alternatives may also be available. For example, staff may be able to access information through a different screen than what they generally use. Despite these problems, implementation of backup alternatives do permit ongoing delivery of care, even if it is at a slower pace.

Calculation of backup costs goes beyond initial setup costs and ongoing expenditures (Fried 1995). One-time recovery costs can be high since they include costs of hiring IS personnel and training staff to use backup alternatives; additional user costs for dual entry; costs for cleanup, repair, or replacement of computer equipment; and payment for backup computing or recovery services. Another cost is the impact on the quality of services rendered during the downtime.

The expense for manual versus automated alternatives varies according to the length of time that the system is down, backup alternatives employed, and the resources they require. Since implementing a backup alternative is costly, administrators must decide if the anticipated downtime merits initiating the alternative. Extremely short down periods are usually not worth the additional time and trouble. Costs include additional labor for IS and other personnel, increased potential for error, and space requirements. Data entry into the system following a manual backup requires additional personnel and a place for them to work. For example, lab tests that were requested but not completed prior to downtime must be requested by nursing again manually. During downtime, lab staff must try to match manual requisitions against those that were entered but not processed prior to downtime. When the system goes live, lab tests that were ordered and completed during downtime, along with results, must be entered so that the client record is not fragmented.

Staff Preparedness The success of a disaster plan is contingent upon the cooperation and support of everyone in the institution, from top management down. One way to ensure this success is through training. Detailed instruction on every aspect of the system, the disaster plan, and implementation of manual alternatives may be incorporated into initial computer training. However, this approach requires a longer training period, and recall of manual procedures is often poor when long periods of time elapse between instruction and implementation. A more effective strategy entails posting plans in conspicuous places, yearly review of IS disaster and recovery plans, mock disasters, and the provision of step-by-step reference guides to help staff implement manual alternatives. Other measures to increase disaster awareness and ensure successful recovery efforts are listed in Box 15–3.

Box 15–3   **Ways to Increase Disaster Awareness and Successful Recovery**

- Display disaster and recovery plans in conspicuous places, and post revised versions as soon as they are available.
- List key contact people responsible for implementing the disaster and recovery plans.
- Provide clear step-by-step reference aids for staff to guide them through manual alternatives.
- Emphasize the importance of disaster preparedness by incorporating mock disaster situations into training.
- Review the disaster and recovery plans yearly along with other mandated programs, such as safe lifting, fire safety, and the materials safety data sheets.
- Schedule mock disasters.
- Test backups periodically.
- Label backup materials and include explicit directions with them.
- Provide up-to-date cold and hot site information to persons responsible for recovery.
- Include 24-hour phone numbers, contracts, and payment authorization numbers.
- Emphasize the need for emergency care arrangements for dependents and pets to personnel involved in disaster and recovery plan implementation.

SOURCE: Adapted from Powell, J. D. (1996). "Murphy's day at the surprise disaster recovery drill." *Disaster Recovery Journal, 9*(3), 35–36, 38, 40, 42.

RECOVERY

The primary focus of disaster recovery is the resumption of operations. It sounds simple, but it is not (Young 1996). Few institutions have actually reconstructed information systems from backups. Organizations may not even verify that backup occurred properly; in this case, problems are not detected until restoration is attempted. Also, large institutions have information located in several areas: the mainframe, networks, PCs, and paper documents. And last, most institutions use a combination of backup formats and programs.

Restoration of system operation may result from one of several techniques. First, materials stored at a cold site can be shipped back to the institution and reloaded onto the system. Second, information may be restored from RBSs. A third option is the use of hot sites. **Hot sites** replicate an organization's information systems, allowing restoration of operations using backup media (Corrigan 1995, Cross 1996, Leary 1998, Strauss 1996). This is accomplished at another location served by a different power grid and central telephone office to avoid the effects of the disaster that affected the health care enterprise. The organization may develop its own hot site or outsource for services. When possible, hot sites should be close enough for practical employee travel, with sufficient space, power, cabling, parking, and satellite dish accommodations to support IS function.

A dedicated hot site usually sits idle when not needed, but is available in the event of an emergency and is compatible with agency systems for ease of system restoration and updates. The creation of redundant computer capabilities and the acquisition of a dedicated hot site is costly, but expenses may be recouped through lease arrangements or sharing the center with other health care alliance partners. A tenant would have to agree to relinquish the site in the event of a disaster. Sharing a site presumes that it is unlikely that two or more partners at separate locations would suffer from a disaster at the same time. A third option is the creation of a backup facility on-site in another building owned by the organization. This option reduces real estate costs but still requires system redundancy.

Commercial hot site services charge monthly reservation fees in addition to restoration charges but are less costly than establishing an independent site (DePompa 1996, Strauss 1996). There is a risk of being bumped by another client who requires services at the same time. Commercial vendors should be able to offer the assurance of a proven track record for mainframe recovery. Unfortunately, the uniqueness of most client–server environments made commercial recovery services unprofitable and unavailable until recently, forcing institutions to develop their own internal recovery options.

An alternative to system restoration is distributed processing (Casey and Kohler 1996, Zeidman 1996). **Distributed processing** uses a group of independent processors that contain the same information but may be at different sites. In the event that one processor is knocked out, information is not lost because remaining processors can continue IS operation with little, or no, interruption. Distributed processing is more expensive up front but eliminates downtime. Rapid replacement of equipment is yet another recovery strategy but it is not always feasible because it is costly to maintain extra hardware.

Salvaging Damaged Records

Once alternative arrangements have been made to access information needed to provide services, restoration of the facility and secondary records becomes a focus. Whether the computing center was without climate control or was physically damaged by an event that exposed it to heat, humidity, and/or smoke damage, there are guidelines to follow to salvage materials. Box 15–4 lists some of these. The first rule is to stabilize the site. Prompt, appropriate action can salvage data and some equipment.

Disaster recovery experts can best ensure data recovery from damaged media, particularly from magnetic media (McDaniel 1996, Moore 1996). Fires, heat, and floods leave behind residues that damage electronic equipment and storage media. Additional damage may occur when media are improperly stored and handled postdisaster and with the passage of time. Degradation of media also impedes recovery efforts. Data integrity is compromised when storage media are damaged. Recovery specialists must verify data bit by bit and reconstruct files before data can be recorded onto new media. Box 15–5 lists some recovery measures.

Box 15–4 General Salvage Rules

- Pump any standing water out of the facility.
- Decrease the temperature to minimize mold and mildew growth and damage.
- Vent the area.
- Do not restore power to wet equipment.
- Open cabinet doors, remove side panels and covers, and pull out chassis to permit water to exit equipment.
- Absorb excess water in equipment with cotton, using care not to damage pins and cables.
- Call in professional decontamination specialists when hazardous chemicals or wastes are present.

SOURCE: Adapted from "First Steps to Take after a Fire," by L. D. D. McDaniel, March 1996, *Communication News, 33*(3), 26, reprinted from CN—Communications News, March 1996; and from "Records Recovery Necessities," by P. Moore, March/April 1996, *Contingency Planning & Management*, 25–29.

Box 15–5	Recommended Storage Media Recovery Techniques

Suggested recovery methods for paper-based materials:

- Initiate recovery within 48 hours of the disaster for best results.
- Separate coated papers such as EKG tracing and ultrasound records to prevent them from permanently fusing together.
- Remove noncoated documents from file cabinets or shelves in blocks—do not pull each page apart, as this increases mold growth.
- Store paper documents in a diesel-powered freezer trailer until proper drying arrangements can be finalized.
- Remove excess mud and dirt before freezing documents.
- Pack wet files or books in a box with a plastic trash liner and allow room for circulation of air.
- Place files with open edges facing up and books with spines down.
- Label all boxes precisely and create a master inventory.
- Freeze-dry priority documents and sterilize and use fungicide as needed.

Suggested magnetic media recovery techniques:

- Initiate recovery within 72–96 hours for best results.
- Consult recovery specialists.
- Open and dry water-damaged floppy disks with isopropyl alcohol, place in empty jackets, and copy files to new disks.
- Clean soot-damaged floppy disks manually. Use recovery software to recover and copy information to new disks.
- Freeze-dry tape cartridges, then use recovery software to recover and copy information to new tape cartridges.
- Dry reel-to-reel tapes on a tape-cleaning machine, using warm air to evaporate moisture. Use recovery software to recover and copy information to new tapes.

SOURCE: Adapted from "Records Recovery Necessities," by P. Moore, March/April 1996, *Contingency Planning & Management*, 25–29.

Recovery Costs

The cost for recovery is frequently overlooked. It should not be. It can be an extremely expensive process, involving the following factors:

- Lost profits
- Temporary computer services, including space rental, equipment, furniture, extra phone lines, and temporary personnel
- Shipping and installation costs
- Postdisaster replacement of equipment
- Postdisaster repairs and bringing the building up to new codes

- Recovery and possible decontamination
- Overtime hours for staff during the disaster for the implementation of manual alternatives, and after the disaster for entering data into the system that was generated during system downtime

Insurance coverage is recommended as a means to help pay for IS disasters (Cox 1996). Table 15–2 lists types of available coverage. One person should be designated to interact with the insurance company and a mechanism should be identified for how disaster-related costs will be documented.

Restarting the System

System restarts after downtime must be planned carefully. All critical data for client management and agency administration should be targeted for restoration first. For example, client admission systems are needed before client-related entries can be made. Therefore, it is logical to make the admissions and discharge functions one of the first areas restored. Users can help identify critical functions. Usage tends to be heavy once the system is live again as users try to catch up on their work. Communication is critical at this point. IS personnel must provide users with a sense of confidence, prevent system overload, and bring the system back on line slowly to prevent further problems. Economic factors should also be considered. For instance, if charges are calculated with the docu-

Table 15–2	Recommended Insurance Coverage

Coverage	Purpose
Business interruption	Provides replacement of lost profits as a result of a covered loss. Must be certain that insurance covers the same period as the event.
Extra expense	Provides financial recovery for out-of-the-ordinary expenses such as a temporary office or center of operations, and additional costs for rent, staff, and rental of equipment and furniture while regular facilities cannot be used.
Code compliance	Often overlooked. Insurance will normally reimburse only for expenses associated with repair or replacement of a damaged building, but not additional costs associated with building code changes implemented since the building was built. This coverage provides for those additional costs.
Electronic data processing	Replaces damaged or lost equipment and media from a covered incident such as storm damage not covered in normal property insurance. May also include coverage for business interruption and extra expenses.

SOURCE: Adapted from Cox, L. P. (1996). "Disaster Recovery: How Do You Pay for It?" *Disaster Recovery Journal, 9*(2), 19–20.

mentation of a medication, or intravenous fluid, this process must be restored as soon as possible. Nonessential functions and reports should be deferred until the system is fully operational to prevent additional downtime.

Decisions Regarding the Extent of Data Re-entry Health care administrators must determine how they will handle late entries and documentation that occurs during system downtimes. One factor that frequently goes unconsidered is the cost for entering information gathered manually into the system once normal operations have resumed. This is a labor-intensive process. The importance of data for inclusion in the

Checklist Item	Yes	No
Are backup(s) available? tested?	❑	❑
Are disaster/recovery plan copies available/accessible?	❑	❑
Are hot-site contract copies available/accessible?	❑	❑
Do key personnel have emergency care arrangements for dependents? pets?	❑	❑
Is home-site staffing coverage adequate?	❑	❑
Are the cold-site storage sites and procedures for retrieval of backups known/arranged?	❑	❑
Are the hot-site locations and access procedures known?	❑	❑
Is travel to the cold and hot sites feasible?	❑	❑
Has authorization for recovery-related expenses been confirmed?	❑	❑
Is shipping information accurate for backup tapes from cold to hot sites and back again?	❑	❑
Is documentation accurate for tape restoration available with starting and ending tape numbers?	❑	❑
Are backup tapes labeled accurately?	❑	❑
Have network/communications persons been sent to the hot site?	❑	❑
Do restoration procedures agree with current software?	❑	❑
Have previous arrangements been made to have persons stay after hours at the remote site?	❑	❑
Are communications links for backup confirmed, appropriate, and available?	❑	❑
Are phone numbers available for all vendor hot sites?	❑	❑
Are stored supplies intact/usable?	❑	❑
Is a timeline for anticipated restoration of operations identified and appropriate?	❑	❑
Are packing materials and labels available to ship media from cold to hot sites and back again?	❑	❑
Is an extra container for reports among supplies?	❑	❑
Are human needs for food and rest adequately included in the plan?	❑	❑

FIGURE 15–2 • **Checklist for Successful Implementation of an IS Disaster and Recovery Plan**

automated record and the possible legal ramifications for data stored only on paper must be weighed. For example, is it necessary to include all vital signs and intake and output in the automated record, particularly if these have been within normal limits? A mechanism must be developed that indicates the availability of additional record information in paper form. Additional considerations include whether the entry of information collected manually and entered into the automated record later might be more prone to error and how the original paper record should be dealt with.

USING POSTDISASTER FEEDBACK TO IMPROVE PLANNING

Postdisaster feedback is invaluable to revising disaster plans for future use (Fried 1995). Personnel input after mock disasters or prolonged downtime should be used to identify what worked and what did not. Systems and organizations change. Plans that looked good before a disaster may not look good after one. Recovery expenses usually exceed anticipated costs, leading to a change in recovery strategies for future use. Figure 15–2 depicts a checklist to evaluate the success of a disaster and recovery plan.

CASE STUDY EXERCISES

As the clinical representative for your unit on the Disaster Planning Committee, you are charged with identifying all forms in your area that require completion of a physical vital records inventory sheet. What forms would you list and why?

• • •

Work crews at Wilmington Hospital inadvertently cut the cable connecting all terminals at the hospital with the computer center. As the on-duty nursing supervisor, what should you tell your employees, and why? Who would you contact for further information? How do you determine whether to initiate manual alternatives?

• • •

An early morning train wreck near St. Luke's Hospital derailed seven freight cars carrying chemicals that can emit toxic fumes. The accident took out power lines for the neighborhood and for St. Luke's. Emergency crews evacuated a seven-block area, stopping just outside of the hospital's main entrance. Power has already been out for 12 hours and restoration is not expected for at least another 12–24 hours. You are on an executive administrative committee charged with determining what information will be brought on line first and what will remain in paper form. What would you restore first? What records, if any, would you not restore? Explain your rationale. How would you document, for record management purposes, that part of the record is automated and part is manual?

· · ·

As IS Project Manager you are responsible for helping the Renal Department select a new database. One of the top vendors must cancel its Web-based demonstration because its server was stolen. What types of questions should this situation raise for disaster planning with the use of vendor-supported applications?

SUMMARY

- Disasters that threaten IS operation may be natural or man-made. Disaster plans help to ensure uninterrupted operation or speedy resumption of services when a catastrophic event occurs.

- Disaster plans must consider potential risks, information vital to the delivery of services, and all factors necessary for restoration of services.

- The identification of information vital to daily operation is best determined through interviewing system users. The purpose, flow, recipients, need for timeliness, and implications of information unavailability must be considered in this process.

- Not all information used in daily operations is automated. A vital records inventory should be conducted to identify additional information that requires protection.

- Documentation is essential to the development and successful implementation of a disaster plan. Plans must be detailed, current, and readily available to be useful.

- Careful attention to backup and storage helps ensure that information may be retrieved, or restored, later. Backup may be handled internally or outsourced. Commercial backup services provide transport or electronic transmission of backup media and special storage conditions until materials are needed.

- Manual alternatives to information systems ensure ongoing delivery of services, although it is at a slower rate. Staff must receive instruction and support as they resort to manual methods.

- Restoration of information services postdisaster is not simple because backup media may be faulty and some information kept on other media is lost forever.

- System restoration may reload backup media stored at cold sites or resort to RBS or hot sites. Distributed processing and rapid replacement of equipment are other alternatives.

- Restoration is costly because it generally requires outside professional services, additional equipment, and extra hours from support staff. Expenses may be partially recouped through insurance coverage.

- Salvage of damaged records is an important aspect of recovery that is best handled by experts.

- System restarts require planning to avoid system overload as users try to catch up on work. Administrators must consider what functions should be restored first and how to integrate backup paper records with automated records.

- Postdisaster feedback is key to the design and implementation of a better plan for future use.

- Disaster planning needs to consider legal and regulatory requirements.

REFERENCES

Amelyn, R. (1996). Record storage: Is it vital to your firm's success? *Disaster Recovery Journal, 9*(1), 57–58.

Carlisle, V. G. (March/April 1996). Make protection a priority, recovery unnecessary. *Contingency Planning & Management,* 28.

Casey, T., and Kohler, S. (1996). Using geographic clustering to build disaster tolerant computing environments. *Disaster Recovery Journal, 9*(3), 23–24, 26.

Cerullo, M. J., and Cerullo, V. (1998). Key factors to strengthen the disaster contingency and recovery planning process security. *Information Strategy: The Executive's Journal, 14*(7), 37, 7p.

Corrigan, P. (1995). Defying disaster. *LAN Magazine, 10*(8), 89.

Cox, L. P. (1996). Disaster recovery: How do you pay for it? *Disaster Recovery Journal, 9*(2), 19–20.

Cross, M. (1996). Disaster planning protects technology investments. *Health Data Management, 4*(9), 66–68, 70.

Defusing the backup bomb. (1995). *Infoworld, 17*(50), 86–87.

Fisher, P. A. P. (1996). How to conduct a business impact analysis. *Disaster Recovery Journal, 9*(3), 64–65, 67–68.

Fried, L. (1995). *Managing information technology in turbulent times.* New York: Wiley.

Hoffman, L. (1995). How safe is your system? *Beyond Computing, 4*(5), 42–44.

Hussong, B. (1996). Corporate executive: Have you cared enough? *Disaster Recovery Journal, 9*(3), 44, 46–48.

Ivancevich, D. M., Hermanson, D. R. and Smith, L. M. (1998). The Association of Perceived Disaster Recovery Plan Strength with Organizational Characteristics. *Journal of Information Systems, 12*(1), 31, 10p.

Jackson, R. (1996). Quantifying a business impact analysis. *Disaster Recovery Journal, 9*(1), 21, 23, 25.

Kutner, M. (1996). Crisis management: Keeping a company strong in times of trouble. *Disaster Recovery Journal, 9*(1), 77–79.

Leary, M. F. (1998). A rescue plan for your LAN. *Security Management, 42*(3), 53(6).

Lee, J., and Hudspeth, L. (1995). Crash-proof your PC. *Home Office Computing, 13*(9), 71+.

Mannion, J., and Persson, J. (1996). Disaster recovery survey from the 1995 Atlanta symposium. *Disaster Recovery Journal, 9*(1), 60–67.

McDaniel, L. D. D. (1996). First steps to take after a fire. *Communication News, 33*(3), 26.

Moore, P. (March/April 1996). Records recovery necessities. *Contingency Planning & Management,* 25–29.

Morrissey, J. (1999). Finding weak links in disaster plans. *Modern Healthcare, 29*(19) 60, 2p.

Nicolet, J. L. (1996). The contingency planning cycle. *Disaster Recovery Journal, 9*(2), 55–57.

Piellucci, R. (1996). The K.I.S.S. method to business resumption planning. *Disaster Recovery Journal, 9*(1), 51–56.

Powell, J. D. (1996). Murphy's day at the surprise disaster recovery drill. *Disaster Recovery Journal, 9*(3), 35–36, 38, 40, 42.

Reshaur, L. M., and Luongo, R. P. (2000). Lessons in business continuity planning: One hospital's response to a disaster. *Disaster Recovery Journal, 13*(2), 12–13.

Sands, G. A. (1996). Lessons learned. *Disaster Recovery Journal, 9*(3), 27.

Simonelli, M. (2000). Lasting effects: The human dimension of disaster recovery. *Contingency Planning & Management, 5*(3), 36–38.

Strauss, R. E. (1996). Real estate aspects of recovery centers. *Disaster Recovery Journal, 9*(3), 30–33.

Young, M. (1996). Backing up is hard to do. *Imaging Magazine, 5*(2), 71–89.

Zeidman, B. (1996). An introduction to remote backup. *Disaster Recovery Journal, 9*(2), 48, 50, 52, 54.

Three

Specialty Applications

16

Using the Computer to Support Health Care Education

After completing this chapter, you will be able to:

- Identify specific ways that computer technology may be used to support education.

- List benefits associated with *computer-assisted instruction (CAI)*, *distance education*, and *Web-based education*.

- Compare and contrast *e-learning* with other educational uses of computers.

- Provide examples of how computer technology may support education in each of the following settings: formal nursing programs, continuing education, and client or consumer education.

- Describe factors that contribute to the successful use of an instructional computer lab.

- Review options for the individual interested in learning more about nursing informatics.

Computer technology can be used to support education in a variety of settings, including formal nursing education, continuing education, and consumer education. This is particularly important as computers become more pervasive in our society and money for health care education shrinks. Educational applications of computers in health care are limited only by imagination. Formal opportunities include continuing and distance education, on-line journals, and programs designed for client education. Informally, individuals may network one-on-one with experts in various clinical specialties via e-mail or participate in special interest group discussions.

There is growing agreement that nursing education models must change to meet the demands of the workplace. Most basic nursing education programs prepare graduates to care for small client loads in acute care settings. This approach ignores the move toward care in the community, the need for graduates to develop and use critical thinking skills, different individual learning styles, and the fact that the explosive growth of information and knowledge renders much of the content presented in nursing school obsolete soon after it is presented. Educational uses of the computer may help to alleviate these problems, since computers offer flexibility as well as opportunities for collaborative and self-paced learning (Mastrian and McGonigle 1999). These features are also valuable in the use of computers for continuing and consumer education. Computers also provide a simulated, but safe, learning environment for the acquisition of skills. Box 16–1 lists some ways that computers may be used to facilitate education.

Some specific educational applications or uses of computers include the following:

- **Web-based instruction (WBI)** uses the attributes and resources of the World Wide Web, such as hypertext links and multimedia, for ed-

Box 16–1 **Applications of Computers in Health Care Education**

Formal opportunities

- Continuing education
- Distance education
- On-line journals
- Client education

Information opportunities

- E-mail
- Listservs
- Support groups
- On-line literature searches and retrieval

Administrative support

- Preparation of presentations, handouts, slides
- Record keeping

SOURCE: Adapted from "Computerized NCLEX-RN preparation programs: A comparative review," by D. Billings et al., 1996, *Computers in Nursing, 14*(5), 262–263, 266; and "Nursing information systems: Applications in nursing curricula," by G. P. Poirrer et al., 1996, *Nurse Educator, 21*(1), 18–22.

ucational purposes. WBI may be offered as a stand-alone course or as a complement to traditional classes. Independent WBI provides access to most or all class materials, resources and interaction via Internet technology. This is in contrast to Web-supported courses that rely on physical meetings of students and teachers but integrate assignments, readings, computer-mediated communications, and/or links to sites into the course activities. Some synonyms for WBI include Web-based training (WBT), Web-assisted instruction (WAI), Internet-based training (IBT), Web-based learning (WBL), Web interactive training (WIT), and on-line courses.

- Computer-assisted instruction (CAI) is the use of the computer to organize and present instructional materials for use by an individual learner. CAI aids learning by actively involving the learner as a participant. In addition, CAI offers 24-hour availability, the ability to proceed at a comfortable pace, and consistency in instructional approach.

- **E-learning** is the delivery of content via electronic media inclusive of the Internet, intranets, extranets, satellite broadcast, audio/video tape, interactive TV, and/or CD-ROM. The basic premise behind e-learning is that it encourages more effective learning. The term is often used to refer to corporate training. It offers flexibility, self-paced instruction, and the ability to focus on needed content or skills. E-learning may or may not incorporate the opportunity to interact with faculty or other students.

- E-mail and Internet access provide formal and informal learning and networking opportunities.

- Administrative support for various aspects of the education process is important. Examples include the development of presentations and audio–visual aids, as well as the maintenance of program attendance records, administration and scoring of examinations, and program evaluations.

The mere presence and use of computers for education does not ensure successful learning, however. Consideration of the following factors and guidelines will enhance the effectiveness of using computers for education:

- *Users are comfortable with the technology*. Not all learners are familiar with computers or know how to use them. Therefore, a basic introduction is required. Once the learner is comfortable with the computer as a tool, other learning needs may be met (Black and Goldstein 1998).

- *Opportunities are provided to ask about material not understood*. Although the computer is an invaluable instructional aid, the ability to question and discuss information presented should also be available.

- *Instruction is well designed and well matched to course objectives*. High-quality Web-based instruction and computer programs for education must maintain learner interest and provide the appropriate information.

- *Evaluation criteria are identified to monitor the effectiveness of the computer as a tool*. These may include increased use of e-mail, increased job satisfaction, and improved student achievement. On-line course evaluations may also be used.

Another issue related to the instructional use of computers is computer resistance on the part of the learner (Henderson and Deane 1995). This may be due to any of the following factors:

- Computer anxiety
- Lack of computer skills
- Previous exposure to poorly designed computer applications
- Fear of job loss secondary to automation
- Administrative failure to consult nurses in the change process, including the selection and implementation of automated information systems or computer labs

POTENTIAL AUDIENCES FOR EDUCATIONAL COMPUTER USES

Educational applications of computers adapt well to a diversity of settings and learners. The majority of current use is seen in formal health care education programs, although computers are also prevalent in continuing education and consumer education.

Formal Nursing Education

Nursing education programs are a logical place to introduce or expand basic computer skills such as word processing, Internet access, and e-mail. These computer literacy skills are increasingly important in the everyday workplace. Providing computer education increases access to information, facilitates the teaching/learning process, decreases anxiety associated with computer use, enhances job skills, and improves record keeping for program attendance, performance, and evaluation. Consequently, most basic nursing programs require an introductory computer course. In addition, instructional use of computers may include programs related to specific topics or the presentation of classes via Web-based instruction, teleconferencing technology, and licensure examination review programs (Canavan 1996). Exposure to National Council Licensure Examination (NCLEX) review programs is particularly important now that all nurses in the United States take their licensure examination via computer. Computers are also used in the clinical setting to document client care on hospital information systems. As a result of this expanding use of computers, most nursing programs have institutional academic computer plans, policies, and facilities.

Applications Related to Specific Topics The benefits associated with computer-supported learning have led to an increased availability of courses and educational software related to nursing and health care topics. It is important to evaluate the quality of these applications and to use them in an effective manner. The nurse educator is responsible for evaluating the merits of available tools prior to their implementation. Nurse educators need not be software experts to do this. Faculty should use the same criteria to evaluate computer uses in education that they apply to any other instructional medium. Box 16–2 lists criteria that may be used to evaluate the quality of instructional software.

Another important consideration is to plan and effectively integrate the use of computer instruction as a component of the overall educational program. Adherence to several factors and guidelines may facilitate successful use of computer technology. For example, hardware and software must be accessible at times and places convenient for learner use. In addition, clients with limited computer experience should receive short, highly interactive training sessions that cover a small amount of information.

Box 16–2 **Evaluation Criteria for Instructional Software**

- Does it support the overall course objectives?
- Is the material presented clearly?
- Is content accurate?
- What is the quality of the design? Does it maintain learner interest and provide the ability to customize learning to individual needs?
- Is information presented in a logical order?
- Does it provide appropriate and immediate feedback?
- Does it make good use of graphics, color, varying letter size, animation, and auditory stimuli at a level appropriate to the audience?

SOURCE: Adapted from "Multimedia training in nursing education," by A. J. Gleydura, C. N. Wilson, and J. E. Michelman, 1995, *Computers in Nursing, 13*(4), 169–175; and "Factors that contribute to computer-assisted instruction effectiveness," by F. Khoiny, 1995, *Computers in Nursing, 13*(4), 165–168.

Licensure Preparation Software Preparation programs for the National Council Licensure Examination for Registered Nurses (NCLEX-RN) are popular now that the licensure exam itself is computerized (Billings et al. 1996). NCLEX-RN preparation programs vary in quality, ranging from simple drill and practice to those that provide rationale for answers. Educators and nursing students need to be discriminating consumers. One question to consider is the approach and intended purpose of the program. For example, some provide a means to decrease anxiety over the NCLEX-RN examination through practice under similar conditions. They may also attempt to simulate the examination experience. Other programs claim to predict student success on the NCLEX-RN examination. Box 16–3 lists some criteria to consider when selecting NCLEX-RN preparation software.

Hospital Information Systems Connectivity with real hospital information systems (HIS) is another important use of computers in nursing education. The incorporation of hospital and nursing information systems into nursing school curricula promotes professional socialization, helps students see the effects of their decision making with care plans or maps, and decreases orientation time for new graduates. Computer-generated care plans or maps allow students to devote to analysis of data the time once spent writing care plans, and allow staff more time to mentor students. This use of information systems ensures that graduates have exposure to computers and possess marketable job skills, and helps students to see the whole clinical picture. Students may be trained in system use by faculty or by hospital-based trainers. Students may retrieve information for use in preparing for client assignments, but should not be able

Box 16–3 | **Features to Look for in NCLEX-RN Preparation Programs**

- Ease of use
- Good feedback for answers. For example, does it provide rationale and scores?
- Effective screen design and keyboard use. If the goal of the program is to simulate the exam, then screen design and keyboard use must be the same as the NCLEX-RN.
- Questions that are high-quality, clear, and in adequate numbers
- Questions presented in a randomized fashion, as in the actual exam
- A match between the preparation program content and NCLEX-RN examination content
- A bookmark feature that allows students to mark the spot where they quit, exit the program, and return to that spot later
- Clear instructions
- Adequate technical support
- A warranty
- An upgrade policy
- Acceptable system requirements (type of computer, memory requirements, etc.)

SOURCE: Adapted from "Computerized NCLEX-RN preparation programs: A comparative review," by D. Billings et al., 1996, *Computers in Nursing, 14*(5), 262–263, 266.

to make changes or add information to the actual client record from remote sites.

Access to hospital information systems as a learning tool in schools of nursing offers the following benefits (Doorley, Renner, and Corron 1994, Poirrier et al. 1996):

- Provides time to analyze clinical information
- Provides the student with adequate time to compose care plans or review critical pathways
- Allows students to review their plans with faculty or hospital nursing staff prior to entry into the system

HIS connectivity can be provided at schools of nursing via modem. This requires negotiation with the vendor for permission and the installation of extra phone lines. Other considerations include increased demands upon the HIS and concerns related to confidentiality of patient information. HIS connectivity allows students to be more familiar with their assigned clients and poses fewer interruptions for staff from students requesting information. Incorporation of hospital and nursing information systems at schools of nursing also facilitates role transition from student to graduate nurse, makes graduates more attractive to prospective employers, and allows hospitals to cut orientation time for graduates with prior HIS training.

Continuing Education

Nationwide budget cuts caused many institutions and employers to reduce or eliminate continuing education program offerings provided by traditional classes, conferences, and workshops. There is now an increased reliance on outside agencies to meet this need. One approach to this problem is home study offered through professional journals. Readers review articles, answer related questions, send in their test form and fee, and wait to find out whether they received credit. The journal approach offers little, if any, interaction with peers. Another approach is the use of the Internet for continuing education courses. This approach offers several benefits. It is available without a subscription 24 hours a day to a large population. Furthermore, it can provide instant feedback and highly individualized instruction, since the incorporation of links allows users to skip familiar content or seek additional information as required. Internet continuing education programs may be found through professional publications and organizations, as well as Web searches. Unfortunately, this option is limited to people with access to a computer (Marks 1996).

Computers can also be used for administrative support of continuing education (Doorley et al. 1994, Poirrier et al. 1996, Simpson 1995, Wilson 1991). For example, computerized records can be searched rapidly to determine if and when a particular student attended a program such as fire safety or cardiopulmonary resuscitation (CPR). It is also possible to administer and score proficiency examinations and evaluation tools. Improved records also help to determine program costs and demonstrate staff development, or continuing education staff, productivity.

E-learning has been suggested as an alternative delivery method for mandatory educational programs as well as other programs that provide employees with opportunities to improve or maintain skill sets. The rationale for this approach is that e-learning allows employees to learn at their own pace and skip material that they already know. There are no costs associated with travel, lodging, or meals. Training is available upon demand and course materials and tests are on-line (Barrett 2000).

Client Education

Although many computer applications directly benefit nurses and other health care professionals, the instructional use of computers for consumers is more prevalent (Miholland 1996). Direct uses include software designed to educate consumers and the availability of information via the Internet, Web sites, and e-mail. Some sites allow consumers to pose questions and then provide an answer within 24 hours. Home pages on the World Wide Web provide information on a variety of topics, including preparation for diagnostic tests. They may even show film clips. Client education materials and discharge instructions by hospital information systems can also be generated by computer. An example of this application may be seen with a client who had heart bypass surgery. Instructions should include the following: when to schedule a follow-up visit with the cardiac surgeon and the primary physician; wound care; signs or symptoms that should be reported to the physician; and discharge medications. Computer generation of discharge instructions can tailor instructions to the individual client and the physician authorizing the discharge, and offers the following advantages (Tronni and Welebob 1996):

- Consistent instruction despite the fact that different nurses provide teaching
- Improved quality and detail
- Speed
- Clarity and legibility
- Eliminates repetition. Nurses no longer need to write the same instructions over and over again.

INSTRUCTIONAL APPLICATIONS OF COMPUTER TECHNOLOGY

Computers may be used in a variety of ways to provide or support instruction. One common application is the ability to perform on-line literature searches through sites such as Sigma Theta Tau's Virginia Henderson library and the National Library of Medicine. Abstracts and occasionally full text articles may be retrieved on-line. Other examples include computer-assisted instruction (CAI), teleconferencing, multimedia presentations, distance learning and Web-based instruction, and computer learning labs.

Computer-Assisted Instruction (CAI)

In computer-assisted instruction, the computer teaches a subject (other than computing) to the student through interactive software. Advocates of CAI allege that it enhances computer literacy, facilitates decision making, reduces computer anxiety, and positively affects student achievement (Gleydura et al. 1995). Although originally designed to promote individualized learning, CAI can enhance group learning as well (Calderone 1994).

CAI offers the following advantages (Glover and Kruse 1995):

- *It may improve reading habits.* Learners can proceed at a pace conducive to comprehension.
- *It is convenient.* CAI can be offered at any site that has computer access. Programs may be available for single users on freestanding PCs or via network connections.
- *It can reduce learning time.* Because learners can proceed at their own pace, they can skim through familiar content and focus on weak areas.

- *Increased retention.* The active nature of the media requires learner participation, which improves retention.
- *Twenty-four-hour access.* CAI is available at any time of the day or night so that learners can use it at times convenient to them.
- *Consistent instruction in a safe environment.* CAI allows learners to practice new skills without fear of harm to themselves or others.

Three major variables influence CAI effectiveness: quality of the software, the environment of computer use, and characteristics of the learner. Some factors that lead to negative attitudes toward CAI include (Gleydura et al. 1995, Khoiny 1995)

- *Poor design.* Many CAI applications do nothing more than automate page turning.
- *Lack of feedback on incorrect answers.* This is frustrating to learners who want to know why their selections were wrong.
- *Lack of control.* Control encompasses the ability to advance, repeat, or review portions of the program, or to quit at any point.
- *Lack of intellectual stimulation.* Programs that fail to maintain interest may cause learners to feel that they wasted their time.

Drug calculation programs are a common CAI application in most nursing schools. These programs are popular because drug calculation is a basic skill needed by all nurses, and, as such, drug calculation programs fit well into the curriculum, while programs on other content areas may not match curriculum objectives. An example is the case of a CAI program that addresses the care of the critically ill client. Concepts from such an offering may be too complex for junior level students in some schools but not others.

Multimedia

Nursing education has always incorporated a multimedia approach with its inclusion of chalkboard diagrams, overheads, slide-tape presentations, video, skill demonstrations, computer-based instruction, interactive video disk (IVD), and CD-ROM (Billings 1995, Calderone 1994, Gleydura et al. 1995). Now it is possible to add video clips from Web sites to the list of examples. Quite simply, **multimedia** refers to presentations that combine text, voice or sound, images, and video, or hardware and software that can support the same. Tools change with technological advances. Multimedia is an excellent approach for nurses because they must learn and communicate complex issues to clients. Research has shown that learning retention is facilitated with an approach that incorporates seeing, hearing, and doing. Group-paced instruction with multimedia decreases costs associated with individual instruction, increases comfort with computers, and improves learning as long as the environment is conducive to group use.

Changing technology now makes tailored compact disc (CD) presentations feasible. Quality multimedia should reduce labor costs for instructor and participant time, improve overall instructional effectiveness, and foster productivity through user satisfaction and enjoyment (Calderone 1994, Gleydura et al. 1995, Goodman and Blake 1996). Recent CD advancements, chiefly increased storage capacity and low costs, and multimedia capability make CD drives standard equipment on PCs. CDs can enhance CAI by using the interactivity, information management, decision making, and multimedia capability of computers (Billings 1994, Cambre and Castner 1993, Goodman and Blake 1996).

Authoring tools allow program design to match learning objectives and foster higher cognitive development. **Authoring tools** are software applications designed to allow persons with little or no programming expertise to create instructional programs. These tools require time for mastery: As many as 50 to 200 hours are needed to prepare 1 hour of instruction and work out the program bugs. Box 16–4 contains some suggestions to enhance the successful use and benefits of multimedia instruction. Faculty who are comfortable with the various forms of multimedia usually do a better job of integrating it into their instruction for optimal student benefit.

Teleconferencing

Teleconferencing is the use of computers, audio and video equipment, and high-grade dedicated telephone lines to provide interactive communication between two or more persons at two or more sites. Recent developments make teleconferencing capability possible from desktop computers. Teleconferencing is particularly useful for graduate and doctoral students and staff nurses because it brings educational opportunities to areas that may not otherwise offer courses or programs. In teleconferencing, learners at one site view and interact with an instructor and other learners at separate locations. Participants can pool resources to establish collaborative programs, thus maximizing resources through shared classes and conferences. Teleconferencing requires start-up funds and an

---

Box 16–4 **Strategies to Maximize the Benefits of Multimedia Instruction**

- Master basic course content before going on to other content.
- Use pretests, content review, case studies, clinical situations or simulations, and post-tests to enhance comprehension of material.
- Use computerized testing that randomly assigns test items so that no two tests are exactly the same.

investment in equipment and transmission media. Classes may be offered entirely on-line along with assignments and feedback. Content may be clinically oriented or focus on nursing informatics. This approach extends the reach of educational programs and continuing education courses by accommodating students who would otherwise be unable to attend programs because of their distance from offered programs (Canavan 1996).

Distance Learning

Improved Internet capabilities, telephone usage, and teleconferencing have virtually eliminated the barriers faced by nurses in remote locations who wish to further their education via formal study or through continuing education programs, or who require additional job training (Billings 1996a, Corwin 2000, Sirota 1995). **Distance learning** is the use of print, audio, video, computer, or teleconferencing capability to connect faculty and students who are located at a minimum of two different locations. Print media is an inexpensive, low-technology approach that may be developed quickly. Audio conferences take place over the telephone. At present, video and teleconferencing are very popular. Video signals may be one-way or two-way transmissions over telephone lines. Distance learning may occur in real, or synchronous, time or via a delay. In real time all parties participate in the activity at the same time. With the delayed, or asynchronous, approach, the learner reviews material at a convenient time. Asynchronous learning can be enhanced with the incorporation of ongoing electronic discussion (Cartwright 2000). Synchrony influences instructional design, delivery, and interaction. Distance learning may require additional course preparation and organization by faculty and a concerted effort on the part of students to remain active participants. It can, however, be an effective means of instruction. Box 16–5 lists key points for the participant in distance learning. Distance learning broadens educational opportunities and eliminates long commutes. For this reason it may serve as a recruitment and retention mechanism for schools of nursing and health care agencies. It may provide access to experts and cut costs by paying faculty to teach at one site rather than multiple sites. Despite these advantages, distance learning may be impeded by budget constraints as well as slow planning and decision making.

Web-Based Instruction (WBI)

WBI is a popular educational use of computers (Buhmann 2000, Clauson 1999, Karupan and Karuppan 1999, Kiser 1999, Krebs, 2000, Santosus 1998, Womack, Lyons, Roskos, et al. 1999). It shares many of the advantages associated with CAI, such as self-paced learning, 24-hour availability, prompt feedback, and interactivity. WBI is also free from geographic constraints and can be revised as needed. The Web provides a user-friendly format along with access to multimedia in a fairly consis-

Box 16–5 **Key Points for Students Involved in Distance Learning**

- Reception sites may be in students' homes or workplaces.
- Increases educational opportunities by decreasing long commutes.
- Class rosters with phone numbers and addresses are generally distributed to all class members (pending individual approval) as a means to encourage interaction among students.
- Faculty can hold office hours on-line and provide feedback by telephone and e-mail as well as during class time.
- Students may remain after class to ask questions via teleconferencing links.
- The sponsoring agency notifies students of information pertaining to reception sites, parking, security, and on-site technical support.
- Additional effort is required from both students and faculty to maintain interactive aspects of the education process.
- Some modifications are required in the use of audiovisual aids. Additional attention must be given to how well audiovisual aids transmit and whether they are visible to persons at other sites.
- Successful offerings are the result of a team effort that involves instructional designers, graphic artists, computing services, faculty training, reception site coordinators, and technical support.

SOURCE: Adapted from "Distance education in nursing: Adapting courses for distance education," by D. M. Billings, 1996, *Computers in Nursing, 14*(5), 262–263, 266; and "CE key career tool, mandatory in some states," by D. Marks, September 1996, *The American Nurse*, 7–8.

tent manner. Most WBI sites provide basic course information, such as syllabus, schedule, announcements, and reading lists (Hazari and Schnorr 1999). Many other sites include synchronous or asynchronous communication, online testing, discussion groups, conferences, whiteboards, streaming audio and video, and in some cases on-line help. WBI can be used as a stand-alone course for distance education or as a complement to traditional courses. Teleconferencing capability is sometimes included. There is debate as to whether WBI is actually cost effective when development and support costs are considered. In the case of course materials, printing costs are shifted from the institution to the student.

It is important to consider a number of issues before Web-based instruction is offered. These include (Kiser 1999, Mills 2000, Zalon 2000) the following:

- *Institutional commitment of resources.* WBI requires human and material resources. It is labor intensive to develop and manage. It requires administrative support for needed equipment, technical staff, and help for faculty interested in using this medium.

- *The technology infrastructure.* Networking and technical support staff should be consulted to determine server and network specifications, technical standards, bandwidth, and software requirements for Web-based instruction. When teleconferencing is used it is important to look at room layout in relationship to equipment capabilities.

- *Web course building tools.* This type of software provides a shell for course layout and administration (Fredrickson 1999, Ganzel 1999, Munger 1999). Common features include tracking, chat capability, a whiteboard, e-mail, the ability to post information, scheduling capability, templates, the ability to share files, grading components, exam and evaluation capability, and administrative and security features that limit access to authorized users. Some examples include First-Class, TopClass, WebCT, LearningSpace, LearnLinc I-Net, Knowledge Soft's Lois, and Centra Software's Symposium.

- *Adaptation of course materials and delivery for on-line instruction.* Successful WBI makes use of the hypertext capabilities of the Web. This includes links to other sites of potential interest. It represents a deviation from traditional class structures and acknowledges that the locus of control for learning lies with the learner.

- *Practice time prior to the actual start of instruction.* One cannot assume that faculty or students come to Web-based instruction with an intuitive grasp of the technology. For this reason it is important to practice using the tool prior to the start of a course. Preparatory tutorials ensure that instructional time is not squandered on technical assistance for a few.

- *Develop and communicate a contingency plan.* While the advantages of WBI include 24-hour availability from any location, there may be instances when access cannot be accomplished. This may be related to an individual's PC or Internet service provider, power outages, or problems with the organization's infrastructure. It is of particular concern when classes are synchronous. Identify alternative means of communicating assignments early in the class.

Box 16–6 includes a few suggestions for faculty who are developing Web-based instruction or considering its use.

Computer Labs

Computer labs have become an important instructional tool and a feature that students look for when they choose an educational facility (Ring and Vander Meer 1994). Box 16–7 identifies features for students to consider when they have the opportunity to evaluate computer labs. There are three types of instructional computer labs: public access, limited access, and computer classrooms. Public access facilities provide a collection of general-purpose software, and are open to all members of the institution on a first-come, first-served basis. Limited access labs are

Box 16–6 **Do's and Don'ts for Developing a Web-Based Course**

Do's

- *Humanize the course.* Encourage students to provide background information about themselves and their goals at the onset of the course.

- *Post materials prior to class and discussions.* This provides reinforcement and promotes active listening when WBI is used as an adjunct to traditional classes.

- *Provide mechanisms for student feedback.* Use threaded discussions, chats, e-mail, and whiteboard capability.

- *Keep lessons short and modular.* Long documents on-line do not facilitate learning.

- *Use methods to develop face-to-face skills.* Include situations and ask participants to identify how they would respond. Encourage discussion among classmates.

- *Incorporate a mechanism to access library resources.*

- *Use formative feedback.* This will allow faculty to modify the course as needed to benefit students.

- *Provide information related to resources for technical support.*

Don'ts

- *Don't assume preexisting knowledge.* Provide a tutorial prior to class or as part of the first class to familiarize students with the technology.

- *Don't assume that everyone has the latest versions of software or fastest processor.* Students who cannot access all documents or portions of the class will become frustrated.

- *Avoid items that take a long time to download.* People won't wait. Large files also place a heavy demand on the server and network.

- *Avoid "plug-ins."* These programs can change the way the user's computer processes tasks as well as place additional demands on the processor.

---

usually located within a particular department and are open only to people associated with that department. Limited-access lab software is determined by subject need. Computer classrooms are used as an instructional tool by faculty who conduct classes in the lab. This arrangement calls for one computer per learner. Computer classrooms may be used as public or limited access facilities when not in use as a classroom. Lab purpose determines the type and amount of hardware and software needed, and has implications for size, the number of hours that it is accessible for use, and how it is staffed. Most computer labs rely on local area networks (LANs) instead of freestanding PCs because LANs are easier to administer, offer lower support costs, and permit sharing of resources, including software, printers, and information (Davis and McGuffin 1995).

A successful computer lab requires careful planning and commitment to its ongoing support (Ring and Vander Meer 1994). It should provide

---

Box 16–7   Evaluation Criteria for a Computer Lab

Lighting

- Windows, if present, are high up on the walls with shades, blinds, and/or curtains to control glare.
- Lighting for the room and at each computer is adjustable to accommodate the use of over-heads, reading, note-taking, and computer work, while avoiding fatigue and headaches.

Heating/Ventilation/Air Conditioning

- Room temperature ranges between 70 and 72°F.

Acoustics

- Outside noise that can decrease concentration is minimal or nonexistent.

Furniture

- Chairs are comfortable and adjustable in height, with good lumbar support, wheels, and arm-rests that fit under tables to minimize restlessness and fatigue.
- Large tables support writing, training materials, and computer equipment while providing knee room.
- Surfaces are free from glare.
- Furniture has rounded corners to decrease risk of injury.
- A separate portable master workstation with room for a PC, mouse pad, and projector provides a place for faculty to demonstrate program features.

Color

- The room is a cheerful medium to light color.

Power/Cabling/Phone Jacks

- There are sufficient electrical outlets and phone jacks to accommodate each workstation.
- Cables are properly secured and out of the way, so as not to pose a safety hazard.

SOURCE: Adapted from "Planning a computer lab: Considerations to ensure success," 1994, *IALL Journal of Language Learning Technologies, 27*(1), 55–59.

---

an orientation for users and be located at a convenient site with hours convenient to users. Equipment and software must be current. Staff should have a working knowledge of PCs and/or networks, software, and peripheral devices in order to provide user support. In addition to taking care of equipment and assisting users, computer lab staff maintain security, create and monitor user accounts, track system use, and back up software to prevent accidental damage. Faculty contribute to computer lab success by encouraging its use and through the selection of high-quality instructional software.

One source of frustration for students using computer labs is when they cannot access or use a particular software program. Careful lab management should limit this problem. Inability to access software may result when installation is improper, when a program is designed for use by one user, or when the number of users permitted by the lab's site license has been met. **Site licenses** are an agreement between the computer lab and the software publisher on the terms of use. For example, the site license for a network version of a word processing package may allow up to 25 users at one time. Additional individuals cannot access the software until another user has logged off. Institutions and lab administrators must estimate software use to negotiate site licenses that meet their needs. Lab users should exit applications and log off of the system so that others may access the software. Publishers may offer special site license agreements for the computer lab market, particularly if a need for special agreements is demonstrated (Happer 1995).

Educational Opportunities in Nursing Informatics

Until recent years the opportunities for nurses and other health care professionals to learn more about informatics were largely limited to programs sponsored by special-interest groups. Only a handful of undergraduate and graduate nursing programs offered introductory nursing informatics courses. This situation is changing, although Hardy et al. (1997) found that nursing informatics has been slow to emerge in nursing curricula. An increased number of schools now also offer a graduate degree or a focus or certificate in nursing informatics. Some of these programs use distance or Web-based education, while others use the traditional classroom setting. Doctoral programs are still limited. There are also a number of programs with a focus on health information management or health informatics.

CASE STUDY EXERCISES

You are on the education committee at your small community hospital. Your staff development department was eliminated several years ago. You and your colleagues are charged with developing strategies to meet the educational needs of agency RNs and LPNs. Limited capital and the isolated location of your community make this a difficult assignment. Your institution does have Internet and WWW access in the medical library, as well as teleconferencing capability. Develop a proposal to meet your charge using available resources. Be prepared to defend your proposal to an administration loathe to part with monies beyond those already budgeted.

• • •

You are the client educator at a medical center in the Pacific Northwest. Your clientele are drawn from a 150-mile radius and beyond. For this reason it is difficult to have clients complete diabetic education or other classes. You have been told to improve client completion of classes or face elimination of your department. The medical center has both teleconferencing capability presently used for consults and an established Web page that provides basic information about the institution. How might you use these resources to develop alternative strategies for client education? Address budget considerations, necessary resources, target populations that might be better served, and how you propose to link distant clients with instructional offerings.

• • •

You recently joined the faculty at a small, private rural college. Because you express an interest in computers and are slightly more knowledgeable about computers than your faculty colleagues, you have been asked to establish a computer lab for the nursing department and incorporate computer use in all of the nursing courses. Current resources are quite limited. Provide a detailed plan of how you would accomplish this charge from start to finish. Identify potential stumbling blocks and ways that you would address them.

SUMMARY

- Computer technology can be used to support education in formal nursing programs, continuing education, and consumer education. It also provides informal opportunities for networking among professionals via e-mail and discussion groups.

- Successful use of computers for education requires careful planning, orientation to the technology, convenient access, opportunities to question what is not understood, and good instructional design.

- Formal nursing education is a logical place to introduce or expand basic computer skills, such as word processing, Internet access, e-mail, and on-line literature searches.

- Educational software should be subject to the same review criteria applied to other instructional materials prior to their adoption.

- Computer instruction should match curriculum level and objectives.

- NCLEX-RN preparation programs are a popular use of computerized test programs in basic nursing programs.

- Connectivity to hospital information systems from schools of nursing allows students more opportunity to analyze client information prior to scheduled clinical experiences and facilitates professional socialization.

- Computers provide invaluable assistance in the preparation of educational materials and presentations, the delivery of instruction, examinations, and evaluations, and the maintenance of educational records.

- CAI is the use of a computer to teach a subject other than computing via direct interaction of the student with the computer. CAI offers the following advantages: convenience, decreased learning time, and increased retention.

- Teleconferencing is the use of computers, audio and video equipment, and high-grade dedicated telephone lines to provide interactive communication between two or more persons at two or more sites.

- Distance learning is the use of print, audio, video, computer, or teleconference capability to connect faculty and students located at a minimum of two different sites. Distance learning may take place in real time or on a delayed basis. It expands educational opportunities without the need for a long commute.

- Web-based instruction (WBI) uses the attributes and resources of the Internet to deliver and support education. It may be used as a stand-alone course or to supplement traditional classes.

- E-learning uses electronic media to present instruction. It is often suggested for corporate training because it is considered to be efficient. It allows users to skip material that they already know.

- Multimedia refers to the ability to deliver presentations that combine text, voice or sound, images, and video. Multimedia presentations tend to improve learning by actively engaging the senses.

- Computer labs are an asset to educational facilities. Most use LAN technology to share information, software, and other resources.

- Educational opportunities in nursing informatics range from the informal to the formal. There are numerous introductory courses on undergraduate and graduate levels. Some institutions offer areas of specialization within a degree on the graduate level or certificate programs. Opportunities for doctoral work in nursing informatics are limited.

REFERENCES

Barrett, A. (2000). E-learning improves training process, cuts costs. *Austin Business Journal, 20*(9), 40.

Billings, D. M. (1994). Effects of BSN student preferences for studying alone or in groups on performance and attitude when using interactive videodisc instruction. *Journal of Nursing Education, 33*(7), 322–324.

Billings, D. M. (1995). Preparing nursing faculty for information age teaching and learning. *Computers in Nursing, 13*(6), 264, 268–270.

Billings, D. M. (1996a). Connecting points: Distance education in nursing. *Computers in Nursing, 14*(4), 211–212.

Billings, D. M. (1996b). Distance education in nursing: Adapting courses for distance education. *Computers in Nursing, 14*(5), 262–263, 266.

Billings, D., Hodson-Carlton, K., Kirkpatrick, J., Aaltonen, P., Dillard, N., Richardson, V., Siktberg, L., and Vinten, S. (1996). Computerized NCLEX-RN preparation programs: A comparative review. *Computers in Nursing, 14*(5), 272–286.

Black, D., and Goldstein, J. (1998). Live and online: A WBT primer. *Training & Development, 52*(9), 34(2).

Buhmann, J. (2000). Electronic education: Authoring software for courses delivered on the Web, part 3: Designer's Edge/Net Synergy. *Nurse Educator, 25*(3), 110–113.

Calderone, A. B. (1994). Computer-assisted instruction: Learning, attitude, and modes of instruction. *Computers in Nursing, 12*(3), 164–170.

Cambre, M., and Castner, L. J. (March 1993). The status of interactive video in nursing education environments. Presented at FITNE: Get in touch with multimedia, Atlanta, GA.

Canavan, K. (November/December 1996). New technologies propel nursing profession forward. *The American Nurse*, 1, 2, 3.

Cartwright, J. (2000). Lessons learned: Using asynchronous computer-mediated conferencing to facilitate group discussion. *Journal of Nursing Education, 39*(2), 87–90.

Clauson, J. (1999). On-line quality courses offer many side benefits. *Quality Progress, 32*(1), 83(7).

Corwin, E. J. (2000). Distance education: An ongoing initiative to reach rural family nurse practitioner students. *Nurse Educator, 25*(3), 114–115.

Davis, P. T., and McGuffin, C. R. (1995). *Wireless local area networks: Technology, issues, and strategies*. New York: McGraw-Hill.

Doorley, J. E., Renner, A. L., and Corron, J. (1994). Creating care plans via modems: Using a hospital information system in nursing education. *Computers in Nursing, 12*(3), 160–163.

Fredrickson, S. (1999). Untangling a tangled Web: An overview of Web-based instruction programs. *T H E Journal, 26*(11), 67.

Ganzel, R. (1999). What price online learning? *Training, 26*(2), 50(5).

Gleydura, A. J., Michelman, J. E., and Wilson, C. N. (1995). Multimedia training in nursing education. *Computers in Nursing, 13*(4), 169–175.

Glover, S. M., and Kruse, M. (1995). Making the most of computer-assisted instruction. *Nursing 95, 25*(9), 32N.

Goodman, J., and Blake, J. (1996). Multimedia courseware: Transforming the classroom. *Computers in Nursing, 14*(5), 287–296.

Happer, S. K. (1995). Software, copyright, and site license agreements: Publishers' perspective of library practice. Thesis. Kent, OH: Kent State University.

Hardy, J. L., Lindqvist, R., Kristofferzon, M. L., and Dahlberg, O. (1997). The current status of nursing informatics in undergraduate nursing programs: Comparative case studies between Sweden and Australia. *Studies Health Technology and Informatics, 46*, 132.

Hazari, S., and Schnorr, D. (1999). Leveraging student feedback to improve teaching in Web-based courses. *T H E Journal, 26*(11), 30.

Henderson, R., and Deane, F. (1995). Assessment of satisfaction with computer training in a healthcare setting. *Journal of Nursing Staff Development, 11*(5), 255–260.

Karupan, C. M., and Karuppan, M. (1999). Empirically based guidelines for developing teaching materials on the Web. *Business Communication Quarterly, 62*(3), 37(9).

Khoiny, F. (1995). Factors that contribute to computer-assisted instruction effectiveness. *Computers in Nursing, 13*(4), 165–168.

Kiser, K. (1999). 10 things we know so far about online training. *Training, 36*(11), 66(6).

Krebs, B. (22 March 2000). Teacher training key to Web-based education initiatives. *Newsbytes*, pNSBT10191044.

Marks, D. (September 1996). CE key career tool, mandatory in some states. *The American Nurse*, 7–8.

Mastrian, K. G., and McGonigle, D. (1999). Using technology-based assignments to promote critical thinking. *Nurse Educator, 24*(1), 45–47.

Miholland, D. K. (September 1996). New information technologies suggest new roles for nurses. *The American Nurse*, 2–3.

Mills, A. C. (2000). Creating Web-based, multimedia, and interactive courses for distance learning. *Computers in Nursing, 18*(3), 123–131.

Munger, R. (1999). Web-based instructional tools. *Technical Communication, 46*(2), 275.

Planning a computer lab: Considerations to ensure success. (1994). *IALL Journal of Language Learning Technologies, 27*(1), 55–59.

Poirrier, G. P., Wills, E. M., Broussard, P. C., and Payne, R. L. (1996). Nursing information systems: Applications in nursing curricula. *Nurse Educator, 21*(1), 18–22.

Ring, D. M., and Vander Meer, P. F. (Summer 1994). Designing a computerized instructional training room for the library. *Special Libraries*, 154–160.

Santosus, M. (1998). Nothing like the real thing: Can courses without discourse really deliver education? *CIO, 12*(4), pM24.

Simpson, R. L. (1995). Getting wired for success. *Nursing Administration Quarterly, 19*(4), 89–91.

Sirota, W. J. (1995). Desktop videoconferencing: Voice, vision, reality. *The Workgroup Computing Report, 18*(5), 19(7).

Tronni, C., and Welebob, E. (1996). End-user satisfaction of a patient education tool: Manual versus computer-generated tool. *Computers in Nursing, 14*(4), 235–238.

Wilson, A. W. (1991). Computer anxiety in nursing students. *Journal of Nursing Education, 30*, 52–56.

Womack, D., Lyons, A., Roskos, J., Byrne, F., and Staggers, N. (1999). *Computers in Nursing, 17*(5), 212–214.

Zalon, M. L. (2000). A prime time primer for distance education. *Nurse Educator, 25*(1), 28–33.

Telehealth

After completing this chapter, you will be able to:

- Define the term *telehealth*.
- List the advantages of telehealth.
- Identify equipment and technology needed to sustain telehealth.
- Discuss present and proposed telehealth applications.
- Describe legal and practice issues that impact telehealth.
- Review the implications of telehealth for nursing and other allied health professions.
- Identify several telenursing applications.
- Discuss some issues pertaining to the practice of telenursing.

Telehealth is the use of telecommunication technologies and computers to provide healthcare information and services to clients at another location. This was once known as **telemedicine** but applications are now widely used by other members of the health care community. Teleconferences and videoconferences are tools used to deliver these services. Electronic, visual, and audio signals sent during these conferences provide information to consultants from remote sites. Distant practitioners and clients benefit from the skills and knowledge of the consultants without the need to travel to regional referral centers. Telehealth is a tool that allows health care professionals to do the following (Davis 1996, Ensminger 1996, McGee and Tangalos 1994, Nelson 1999, Perednia and Allen 1995, Zurier 1995):

- Consult with colleagues
- Conduct interviews
- Assess and monitor clients
- View diagnostic images
- Review slides and lab reports

Telehealth-related terms describing these capabilities have proliferated (see Box 17–1 for a partial listing).

TERMS RELATED TO TELEHEALTH

While *telemedicine* formerly was the predominant term, it has largely been supplanted by the term **telehealth** (Montgomery 1996, Zurier 1995). Telehealth encompasses telemedicine but is a broader term that emphasizes both the delivery of services and the provision of information to health care providers and consumers. For example, federal agencies use the Internet to provide health care professionals and consumers with medical information.

Box 17–1 Some Common Telehealth Terms

- *E-care.* The provision of health information, products, and services on-line as well as the automation of administrative and clinical aspects of care delivery.

- *E-health.* A broad term often used interchangeably with the term telehealth to refer to the provision of health information, products, and services on-line.

- *E-medicine.* The use of telecommunication and computer technology for the delivery of medical care.

- *Telecardiology.* Transmission of cardiac catheterization studies, echocardiograms, and other diagnostic tests in conjunction with electronic stethoscope examinations for second opinions by cardiologists at another site.

- *Teleconsultation.* Videoconferencing between two health care professionals or a health care professional and a client.

- *Telementoring.* Real-time advice is offered during a procedure to a practitioner in a remote site via a telecommunication system.

- *Telenursing.* The use of telecommunication and computer technology for the delivery of nursing care.

- *Telepathology.* Transmission of high-resolution still images, often via a robotic microscope, for interpretation by a pathologist at a remote site.

- *Telepsychiatry.* Variant of teleconsultation that allows observation and interviews of clients at one site by a psychiatrist at another site.

- *Teleradiology.* Transmission of high-resolution still images for interpretation by a radiologist at a distant location.

- *Telesurgery.* Surgeons at a remote site can collaborate with experts at a referral center on techniques.

- *Teleultrasound.* Transmission of ultrasound images for interpretation at a remote site.

The Public Health Service's Agency for Health Care Policy and Research (AHCPR) places clinical practice guidelines on-line, and the *Journal of the National Cancer Institute* is available on the World Wide Web. As a consequence of this information explosion, health care professionals and clients gain access to the most current treatment options at essentially the same time. No matter what term is used, the basic premise of telehealth is that it can provide services to underserved communities. Another frequently used term is **e-health.** E-health is often used interchangeably with the term telehealth. **Telenursing** is the use of telecommunications and computer technology for the delivery of nursing care.

Teleconferencing

Teleconferencing implies that people at different locations have audio, and possibly video, contact, which is used to carry out telehealth applications. The terms *teleconference* and *videoconference* may be used synonymously, since both use telecommunications and computer technology.

Videoconferencing

Videoconferencing implies that people meet face-to-face and view the same images through the use of telecommunications and computer technology even though they are not in the same location (Condon 1995, Davis 1996, Sirota 1995). It saves travel time and costs, which actually encourages people to meet more frequently. Videoconferencing is an appealing concept that can be used for many applications, especially distance learning and telehealth (although some applications may require high resolution and audio quality and high-speed transmission).

Desktop Videoconferencing

Desktop videoconferencing (**DTV**) is a synchronous, or real-time, encounter that uses a specially equipped personal computer with telephone line hookup to allow people to meet face-to-face and/or view papers and images simultaneously (Holmes 1994, Robinson 1995, Sirota 1995). DTV is less expensive than custom-designed videoconference systems, but as of this writing it is not acceptable for telehealth applications that require high resolution or high-speed transmission, such as interpretation of diagnostic images where slower frame rates produce a jerky image or lengthy transmission times.

HISTORICAL BACKGROUND

Telehealth began with the use of telephone consults and became more sophisticated with each advance in technology (McGee and Tangelos 1994, Perednia 1995, Perednia and Allen 1995, "Rural America" 1995, Silver 1995). During the past four decades the U.S. government has played a major role in the development and promotion of telehealth through various agencies. Although interest waned as funds were depleted in the 1980s, technological advancements during the 1980s made it a more attractive prospect. Federal monies and the Agriculture Department's 1991 Rural Development Act laid the groundwork to bring the information superhighway to rural areas for education and telehealth purposes.

The most aggressive development of telehealth in the United States has been by NASA and the military (Brewin 1995, Green 1995, Telehealth Research Center 1996). NASA provided international telehealth consults for Armenian earthquake victims in 1989, while more recently the military has been working on several projects to feed medical images from the battlefield to physicians in hospitals for improved treatment of casualties.

The single largest U.S. project is at the University of Texas at Galveston, where the medical branch provides care to inmates across the state (Condon 1995, "Telehealth helps Texas" 1995). Other states also use telehealth to treat prisoners.

One major barrier to telehealth was removed with the passage of the Telecommunications Act of 1995, which allowed vendors of cable and telephone services to compete in each others' markets (Schneider 1996). Investment in the telecommunications technologies needed to create the information superhighway should result from the ensuing competition. The Snowe–Rockefeller Amendment requires telecommunications carriers to offer services to rural health providers at rates comparable to those charged in urban areas so that affordable health care may be available to rural residents.

Grant monies are now targeted for projects likely to succeed (Office of Public Information 1996). The National Library of Medicine recently announced funding for several projects that will evaluate the impact of telemedicine on costs, quality, and access to health care; test emerging data standards; and examine the issue of confidentiality of health data sent across networks. Despite the emphasis in this text on U.S. development of telehealth, it is an international phenomenon that has been used successfully to serve sparsely populated regions in Australia and Canada, and for various applications around the world (Telemedicine Research Center 1996).

DRIVING FORCES

Recent attention to cost containment, managed care, and uneven access to health care services make telehealth an attractive tool to save health care dollars (McGee and Tangalos 1994, Perednia 1995, Robinson 1995, Slipy 1995, "To your health" 1995, Weaver 1996, Zurier 1995). Savings may be realized via the following measures:

- Improved access to care, which allows clients to be treated earlier when fewer interventions are required.
- Clients may receive treatment in their own community where services cost less.
- Improved quality of care. Expert advice is more easily available.
- Extending the services of nurse practitioners and physician assistants through ready accessibility to physician services.
- Improved continuity of care through convenient follow-up care.

Telehealth is also a marketing tool. Large institutions offer links with the understanding that additional services will be rendered at their facilities. For example, imagine that a client with symptoms of coronary artery disease is seen at a community hospital that has no facilities for cardiac surgery. The client is more likely to follow up at the larger institution that has established links to the community hospital, because a rapport has been established with the consulting physician. As a result of the above factors, many agencies offer telehealth or plan to do so in the near future. Box 17–2 lists some additional benefits associated with telehealth.

Box 17–2 Telehealth Benefits

- *Continuity of care.* Clients can stay in the community and use their regular health care providers.
- *Centralized health records.* Clients remain in the same health care system.
- *Incorporation of the health care consumer as an active member of the health team.* The client is an active participant in videoconferences.
- *Collaboration among health care professionals.* Cooperation is fostered among interdisciplinary members of the health care team.
- *Improved decision making.* Experts are readily available.
- *Education of health care consumers and professionals.* Offerings are readily available.
- *Higher quality of care.* Access to care and access to specialists is improved.
- *Removes geographic barriers to care.* Clients living away from major population centers or in economically disadvantaged areas can access care more readily.
- *May result in lower costs for health care.* Eliminates travel costs. Clients are seen earlier when they are not as ill. Treatment may take place in local hospitals, which are less costly.

APPLICATIONS

Telehealth applications vary greatly and include client monitoring, diagnostic evaluations, decision support systems, storage and dissemination of records for diagnostic purposes, image compression for efficient storage and retrieval, research, voice recognition for dictation, and education of health care professionals and consumers (Ensminger 1996, Perednia 1995). Sophisticated equipment is not always necessary. Some applications are "high tech," while others are relatively "low tech." Real-time videoconferencing between physicians or health care professionals and clients and the transmission of diagnostic images and biometric data are examples of high-tech applications. An example of a low-tech application is a home glucose-monitoring program that uses a touch-tone phone to report glucose results. Desktop PCs outfitted with video cameras can provide telehealth opportunities for applications that do not require high resolution. Telemedicine can be divided into four types of applications: interactive video, store-and-forward consultations, video on the Internet, and cable-based video. Box 17–3 lists some other actual and proposed applications.

On-Line Databases and Tools

On-line resources can include the following:

- *Standards of care.* These may include recommended guidelines for care for a particular diagnosis.

Box 17–3 **Current and Proposed Telehealth Applications**

- *Cardiology.* EKG strips can be transmitted for interpretation by experts at a regional referral center, and pacemakers can be reset from a remote location.
- *Counseling.* Clients may be seen at home or in outpatient settings by a counselor at another site.
- *Data mining.* Research may be conducted on large databases for educational, diagnostic, and cost/benefit analysis.
- *Dermatology.* Primary physicians may ask specialists to see a client without the client waiting for an appointment with the specialist and traveling to a distant site.
- *Diabetes management.* Clients may report blood glucose readings by using the touch-tone telephone.
- *Mobile unit postdisaster care.* Emergency medical technicians (EMTs) and nurses at the site of a disaster can consult with physicians about the health needs of victims.
- *Education.* Health care professionals in geographically remote areas can attend seminars to update their knowledge without extensive travel, expense, or time away from home.
- *Emergency care.* Community hospitals can share information with trauma centers so that the centers can better care for clients and prepare them for transport.
- *Fetal monitoring.* Some high-risk antepartum clients can be monitored from home with greater comfort and decreased expense.
- *Geriatrics.* Videoconference equipment in the home permits home monitoring of medication administration for the client with memory deficits who is otherwise able to stay at home.
- *Home care.* Once equipment is in the client's home, nurses and physicians may evaluate the client at home without leaving their offices.
- *Military.* Physicians at remote sites can evaluate injured soldiers in the field via the medic's equipment.
- *Pharmacy.* Data can be accessed at a centralized location.
- *Pathology.* The transmission of slide and tissue samples to other sites makes it easier to obtain a second opinion on biopsy findings.
- *Radiology.* Radiologists can take calls from home that receive images from the hospital on equipment they have in place. Rural hospitals do not need to have a radiologist on site.
- *School clinics.* School nurses, particularly in remote areas, can quickly consult with other professionals about problems observed.
- *Speech–language pathology.* More efficient use can be made of scarce speech–language pathologists.

- *Critical pathways and client outcomes.* A **critical pathway** is a suggested blueprint for the care of a client with a particular diagnosis such as pneumonia. The pathway outlines recommended multidisciplinary interventions and outcomes for the expected length of stay.

- *Computerized medical diagnosis*. This database assists the physician to match symptoms against suspected diagnoses.
- *Drug information*. One important application is the determination of the most effective, least expensive antibiotic for a particular infection.
- *Electronic prescription filing*. This permits the physician to "write" a prescription that is sent automatically to the pharmacy.
- *Abstracts and full text retrieval of literature*. These can be retrieved easily at any time of the day.
- *Research data*. This information is available via literature searches and Web access.
- *Bulletin boards, reference files, and discussion groups on various specialty subjects*.

Ready access to information improves care delivery and decreases related costs (Betts 1994, Zurier 1995). For example, the incorporation of national standards of care and drug information eliminates redundant efforts by individual institutions to prepare their own standards and formularies. It also decreases malpractice claims through adherence to standards of care. On-line research databases facilitate research through the systematic collection of information on large populations, with potential for data mining at a later time. Further benefits from on-line resources will be accrued as projects are implemented to develop common terms to facilitate sharing of data, such as the National Library of Medicine's Unified Medical Language System.

Education

Telehealth affords opportunities to educate health care consumers and professionals through increased information accessibility via on-line resources, including the World Wide Web, distance learning, and clinical instruction. Grand rounds and continuing education comprise two of the most touted applications for education.

Grand rounds are a traditional teaching tool for health professionals in training (Siwicki 1996a). As the name indicates, a group of practitioners review a client's case history and present condition, at which time they mutually determine the best treatment options. Grand rounds help to maintain clinical knowledge and expertise but are not always available in smaller institutions. Telehealth facilities allow the incorporation of diagnostic images, client interviews, and biometric measurements from outlying hospitals into medical center grand rounds, thereby allowing practitioners from two or more sites to participate. In like fashion, consultations and images from major teaching centers may be made available to remote facilities to enhance the practice of professionals in outlying areas.

Continuing Education

Telehealth offers direct access to traditional continuing education and extemporaneous teaching opportunities with every teleconsultation (Karon 1996, McGee and Tangalos 1994). Training costs for continuing education may be decreased by bringing people together from many distant sites without travel or lodging expenses or extended time away from their responsibilities.

Home Health Care

Telecommunication technology can reduce home health care costs and increase availability of services and support (Brennan 1996, D'Amico 1995, Dansky, Bowles, and Britt 1999). For example, use of a home monitoring system in Japan provides 24-hour contact and medical response for clients as needed in addition to regularly scheduled visits. Biometric measurements such as heart rate and pattern, blood pressure, respiratory rate, and fetal heart rate can be monitored at another site, with electronic or actual house calls provided as needed. Women with high-risk pregnancies, diabetics, and cardiac and postoperative clients can be monitored at home. Internet access for home health clients and their families provides convenient access to support groups, treatment information, and electronic communication with their health care providers, while decreasing feelings of isolation. Required equipment is dictated by the nature of the monitoring. For example, telemetry and fetal heart sounds require continuous monitoring, necessitating a dedicated phone line as well as the monitoring devices supplied by the home health care agency. Figure 17–1 depicts a teleconference that connects a home health care client, a nurse, and a physician.

LEGAL AND PRIVACY ISSUES

Reimbursement and licensure issues are two of the major barriers to the practice of telehealth and telenursing (Schneider 1996). Both are expected to become nonissues as telehealth becomes more prevalent. There are also concerns about the impact of telehealth on record privacy, particularly with the implementation of the Health Insurance Portability and Accountability Act (HIPAA).

Referral and Payment

Except for a limited experimental basis, present Medicare, Medicaid, and most third-party payers will reimburse providers only for face-to-face meetings with clients (Perednia 1995, Schneider 1996, Siwicki 1996a, Siwicki 1996b, Zurier 1995). This means that physicians as well as some other providers who do teleconsultation are not paid for their services. This rule does not apply to interpretation of diagnostic tests. This lack of

FIGURE 17–1 • Diagram of a Teleconference Involving Client, Nurse, and Physician at Separate Sites

reimbursement may be offset by increased client volume at referral centers because clients who receive telehealth services will most likely go to this site for additional services. Remote sites that do not have specialists or 24-hour specialty coverage gain coverage without retaining additional staff, reduce treatment times for clients, and strengthen relationships with referral centers.

Support Personnel

While the technology behind telehealth should be easy to use, technical support may be required. Support staff should be capable, flexible, and preferably experienced. At present, questions have not been resolved as to who will train health care professionals to participate in telehealth and how compensation will be derived for the additional person hours associated with installation, training, and use of telehealth technology. There is also an issue of confidentiality. Technical support staff that are present during the exchange of patient information need to be aware of institutional policies as well as laws designed to protect patient privacy. These personnel should sign the same sort of statement that clinical personnel sign upon the receipt of their information system access codes.

Liability

Telehealth is plagued by a number of liability issues (Braly 1995, Bulkeley 1995, McGee and Tangalos 1994, Perednia and Allen 1995, Zurier 1995). First, there is the possibility that the client may perceive it as inferior because the consulting professional does not perform a hands-on examination. Second, professionals who practice across state lines may be subject to malpractice lawsuits in multiple jurisdictions, raising questions about how that liability might be distributed or which state's practice standards would apply. Theoretically, clients could choose to file suit in the jurisdiction most likely to award damages. And, third, how might liability be spread among physicians, other health care professionals, and technical support persons? Practice guidelines are needed.

Telehealth has the potential to raise or lower malpractice costs. For example, Pennsylvania's HealthNet records teleconferences to provide a complete transcript of the session. Clients receive a videotape for later review and as a means to clarify their comprehension, and the original videotape is kept as part of the client record. The American Nurses Association (1999) also calls for the development of documentation requirements for telehealth services that address treatment recommendations as well as any communication that occurs with other health care providers. This strategy should decrease malpractice claims through better documentation and improved client understanding. On the other hand, liability costs may increase if health care professionals can be sued in more than one jurisdiction.

Major issues for nurses include questions of liability when information provided over the telephone is misinterpreted, when advice is given across state lines without a license in the state where the client resides, or, particularly, when an unintentional diagnosis comes from the use of an Internet chat room ("Troubled waters" 1997). Liability is unclear in these areas. Regulation of telenursing practice by boards of nursing is difficult when practice crosses state lines. Unless nurses are licensed in every state in which they practice telenursing, respective regulatory boards are unaware of their presence. Authority to practice telenursing across state lines provides the following advantages (National Council of State Boards 1996):

- It establishes the nurse's responsibility and accountability to the board of nursing.
- It establishes legitimacy and availability to practice telenursing.
- It provides jurisdictional authority over the discipline of telenursing in the event that unsafe delivery becomes an issue.

Until this issue has been resolved nurses must also be cautious when providers from other states give them directions. Several state boards of nursing specifically forbid taking instructions from providers not licensed in the current state. Box 17–4 summarizes barriers to the practice of telehealth.

Box 17–4

Barriers to the Use of Telehealth Applications

- *Regulatory barriers.* State laws are either unclear or may forbid practice across state lines.

- *Lack of reimbursement for consultative services.* Most third-party payers do not provide reimbursement unless the client is seen in person.

- *Costs for equipment, network services, and training time.* Equipment capable of transmitting and receiving diagnostic-grade images is still expensive, though costs are declining.

- *Fear of health care system changes.* Personnel may fear job loss as more clients can be treated at home and hospital units close.

- *Lack of acceptance by health care professionals.* May stem from liability concerns and discomfort over not seeing a client face-to-face.

Licensure Issues

In general, current laws require health care professionals to be licensed in the state in which they practice (Braly 1995, National Council of State Boards 1996, Sandberg 1995a). Application for licensure in additional states can be lengthy and expensive. Telehealth and telenursing advocates want to remove legal barriers to practice through nationwide licensing or changes in practice acts that permit practitioners from any state to consult with practitioners from another state without the need to be licensed in that second state. The Federation of State Medical Boards drafted legislation to address this issue that calls for the establishment of a registry for telehealth physicians, who would enjoy shorter license application periods and lower fees, but with some practice restrictions. Some licensing laws pertaining to telehealth have been enacted or are under consideration but these still primarily address physicians, not other health professionals (Stone 1999). Task forces of the National Council of Nurses are looking at the issue of multistate licensure as a means to support telenursing. Until changes are implemented, delivery of services across some state lines via telehealth may be illegal and practitioners must proceed cautiously.

Confidentiality/Privacy

Although telehealth should not create any greater concerns or risks to medical record privacy than any other form of consultation, records that cross state lines are subject to different privacy laws in different states (Ensminger 1996, McGee and Tangalos 1994, Office of Public Information 1996, Sandberg 1995a). Practitioners also need to consider the impact of federal legislation, including HIPAA, on telehealth. There should be other ways to safeguard records as well. In 1993 the United States

Congress asked the National Research Council's Computer Science and Telecommunications Board (Dam and Lin 1996) to study national cryptography policy as a tool to protect the increasing amounts of information that are sent via electronic networks. The Committee to Study National Cryptography Policy was created for this purpose. Their report was issued in 1996 with a recommendation for a strong national policy on data encryption to protect information sent over a national information infrastructure, such as the Internet, from unauthorized access and as a means to promote commercial use of the Internet as a link in the information highway.

ESTABLISHING A TELEHEALTH LINK

Successful establishment and use of a telehealth link requires strategic planning as well as consideration of the following factors: necessary infrastructure, costs and reimbursement, human factors, equipment, and technology issues.

Formulating a Telehealth Plan

Any plans for the use of telehealth applications should be in concert with the overall strategic plan of the organization (Burns 1999). A telehealth plan minimizes duplicate effort and helps to ensure success (Perednia and Allen 1995). Goals should address the following:

- Current services and deficits
- Telehealth objectives
- Compliance with standards
- Reimbursement policies that favor desired outcomes rather than specific processes
- Periodic review of goals and accomplishments in light of changing technology and needs
- How telecommunication breakdowns will be handled. Will backup be provided? What happens when a power outage in the home severs a link?

The people who will use the system need to be involved in its design from the very beginning (Davis 1996). It is wise to start small and expand offerings. Most institutions begin with continuing education and later expand capability. Educational teleconferences require larger rooms that are not suitable for client examinations. Selection of equipment should be based on transmission speed, image resolution, storage capacity, mobility, and ease of use. Higher bandwidth generally improves performance. Equipment should match defined telehealth goals. Box 17–5 lists some strategies to ensure successful teleconferences.

> ### Box 17–5 Strategies to Ensure Successful Teleconferences
>
> - Select a videoconferencing system to fit your needs, such as a desktop or mobile system or customized room.
> - Locate videoconferencing facilities near where they will be used, yet in a quiet, low-traffic area.
> - Schedule sessions in advance to avoid time conflicts.
> - Establish a working knowledge of interactive conferencing features.
> - Create an agenda to keep the conference on track.
> - Set time limits.
> - Send materials needed in advance to maintain focus and involve participants.
> - Participate in a conference call as if it were a face-to-face meeting. Enunciate clearly.
> - Minimize background noise or use the mute feature.
> - Promote interactivity through questions and answers.
> - Have a facilitator available to resolve any technical problems that might arise.
>
> Source: Adapted from "The Big Picture: Videoconferencing Today–Seeing Is Believing," by P. A. Staino, 1995, *Teleconnect, 13*(5), *79*(5); and "User Tips: 9 Steps to More Effective Teleconferences," 1996, *Communication News, 33*(10), 72.

Building the Supporting Framework

Another consideration in telehealth is the question of who will build the infrastructure to support telehealth and what role the federal government should take ("NIIT demos" 1994, Perednia and Allen 1995). Federal and state governments already commit considerable resources to telehealth and related technology. The Department of Commerce, Health Care Financing Administration (HCFA), Office of Rural Health Policy, and Department of Defense are some federal agencies that have done telehealth research and demo programs. Most states have projects in process. The National Information Infrastructure Testbed (NIIT) is a consortium of corporations, universities, and government agencies that sees the development of a national information infrastructure as a means to create jobs, promote prosperity, and improve health care by reducing redundant procedures and creating an electronic record repository.

Telehealth transmissions can be supported by satellite or microwave, telephone lines, or the Internet (Braly 1995, Cannavo 1995, Davis 1996, Ensminger 1996, Sandberg 1995b, Slipy 1995, "To your health" 1995, Weinberg 1995). Cost and speed of the service are interrelated. Satellite and microwave transmission is not feasible for most users. **Asynchronous Transfer Mode (ATM)** service is a high-speed data transmission link that can carry large amounts of data quickly. Speeds range from 0.45 megabits per second (Mbps) to 2.48 gigabits per second (Gbps).

ATM works well when large sets of data, such as MRIs, need to be exchanged and discussed. Present ATM use is limited for reasons of cost, availability, and lack of standards. Another option for data transmission is **switched multimegabit data service (SMDS),** better known as a T1 line. T1 lines are high-speed telephone lines that may be used to transmit high-quality, full-motion video at speeds up to 1.544 Mbps. T1 services are leased monthly at a fixed charge independent of use. Next in descending order of speed are **DSL (digital subscriber lines)** and **integrated service digital network (ISDN)** lines. DSL uses existing copper telephone wires to transfer high bandwidth data for distances less than 20,000 feet from the central telephone office. Variants of DSL technology can rival T1 lines for speed of data transmission. ISDN lines carry 128 kilobits per second (kbps), although lines can be bundled for faster speeds. Each ISDN line costs approximately $30 per month plus costs for calls. ISDN lines support medical imaging, database sharing, desktop videoconferencing, and access to the Internet. Telehealth's identification of 384 kbps as its practical minimum bandwidth renders plain old telephone service (POTS) unsuitable for most applications. Faster access speeds are required for continuing medical education, telemetry, remote consults, and network-based services.

The Internet already carries e-mail for many health care professionals and is a powerful tool for obtaining and publishing information ("To your health" 1995). Security and access issues will determine the extent to which client-specific information is interchanged on the Internet.

Cable TV also has the potential to bring high-resolution x-ray images to on-call radiologists at home (Lutkowitz 1995). Its one-way broadband capabilities are suited for incoming images. Less capability is required to send the interpretation of the image back quickly.

Human Factors

On-site support and commitment from administrators and health care professionals are necessary for successful telehealth (Chin 1996, Perednia 1995). Acceptance is frequently more difficult to obtain from health care providers than it is from clients. Overall patient satisfaction is high, particularly when clients perceive that care is easier to obtain (Gustke, Balch, West, and Rogers 2000). Health care professionals should provide input about the type of telehealth applications that they would like to see to their professional organizations and health care providers. One application, continuing education distance learning programs, is well received and serves to introduce other applications. Adequate training time is needed to learn how to use equipment, and support staff must be available. Telehealth, and all of its applications, is new to most people and time is needed to get accustomed to it. An example of this may be seen in teleradiology, where radiologists must learn how to interpret images using a monitor.

Equipment

Equipment must be reliable, accurate, and flexible enough to meet varying needs (Perednia and Allen 1995, Siwicki 1996c). One example of this principle may be seen when equipment purchased for continuing education also supports high-resolution images needed for diagnostic images. However, it is not necessary to have all the latest, most expensive technology to start telehealth. Desktop videoconferencing uses specially adapted personal computers to operate over telephone lines. These PCs may be merged with existing diagnostic imaging systems and other information systems. While it usually lacks broadcast picture quality, DTV provides an opportunity to practice some telehealth applications at a fairly low cost. Consulting parties may be able to see each other and diagnostic images by splitting the PC screen into segments. Box 17–6 lists components needed to support DTV.

Telehealth Costs

Estimates for setting up videoconferencing vary greatly, depending on the type of system and applications chosen (Hatlestad 1996, Montgomery 1996, Perednia 1995, Sirota 1995). Desktop systems are fairly inexpensive. Better resolution increases costs. Costs include equipment purchase, operation, and maintenance; network services; and time to learn a new skills. Time needed to learn how to use telehealth applications is often underestimated. Installation of DTV in doctors' offices and ambulatory care settings is now feasible.

Technology Issues

Many of the early technical problems associated with telehealth have been resolved. Present issues include resolution, frame rate, standards, and record storage and location. **Resolution** is the sharpness or clarity of an image. The resolution needed for interpretation of diagnostic images re-

---

Box 17–6 **Basic DTV Components for Telehealth Applications**

- PC
- PC adapter cards
- Camera
- Microphones
- Video overlay cards
- External speakers on existing PCs with broadband switches
- Special adapative tools, such as an electronic stethoscope

quires a broad bandwidth that is at least 384 kilobits and 30 frames per second (FPS) (Cannavo 1995). Video systems work by rapidly displaying a series of still images referred to as frames (Staino 1995). **Frames per second** (FPS), or the **frame rate,** refers to the number of these images that are captured, transmitted, and displayed in one second. The higher the FPS, the smoother the picture. Broadcast quality transmission is 30 FPS. Lower FPS rates produce marginally acceptable video that may be suitable for purposes other than interpretation of diagnostic images. Many DTV systems do not offer broadcast quality at this time. Bandwidth, the efficiency of compression, and hardware and software limitations all determine videoconference frame rates. Another issue related to frame rate is the delay that is noted for one videoconferencing party to respond to another. Although this period is only a few seconds long, it must be factored into teleconferences. Another issue related to resolution is the need to digitize x-rays for transmission and storage. For these reasons, teleradiology applications require more costly equipment and telecommunication services.

Health care personnel need to shape the development of technological standards by determining the minimal acceptable standards to ensure quality at the lowest possible costs (Cannavo 1995, Ensminger 1996, McGee and Tangalos 1994). Acceptance of **international standard H.320** for passing audio and video data streams across networks allowed videoconferencing systems from different manufacturers to communicate. H.320 is a standard for the connection and transfer of multimedia data that allows the transmission and reception of image and sound. It supports a wide range of transmission rates. Prior to the adoption of H.320, only systems produced by the same vendor could communicate. Work continues in this area so that continued improvements can be expected. Other important standards for telehealth include the **Digital Image Communication in Medicine (DICOM) standard** and the **Joint Photographic Experts Group (JPEG) compression standard** for digital images. DICOM seeks to promote the communication, storage, and integration of digital image information with other hospital information systems, while JPEG is used to compress images as a means to decrease transmission time and storage requirements.

Most discussions of telehealth include the computer-based patient record (CPR) as a means to make client data readily available and store diagnostic images (Braly 1995). **Picture archiving communications systems (PACS)** are storage systems that permit remote access to diagnostic images at a time convenient to the physician. While PACS technology has been available for a number of years, its early history was troubled. Recent technological improvements make PACS feasible.

TELENURSING

Until recently the number of references noted in the literature relative to telenursing was limited (National Council of State Boards 1996, Yensen

1996), but telenursing has been in existence for decades, using available technology to serve its purposes. For example, the telephone has long been used as a communication tool between nurses and health care consumers as well as other professionals. As new technology became available it was also adapted to educate consumers and peers, maintain professional contacts, and provide care to clients at other sites. As a result, nurses currently use telephones, faxes, computers, teleconferences, and the Internet in the practice of telenursing. Potential applications are varied, but common uses are telephone triage, follow-up calls, and checking biometric measurements. Other examples include education, professional consultations, obtaining test results, and taking physician instructions over the phone. Interactive television or teleconferences enable home health nurses to make electronic house calls to clients in their homes; thus nurses can see more clients per day than would be possible via on-site visits. Another instance of telenursing is the Telenurse project in Europe, which seeks to standardize the mechanism for describing and communicating nursing care as a means to enable comparisons of nursing practice from one site to another without regard to region or country.

The International TeleNurses Association (ITNA) was founded in 1995 to promote and support nursing involvement in telehealth and serve as a resource for nurses. There is also an electronic magazine for telephone nursing called *Telephone Nursing Telezine*. While practice standards have not yet been developed for telenursing, the American Nurses Association published their Core Principles on Telehealth in 1999. These guidelines are intended to help nurses to protect client privacy during the delivery of telehealth services (Chaffee 1999, American Nurses Association 1999).

Future Development

Many providers expect that telehealth will revolutionize health care (Brown 1995, Ensminger 1996, McGee and Tangalos 1994, Perednia and Allen 1995). It does promise to improve the speed and accuracy of communicating medical information. Telehealth will continue to grow and become commonplace as technical, reimbursement, and legal barriers are removed. It will facilitate the move from health maintenance to health promotion, and improve the quality of care delivered.

The Federal Communications Commission (FCC) Advisory Committee on Telecommunications and Health Care calls for an expansion of telehealth applications and recommends the following measures to facilitate its growth:

- Higher bandwidth services
- Funding for higher bandwidth services to rural areas
- The creation of a joint advisory committee consisting of representatives of the FDA, FCC, and Department of Health and Human Ser-

vices to share information related to standards and interoperability of equipment

- The creation of an international working group to promote international telehealth

Additional measures include real-time transmission of video for consultation use; direct transmission of client information to hospitals from remote devices in homes; virtual surgery for teaching purposes, data mining of records for educational, diagnostic, and/or cost–benefit analysis; and equipment control through virtual reality. Demands for cost containment will move telehealth increasingly into the community and long-term care facilities, with greater involvement required from nurses. Effective telehealth will improve the abilities of mid-level practitioners such as nurse practitioners and physician assistants to provide care to underserved populations. Telehealth will also permit more individuals to be monitored at home, avoiding hospital stays. Eventually remote adjustments in oxygen therapy, patient-controlled analgesia (PCA) pumps, and other equipment will become commonplace.

CASE STUDY EXERCISES

You are the nurse practitioner in St. Theresa's emergency department. A client is brought in with obvious psychiatric problems. You have no psychiatrist available and the nearest psychiatric facility is a 1-hour drive away. St. Theresa is a Tri-State Health Care Alliance Member. Tri-State has telehealth links with the regional hospital, where a psychiatrist is in the emergency department. What steps would you take to initiate a productive teleconference? Justify your response.

•   •   •

Erin O'Shell, home health nurse, just set up teleconference equipment for Dr. Bobby to evaluate Mr. Richard Goldstein for possible hospitalization for congestive heart failure. Dr. Bobby and the hospital are a 1-hour drive away. Just as the teleconference started, but before Dr. Bobby could listen to Mr. Goldstein's lungs or complete other key portions of the exam, a power outage severed the teleconference link. How should Ms. O'Shell handle this situation? Provide your rationale.

SUMMARY

- Telehealth is the use of telecommunication technologies and computers to provide medical information and services to clients at another location.
- *Telehealth* is a broad term that encompasses telemedicine but in-

cludes the provision of care and the distribution of information to health care providers and consumers.

- Efforts to contain costs and improve the delivery of care to all segments of the population make telehealth an attractive tool. Telehealth can help health care providers treat clients earlier when they are not as ill and care costs less, provide services in the local community where it is less expensive, improve follow-up care, and improve client access to services.

- Telehealth applications vary greatly and include client monitoring, diagnostic evaluation, decision support and expert systems, storage and dissemination of records, and education of health care professionals.

- Teleconferencing and videoconferencing are tools that facilitate the delivery of telehealth services.

- Desktop videoconferencing (DTV) is an important development that enables the expansion of telehealth applications into new areas. DTV uses specially adapted personal computers to link persons at two or more sites.

- Telenursing uses telecommunications and computer technology for the delivery of nursing care and services to clients at other sites.

- Despite limited references in the literature, telenursing is not new. Its applications include education of health care consumers and nurses as well as the provision of care. In addition to the use of the telephone for triage and information, clients may be monitored at home via telephone or teleconferences. Telenursing is a tool that helps nurses to work more efficiently.

- Major issues associated with the practice of telehealth and telenursing include reimbursement, licensure, technical support, liability, and safeguards for client privacy and confidentiality.

- The successful use of telehealth and telenursing is best ensured through the development and implementation of a plan that addresses current services and deficits, goals, technical requirements, compliance with standards and laws, reimbursement, and strategies to handle telecommunication breakdowns.

- Telehealth and telenursing applications are expected to become more commonplace as licensure and technical barriers are removed.

REFERENCES

American Nurses Association. (1999). *Core principles on telehealth*. Washington, DC: American Nurses Publishing.

Betts, M. (1994). Doctors get HELP to fight infections: Expert system at LDS Hospital assists doctors with selection of best antibiotics for patients. *Computerworld, 28*(23), 67.

Braly, D. (1995). Remote image access expands services. *Health Management Technology, 16*(12), 20+.

Brennan, P. (October 1996). *Nursing informatics: Technology in the service of patient care*. Paper presented at the meeting of Alpha Rho Chapter of Sigma Theta Tau, Morgantown, WV.

Brewin, B. (1995). Expo showcases move toward digitized force. *Federal Computer Week, 9*(31), 20+.

Brown, J. (28 August 1995). Running with a winning team: VARs are captaining corporate America's embrace of collaborative solutions. *Computer Reseller News*, S6+.

Bulkeley, D. (1995). Teleconferencing turns city slicker into country doctor. *Government Computer News, 14*(9), 44.

Burns, P. (1999). Telehealth or telehype? Some observations and thoughts on the current status and future of telehealth. *Journal of Healthcare Information Management, 13*(4, Suppl), 1–10.

Cannavo, M. (1995). Fastest is always best and other PACS fallacies. *Health Management Technology, 16*(12), 27+.

Chaffee, M. (1999). A telehealth odyssey. *American Journal of Nursing, 99*(7), 26–32.

Chin, T. L. (1996). Solving a rural hospital problem. *Health Data Management, 4*(11), 33–36.

Condon, R. (1995). Manager's bulletin board. *InfoWorld, 17*(39), 96.

Dam, K., and Lin, H. (1996). *Cryptography's role in securing the information society*. A report of the Committee to Study National Cryptography Policies. Washington, DC: National Academy Press.

D'Amico, M. (1995). Mythical computer curmudgeons. *Digital Media, 5*(4), 25+.

Dansky, K. H., Bowles, K. H., and Britt, T. (1999). Nurses' responses to telemedicine in home healthcare. *Journal of Healthcare Information Management, 13*(4), 27–38.

Davis, A. W. (1996). Remote control medicine: VARs help doctors make house calls. *Reseller Management, 19*(7), 170–174.

Ensminger, P. A. (3 April 1996). Telehealth. On the Web at: *http://www.npac.syr.edu/users/ensminger/TMED.html#issue1*.

Green, R. (1995). Joint readiness training reaches beyond boundaries. *Government Computer News, 14*(14), 68+.

Gustke, S. S., Balch, D. C., West, V. L., and Rogers, L. O. (2000). Patient satisfaction with telemedicine. *Telemedicine Journal, 6*(1), 5–13.

Hatlestad, L. (1996). Videoconferencing system offers TV quality video on LANs. *InfoWorld, 18*(11), 45.

Holmes, P. (December 1994). Hypermedia, desktop conferencing and PACs. *EuroPACS Newsletter* [On-line], *9*, pp. 1–6. On the Web at: *http://www.bazis.nl/research-dept/europacs/article-holmes.html*.

Karon, P. (1996). Videoconferencing tools are finally ready for prime time. *InfoWorld, 18*(11), 67.

Lutkowitz, M. (1995). CATV providers: Can they succeed with business users? *Telecommunications, 29*(6), 27+.

McGee, R., and Tangalos, E. G. (1994). Delivery of health care to the under-served. *Mayo Clinic Proceedings, 69*(12), 1131–1136.

Montgomery, W. L. (March 1996). Advances in telehealth. *Healthcare Informatics, 12*(3), 91.

National Council of State Boards of Nursing, Inc. (1996). Telenursing: The regulatory implications for multistate regulation [On-line]. *Issues, 17*(3). On the Web at: *http://www.ncsbn.org/pfiles/issues/vol173/telenurs173.html.*

Nelson, R. (1999). Building telehealth communities and exploiting the possibilities. *Journal of Healthcare Information Management, 13*(4), 1–3.

NIIT demos national high-speed medical network infrastructure. (1994). *OSINetter Newsletter, 9*(10), 6.

Office of Public Information. (8 October 1996). National telehealth initiative. On the Web at: *http://www.nlm.nih.gov/new_noteworthy/press_releases/telemed.html.*

Perednia, D. A. (9 May 1995). Telehealth: Remote access to health services and information. In *Bringing health care on-line: The role of information technologies,* pp. 1–41. On the Web at: *http://www.acl.lanl.gov/sunrise/Medical/ota/09ch5.txt.*

Perednia, D. A., and Allen, A. (1995). Telehealth technology and clinical applications. *Journal of the American Medical Association, 273*(6), 483–488.

Robinson, T. (10 July 1995). Medical center prescribes healthy dose of networked computing. *CommunicationsWeek,* 47.

Rural America gets Infobahn. (1995). *Government Computer News, 14*(22), 18+.

Sandberg, L. (1995a). Legal and policy issues challenge telehealth. *Health Management Technology, 16*(13), 30+.

Sandberg, L. (1995b). Techno jargon: A telecom technology primer. *Health Management Technology, 16*(10), 31(2).

Schneider, P. (1996). Washington word: Telecom reform. *Healthcare Informatics, 12*(3), 93.

Silver, J. (1995). States take the initiative in getting programs on the road. *Government Computer News, 14*(21), 54.

Sirota, W. J. (1995). Desktop videoconferencing: Voice, vision, reality. *The Workgroup Computing Report, 18*(5), 19+.

Siwicki, B. (1996a). Have a heart. *Health Data Management, 4*(10), 62, 64.

Siwicki, B. (1996b). Reading tissues from a distance. *Health Data Management, 4*(10), 66, 68.

Siwicki, B. (1996c). Bringing medical expertise to the desktop. *Health Data Management, 4*(10), 55–58, 60.

Slipy, S. M. (1995). Telehealth and interconnection services reduce costs at several facilities. *Health Management Technology, 16*(8), 52+.

Staino, P. A. (1995). The big picture: Videoconferencing today—seeing is believing. *Teleconnect, 13*(5), 79(5).

Stone, T. H. (1999). Patient health information confidentiality in telehealth applications. *Journal of Healthcare Information Management, 13*(4), 79–88.

Telemedicine helps Texas prison inmates. (24 July 1995). *Newsbytes,* pNEW07240001.

Telemedicine Research Center. (9 October 1996). History of telemedicine. *Telemedicine Information Exchange.* On the Web at: *http://tie.telemed.org/scripts/getpage.pl?client=text&age=history.*

To your health. (1995). *Computer Letter, 11*(32), 1+.

Troubled waters. (1997). *Nursing 97, 27*(2), 10.

User tips: 9 steps to more effective teleconferences. (1996). *Communication News, 33*(10), 72.

Weaver, C. (Spring 1996). HIS in Australia: A view from down under. *Advances,* 14–16.

Weinberg, N. (1995). Hospitals call ATM good medicine. *Computerworld, 29*(49), 20.

Yensen, J. (1996). Telenursing: Virtual nursing and beyond. *Computers in Nursing, 14*(4), 213–214.

Zurier, S. (1995). Telehealth is bringing electronic doctors closer. *Government Computer News, 14*(21), 56+.

18

Research

After completing this chapter, you should be able to:

- Describe ways that computers can support all steps of the research process.
- Discuss the advantages of computerized literature searches over manual methods.
- Identify several well-known statistical analysis software programs.
- Relate the significance of computational nursing models for future health care delivery.
- Name several impediments to health care research.
- Discuss the anticipated effects of increased automation and the computer-based patient record (CPR) on research efforts.
- Explain how students in health care professions may reap the benefits of research tools.

C omputer use in nursing research was once limited to data analysis (Ryan and Nagle 1994). However, increased access to computers and the availability of software packages in the workplace, schools, and at home now make research feasible for nurses in many settings and facilitate the process from start to finish. Fortunately, this phenomenon coincides with a growing need to use research findings to justify actions in health care education and in the administration and direct provision of health care. Research provides data that allows better allocation of scarce resources and supports knowledge development, which in turn enhances the theoretical underpinnings of nursing. Box 18–1 summarizes some ways that computers facilitate the research process.

USING COMPUTERS TO SUPPORT RESEARCH

Computers can assist with every phase of the research process from beginning to end. This is equally true for the student conducting informal research for a class assignment, the staff nurse seeking information about a particular client's diagnosis and treatment, and the nurse researcher embarking upon a funded study. All health care professionals should be aware of how computers can support them in their educational endeavors, clinical practice, and research.

Identification of Research Topics

Constant changes in health care and the health care delivery system make it difficult to keep up with the latest findings and identify areas in need of further research. On-line discussion groups and communities and publication of research findings help solve this problem. The NURSERES listserv group, at *listserv@listserv.kent.edu*, is a discussion list for nurse researchers. There are also discussion groups for specialty practice areas,

Box 18–1	Computer Applications That Support Nursing Research

- *Topic identification.* On-line literature searches, research reports, e-mail, on-line communities, and discussion groups can be used to identify areas in need of research.

- *On-line and CD-ROM literature searches.* Electronic searches enable the researcher to identify prior research in the area as well as articles pertaining to the theoretical framework for proposed studies.

- *Full text retrieval of articles.* This eliminates the need to physically locate journals and photocopy them.

- *Development of resource files.* Computer files that take the place of index cards and handwritten notes may be searched quickly, allowing researchers to spend valuable time performing research and writing reports instead of performing clerical tasks.

- *Selection or development and revision of a data collection tool.* On-line literature searches help researchers locate developed data collection tools. If no suitable tool is found, researchers can develop their own tool using a word processing package and trial it by sending it out via e-mail or the Web.

- *Preparation of the grant/study proposal.* Word processing aids the writing process because revisions can be made quickly.

- *Budget preparation and maintenance.* Spreadsheets and financial planning software assist with this process.

- *Determination of appropriate sample size.* The ability to generalize study findings is related to the size of the sample. Power analysis is the process by which an appropriate sample size may be determined. Software is available for this purpose.

- *Data collection.* Computers aid in the collection of data in several ways. Data may be input into a computer through scanned questionnaires, direct entry of field observations, or the use of an on-line data collection tool.

- *Database utilization.* Databases allow organization and manipulation of collected data.

- *Statistical analysis/qualitative text analysis.* Statistical analysis software performs complex computations, while qualitative text analysis allows searches for particular words and phrases in text, noting frequency of appearance and context.

- *Preparation of the research findings for report.* Word processing and graphics programs enable researchers to present their findings without the need for clerical assistance or graphic artists.

- *Electronic dissemination of findings.* On-line journals, Web pages, and e-mail permit researchers to share their findings quickly. This contrasts with the traditional publication of study findings in print media that might take a year or more from the time of submission until distribution.

SOURCE: Adapted from "Computers and nursing research in acute care settings," by J. A. DePalma (1994), and from "Computer support for power analysis in nursing research," by S. M. Paul (1994). In S. J. Grobe and E. S. P. Pluyter-Wenting (Eds.). *Nursing Informatics: An International Overview for Nursing in a Technological Era, Proceedings of the Fifth IMIA International Conference on Nursing Uses of Computers and Information Science*, with kind permission from Elsevier Science-NL, Sara Burgerhartstraat 25, 1055 K.V. Amsterdam, The Netherlands. Also adapted from "Nurses' Computer-Mediated Communications on NURSENET," by P. J. Murray (1996).

education, and informatics. Appendix C lists several such groups. Timely and ongoing studies allow health care educators, providers, agencies, and alliances to find trends in information and react to market changes proactively. Box 18–2 lists a few suggested health care informatics topics for research based on reading and discussions with health care professionals.

Literature Searches

The primary databases for searching nursing literature are the Cumulative Index for Nursing and Allied Health Literature (CINAHL) and Medline. Both are available in health care libraries in either CD-ROM or on-line form. Literature searches may also be conducted over the Internet. Both the CD-ROM and on-line versions of CINAHL and Medline allow users to enter their search subjects and then narrow the search by language, journal subset, and publication year. For example, users can limit a search to nursing journals and/or research reports. These features allow potential researchers to quickly determine whether research has been conducted in their area of interest and peruse the reported findings. The user may view article abstracts with both CINAHL and Medline. In some cases full text article retrieval is available with on-line searches. Box

---

Box 18–2   **Suggested Health Care Informatics Research Topics**

Attitudes toward computers

- Student/health care provider concepts of health care informatics
- Staff attitudes

Clinical data

- Development and efficacy of acuity and classification systems
- Use of point-of-care
- The impact of informatics on clients, nursing, and nurses
- Critical pathway and database development and use, including outcome assessment
- Expert systems, decision trees and support, and artificial intelligence and knowledge engineering
- Client education
- Quality assurance
- International classifications for nursing practice and work in other countries

Education

- Effectiveness of computer-assisted and/or Web-based instruction (CAI)
- Computerized testing

Box 18–3   **Pros and Cons of On-Line Literature Searches**

Pros

- Searches may be completed quickly.
- Searches may be done without the aid of a librarian.
- Searches may be limited to specific years, languages, or journal subsets.
- Searches may be general or limited to requesting research reports.
- On-line abstracts allow researchers to quickly determine if a particular article suits their purpose.
- When available, full text retrieval allows the researcher to obtain articles without searching for volumes on a shelf or waiting for copies to arrive from other sites.

Cons

- Searches require a basic level of comfort with computers.
- The person conducting the search must be able to narrow the topic area.
- Search results are directly related to the selection of search terms. Poor selection of terms may falsely indicate no or few articles on a given topic or provide an overwhelming number of articles of limited use.
- Researchers may need the services of a librarian to start the programs and for assistance with search terms and limiters.
- On-line searches may not entirely eliminate the need to locate volumes and photocopy articles or wait for copies to arrive from other libraries unless full text retrieval is available.

18–3 summarizes a few advantages and disadvantages associated with on-line literature searches. Figure 18–1 displays a printout obtained from a CINAHL search.

Data Collection Tools

Data collection tools may be located via CD-ROM or on-line literature searches and discussion lists. The use of an existing data collection tool offers the researcher the benefits of established validity and consistency, and the ability to commence research sooner without spending time to devise and test an instrument. A **data collection tool** is a device that has been created for the purpose of accumulating specific details in an organized fashion. Some examples include a physical assessment form, a graphics record, and opinion questionnaires. Once a suitable tool is found, permission for its use often may be obtained more quickly through e-mail than through traditional mail. In the event that a suitable tool is not located, the construction of a data collection tool via word processing software makes revision easy, while on-line construction yields immediate feedback.

Once the data collection instrument is constructed, discussion lists may be used to solicit study participants, and even as a means to collect data. E-mail interviews may also be used to collect research data (Murray 1996). E-mail allows varying degrees of structure in the interview process, as well as ease of transcription via downloading without interpretation error secondary to pauses and inflection. Other options for data collection include the use of **computer-assisted self-interview soft-**

Go to ... Help | Logoff

☐**Citation 3**

Accession Number
  2000019976.
Special Fields Contained
  Fields available in this record: abstract, cited references.
Authors
  Payne J.
Institution
  University of New Mexico Cancer **Research** and Treatment
  Center, Albuquerque.
Title
  Nursing perspectives. The Nursing Interventions Classification: a language to
  define nursing.
Source
  Oncology Nursing Forum, 27(1):99-103, 2000 Jan-Feb. (13 ref)
Abbreviated Source
  ONCOL NURS FORUM. 27(1):99-103, 2000 Jan-Feb. (13 ref)
Document Delivery
  NLM Serial Identifier: O06740000.
Journal Subset
  Core Nursing Journals. Nursing Journals. Peer Reviewed Journals. USA
  Journals.
Special Interest Category
  Oncologic Care
Local Messages
  Current AGH HSL subscription, since 1984. Fiche 1984-1989.
Cinahl Subject Headings
  Association of Pediatric Oncology Nurses
  *Iowa Nursing Interventions Classification
  Nursing Informatics
  *Oncologic Nursing
  Oncology Nursing Society
Abstract
  PURPOSE/OBJECTIVES: To discuss the Nursing Interventions Classification (NIC) framework
  and its relationship to oncology nursing. **DATA SYNTHESIS:** NIC is a standardized language that
  identifies all interventions performed by nurses. The three-tiered taxonomy consists of six domains,
  27 classes, and 433 interventions with related nursing activities. Each intervention consists of a
  label describing the concept, the definition of the concept, and a set of representative activities or
  actions. **CONCLUSIONS:** Although differences exist in the core interventions identified by the
  Oncology Nursing Society and the Association of Pediatric Oncology Nurses as critical to their
  practice, the NIC **research** team, after surveying both organizations, found numerous similarities in
  the possibilities for clinical application. **IMPLICATIONS FOR NURSING PRACTICE:** NIC
  provides a standardized language to enable oncology nurses to describe and demonstrate their work
  and contributions to lawmakers, healthcare policy makers, and the public. (13 ref)
ISSN
  0190-535X
Publication Type
  Journal Article. Tables/Charts.
Language
  English.
Entry Month

FIGURE 18–1 • Results of a CINAHL Search. Extracts from the CINAHL® database reprinted by kind permission of Cinahl Information Systems, Glendale, California, telephone (818) 409-8005 ext. 4483.

200003
Cited References

Boyle D. New identities: The changing profile of patients with cancer, their families, and their professional caregivers. Oncology Nursing Forum 1994; 21, 55-61.

Cooley M, Lin E, Hunter S. The ambulatory oncology nurse's role. Seminars in Oncology Nursing 1994; 10, 245-253.

Engelking C. New approaches: Innovations in cancer prevention, diagnosis, treatment, and support. Oncology Nursing Forum 1994; 21, 62-67.

Henry SB, Holzemer WL, Randell C, Hsieh SF, Miller TJ. Comparison of nursing interventions classification and current procedural terminology codes for categorizing nursing activities. Image: Journal of Nursing Scholarship 1997; 29, 133-138.

Iowa Intervention Project Team. The NIC taxonomy structure. Image: Journal of Nursing Scholarship 1993; 25, 187-192.

Krebs L, Myers J, Decker G, Kinzler J, Asfahani P, Jackson J. The oncology nursing image: Lifting the mist. Oncology Nursing Forum 1996; 23, 1297-1304.

McCloskey J, Bulechek G (Eds). Nursing interventions classification. St. Louis: Mosby Yearbook; 1992.

McCloskey J, Bulechek G. Standardizing the language for nursing treatments: An overview of the issues. Nursing Outlook 1994; 42(2), 56-63.

McCloskey J, Bulechek G (Eds). Nursing interventions classification (2nd ed). St. Louis: Mosby Yearbook; 1996.

McCloskey J, Bulechek G, Donahue W. Nursing interventions core to specialty practice. Nursing Outlook 1998; 46(2), 67-76.

Rakel B. Interventions related to patient teaching. Nursing Clinics of North America 1992; 27, 397-423.

Simons M. Interventions related to compliance. Nursing Clinics of North America 1992; 27, 477-494.

Steelman V, Bulechek G, McCloskey J. Toward a standardized language to describe perioperative nursing. AORN Journal 1994; 60, 786-790, 793-795.

FIGURE 18–1 • Continued

ware (CASI) and data collection tools on the Internet. CASI has been successfully used to interview clients on highly personal behavior. An example of CASI use is the survey done by Jones and Jedrasik (2000) on sexual behavior of clients. These researchers augmented CASI with digitally recorded audio to allow clients with varying degrees of literacy to see and hear questions as a means to improve their overall response, while providing them privacy. Data collection via the Internet can offer several advantages (Houston and Fiore 1998). These can include

- Interactive forms that can be evaluated for completeness and accuracy of data prior to submission
- Automated data compilation and exportation to other software
- Fast, cost-effective administration of surveys

The single biggest disadvantage associated with the Internet as a modal-

Box 18–4	Tips for Design and Administration of Web-Based Data Collection Tools

- Determine the objectives for the tool.
- Write then edit the questions.
- Include the title, introduction, purpose of the tool, and an anonymity statement.
- Critique the tool for reading level.
- Ensure that the tool is visually attractive.
- Limit the amount of information on a page.
- Ask evaluators to rate the tool for readability and time required for completion as well as their suggestions.
- Test the automated data collection process prior to public posting.
- Pretest the tool prior to public posting.
- Include a few open-ended questions, and provide a wrap-up.

ity for data collection is that it is still not widely available to some populations. Box 18–4 provides some suggestions for the design and administration of Web-based data collection tools.

Data Analysis

Data analysis is the processing of data collected during the course of a study to identify trends and patterns of relationships. This task begins with descriptive statistics in quantitative, and some qualitative, studies. Descriptive statistics permit the researcher to organize the data in meaningful ways that facilitate insight (Burns and Grove 1997). Theory development and the generation of hypotheses may emerge from descriptive analysis. In addition to descriptive analysis, there are a number of statistical procedures that a researcher must choose when conducting a study. Until recently, researchers embarking upon large studies needed the services of statisticians and large computing centers for data analysis. Many practitioners and students in the health care professions felt they were unable to perform meaningful research without these supports. Personal computers now rival larger systems in abilities and can easily link with larger computers, making it easier to conduct research in any setting.

In recent years there has been a growing recognition that the huge amounts of data collected within health care systems might be better used and tapped for a variety of purposes (DeGruy 2000). The overwhelming volume of data requires computer processing to turn data into useful information. A variety of terms exist to refer to the use and processing of this data. **Knowledge discovery in databases (KDD)** is a term that has been used in other industries. KDD identifies complex patterns and relationships in collected data. It provides a powerful tool suitable for the analysis of large amounts of data. Commercial packages are available in a range of prices and platforms. KDD may be used to identify risk factors for diseases or efficacy of particular treatment modalities. A more popular term seen in recent literature is **data mining.** Data mining is the use of database applications to look for previously hidden patterns. In general terms data mining may be considered a tool of KDD.

Quantitative Analysis The computational abilities of computers readily lend themselves to statistical analysis of qualitative data and render more accurate results than might be available from hand-calculated statistics. Several software packages are available for quantitative analysis (Wegman et al. 1996). Most evolved during the 1960s and 1970s and permit the importation of data from spreadsheet or database software, and sometimes ASCII files. The majority provide versions of their products for a variety of computer platforms. A partial list follows:

- The SAS System for Statistical Analysis comprises several products for the management and analysis of data. It is considered an industry standard.

- MINITAB Statistical Software offers an alternative to SAS. Geared to users at every level, it is widely used by high school and college students and incorporates pull-down menus for ease of use.

- BMDP evolved as a biomedical analysis package. It comes in personal and professional editions and offers an easy-to-use interface for data analysis. BMDP also prompts the user until analysis is complete. It offers a comprehensive library of statistical routines.

- SPSS is another well-known software company. SPSS provides products for most computer platforms. SPSS provides statistics, graphics, and data management and reporting capabilities.

- S-Plus is known for its flexibility in allowing users to define and customize functions. It also offers extensive graphics.

- SYSTAT, unlike the packages discussed above, was first developed for PC use. It is now available through SPSS.

- DataDesk is a Mac product.

- JMP started as a Mac product and resembles DataDesk. It is now available for use on PCs as well.

Other available packages offer statistical capability, although many are primarily mathematical applications.

Despite the increased use of statistical analysis packages by nurses, some researchers still argue that nurses should work with the traditional users of supercomputers to develop skills needed to use these resources and to access large data archives held by government and private agencies (Meintz 1994). Supercomputers offer the ability to peruse huge databases quickly. This belief gives rise to a new branch of nursing science, nurmetrics. **Nurmetrics** uses mathematical form and statistics to test, estimate, and quantify nursing theories and solutions to problems.

Computer Models **Computational nursing,** a branch of nurmetrics, uses models and simulation for the application of existing theory and numerical methods to new solutions for nursing problems, or the development of new computational methods (Meintz 1994). One proposed use of nurmetrics and computational nursing is the formulation and testing of new models for health care delivery by using computers. This application is cost effective and can demonstrate how factors such as education may affect health practices and outcomes over time without the need to first implement the program and wait for results. Nursing informatics employs computer science and informatics principles to understand how the structure and function of information may be used to solve problems in nursing administration, nursing education, practice, and research. Both graphical user interfaces (GUIs) and global data analysis facilitate modeling and simulation.

Qualitative Analysis Computers also aid the organized storage, tabulation, and retrieval of qualitative data (Pilkington 1996). For example, databases can be used like electronic filing cabinets to store data; software can locate key words or phrases in a database, sort data in a prescribed fashion, code observations or comments for later retrieval, support researcher notes, and help create and represent conceptual schemes. As notes, coding, sorting, and pasting are automated, researchers have more time to analyze data. Despite these benefits, critics cite the following dangers:

- Qualitative research may be molded to fit the computer program.
- Computers tempt researchers to use large populations, thus sacrificing in-depth study for breadth.

Two examples of software applications for qualitative text analysis include Textbase Alpha and AQUAD ("SIByl Program information" 1995). Textbase Alpha is geared for beginners and has no special formatting requirements for imported text. It is designed for descriptive and interpretative analysis. AQUAD is a specialized program for users with an advanced knowledge of qualitative research. Text must first be entered or scanned into a word processor and converted into ASCII. AQUAD permits coding on the screen and researchers may define linkages they wish to explore. Words or phrases in text and their frequency may be noted.

Data Presentation: Graphics

Once data analysis is complete, graphics presentation software helps the researcher put study findings into a form that is easy for the reader to

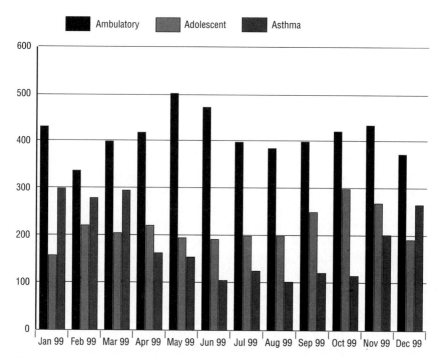

FIGURE 18–2 • **Bar Graph Depicting the Number of Clinic Visits per Month for January 1999 Through December 1999**

follow in written study reports and for the listener to follow when findings are presented at professional meetings and conferences (DePalma 1994). Graphics presentation software allows the researcher to design and make slides for use at presentations without the services of a media department. Harvard Graphics and PowerPoint are two well-known commercial packages. Figure 18–2 shows a bar graph prepared using a graphics application.

Computer-Aided Research in Nursing (CARIN)

Computer software can aid the research process and potentially channel data collected from clinical systems into databases according to defined study protocols and for future research. Computer-aided research also facilitates student learning. An example of this was seen with a computer program that was developed to help graduate students improve assessment skills and identify appropriate nursing diagnosis by completing an automated assessment guide at the bedside (Hirsch, Chang, and Gilbert 1989). Students submitted their assessment data for faculty review and comment. This effort was part of the larger CARIN (computer-aided research in nursing) effort. CARIN has been used subsequently to collect and download data about the probability of a nursing diagnosis given the presence of one or more defining characteristics (Chang 1993). This method could be applied to other databases and settings as well.

On-Line Access to Databases

The National Institutes of Health (NIH) offers access to several databases useful to nurses interested in research, health policy, and the identification of funded research projects (Bair et al. 1996). One of these databases, the Computer Retrieval of Information on Scientific Projects (CRISP), provides information on research grants supported by government agencies. CRISP lists the following data for each project: title, grant number, abstract, principal investigator, thesaurus terms, and key words. CRISP is available on CD-ROM and on the Web at *http://www.nih.gov/grants*. Search results may be printed or saved to disk.

Several other agencies provide on-line databases useful to nurse researchers (Prohaska and Chang 1996). These include the following:

- The National Library of Medicine (NLM) at Web site *http://www.nlm.nih.gov*.

- NursingCenter.com at Web site *http://www.nursingcenter.com/resources/index.cfm*.

- Sigma Theta Tau's Virginia Henderson International Nursing Library (INL). The INL provides information on nurse researchers, meeting proceedings, and access to databases that pertain to nursing research.

Box 18–5 lists some other sources to consider when seeking research funds.

IMPEDIMENTS TO HEALTH CARE RESEARCH

Nursing and health care presently lack information required to deliver more effective health care at a lower cost (Amatayakul 1995, Frawley 1995, Murphy 1994). The computer-based patient record (CPR) will help to provide the database needed to accomplish this feat. The CPR will change the way in which information is collected and used and will help to ensure the survival of enterprises that have CPR capability. Unfortunately, the CPR does not yet exist. In the meantime, automated health care providers can accrue some benefits by tracking information on an ongoing basis and noting emerging patterns. Costs containment may be achieved by decreasing operating expenses, eliminating duplication, and improving quality of care. Client care can be improved by making clinical and financial data available for individual and aggregate profiles and outcome assessments.

Impediments to the realization of the CPR as a source of data to improve health care include competition among health care providers, a lack of common language or data elements, and unresolved technical issues. Hospital mergers and affiliations foster the sharing of data. Compe-

Box 18–5 **Possible Funding Sources for Nursing Research**

Government Agencies
- National Institutes of Health
- National Institute of Nursing Research
- National Library of Medicine
- Substance Abuse and Mental Health Services Administration
- Centers for Disease Control and Prevention
- Food and Drug Administration
- Agency for Health Care Policy and Research

Professional Organizations
- Sigma Theta Tau
- American Nurses Association
- Oncology Nursing Foundation
- Specialty Groups

Foundations and Organizations
- Robert Wood Johnson Foundation
- Skin Cancer Foundation
- Epilepsy Foundation
- Myasthenia Gravis Foundation
- American Cancer Society
- March of Dimes
- Arthritis Foundation

tition does not. This presents an obstacle to the creation of large databases required to accurately find trends in health care problems and successful treatment options.

Unified Language Efforts

The lack of a common language to facilitate data collection and decision making was recognized as a problem in nursing several years ago (Daly et al. 1997). The **Unified Medical Language System** project represents an attempt to standardize terms used in health care delivery. The American Nurses Association has a database steering committee that is working on the **Unified Nursing Language System** as a means to develop and use other clinical databases that will extend nursing knowledge. This committee approved the inclusion of the Nursing Interventions Classification (NIC) and its linkage to the North American Nursing Diagnosis Association (NANDA) diagnoses for inclusion in the Unified Nursing Language System.

At present, the **Uniform Hospital Data Set (UHDS)** is the most commonly used data set in the United States, but it does not include data on nursing care and outcomes (Delaney et al. 1994, Ryan et al. 1994, Sheil and Wierenga 1994). The **Nursing Minimum Data Set (NMDS)** has been defined as a consistent collection of data comprising nursing diagnoses, nursing interventions, nursing outcomes, intensity of care, and demographic and service elements. The NMDS was devised as a means to

• Collect essential and comparable nursing data across different health care settings
• Describe care
• Demonstrate or project trends for care and allocation of resources
• Stimulate nursing research through links to data existing in hospital information systems

Despite efforts to arrive at a common nursing language, several vocabularies and classification schemes exist. The American Nurses Association's Congress of Nursing Practice Steering Committee on Data-bases supports the use of multiple vocabularies and classification schemes as a means to support the diversity in nursing practice ("ANA revises criteria" 1996). This body also advocates the development of links, or mapping of similar terms, among the different schemes and vocabularies. All schemes must be clinically useful and stated in unambiguous terms, and have an associated unique identifier that leaves a machine-readable audit trail. Box 18–6 lists some databases that support nursing practice.

In addition to facilitating data collection, a uniform language will set the definition of key terms, thus ensuring that studies can be replicated. Implementation of uniform language first requires the following (Daly et al. 1997):

• Education of staff who are unfamiliar with standardized terms
• Elimination of computer restraints, such as limited characters and lines per field found with some computer systems
• Database coordination among various clinicians and departments who use terms differently but require access to shared data repositories
• A strategy to code responses when using Nursing Intervention Classifications, given that there is no uniform number of activities per intervention

Multi-Institutional Research

Automation and a uniform language also aid the collection of data from multiple sources simultaneously. At present this capability is limited to health care alliances that can, and already do, share data. This feature will become more important once the CPR is realized. Multi-institutional re-

Box 18–6 Some Databases That Support Nursing

OMAHA

- Model for capturing, sorting, and analyzing client data
- Used as a component of Nursing Minimum Data Set (NMDS)
- Represents community health nursing
- Consists of problem classification scheme, intervention scheme, and problem rating scale for outcomes
- Represents a step in transforming data into information and information into knowledge
- Provides ability to describe client population and level of service provided

North American Nursing Diagnosis Association (NANDA)

- Classification system for nursing diagnosis
- Establishes a common language for client problems
- Gives diagnostic label, contributing factors, and signs and symptoms
- Each diagnostic category is defined
- Each diagnostic category lists major and minor defining characteristics
- Major defining characteristics must be present to validate use of the diagnosis

Nursing Interventions Classification (NIC)

- Three-level taxonomy of nursing interventions
- Domains and classes help care providers locate interventions most appropriate for their clients
- Provides a structure that can be numerically coded for computer use and data manipulation
- Standardizes language as a means to facilitate decision making and cost determinations

SOURCE: Adapted from "The Omaha System: A Model for Nursing Care Information Systems," by K. S. Martin (1994). In S. J. Grobe and E. S. P. Pluyter-Wenting (Eds.), *Nursing Informatics: An International Overview for Nursing in a Technological Era, Proceedings of the Fifth IMIA International Conference on Nursing Use of Computing and Information Science,* with kind permission from Elsevier Science-NL, Sara Burgerhartstraat 25, 1055 KV Amsterdam, The Netherlands. Also adapted from "The NIC taxonomy structure," by J. McCloskey and G. Bulecheck (1993). *Image: Journal of Nursing Scholarship, 25*(3), 187–192; reprinted by permission of Sigma Theta Tau International.

search offers researchers the opportunity to increase the size of their study populations and eliminate idiosyncrasies associated with a particular place as a contributing factor to the findings. In short, multi-institutional research ensures that findings can be applied to a larger population.

Research in Real Time

The potential of hospital information systems to collect large amounts of data almost instantly allows for research in "real time," or essentially as events occur. This ability helps institutions react quickly to changes noted in client populations. Some systems can perform routine work while automatically channeling study information into an appropriate database according to particular study protocols. This is a desirable feature that would eliminate redundant data entry; however, at present, few information systems are flexible enough to do this. This lack of flexibility creates the need to collect data that is already available on information systems to be gathered and formated separately each time it is needed for a research study.

Collaborative Research

Collaborative computing and research fosters productivity by allowing individuals at dispersed sites to share ideas and information in real time (Kouzes 1997). Collaborative computing may use e-mail, desktop video-conferencing, other telecommunication tools, or shared databases to join persons of like interests together. The biggest obstacle to collaborative computing and research is the immaturity of some of the tools that are in present use.

STUDENTS USING COMPUTERS FOR RESEARCH

Students in the health care professions often feel that research has little significance for them, and few carry out the entire research process. This is an unfortunate attitude because students can benefit greatly from information accessed via computers. One of the most obvious applications for student use is the electronic literature search. Despite the availability and merits of this type of search, many students claim that they tried and failed to find anything when in fact they did not enter search limiters or appropriate terms. Both CD-ROM and on-line searches yield information that is more current than most of the reference books students use.

A more popular resource is the World Wide Web. It offers a wealth of information for both health care professionals and consumers. It is widely accessible at educational institutions for students who have no home access. It even has sites of particular interest to students in the health care professions. Students might choose to prepare for a community health teaching project by searching for materials on the Web as long as they are attentive to distribution and revision dates.

Students enrolled in research courses may have occasion to use software for statistical analysis, presentation of graphics, and proposal and report preparation. Many texts include software with study questions for mastery of research content.

Despite the fact that computer literacy is an expectation for nursing students, not all students are equally comfortable with computers. For this reason computer skills should be presented early and reinforced as a measure to get students to make good use of computers for research as well as other applications.

CASE STUDY EXERCISES

You are the staff nurse in a busy medical–surgical department at your community hospital. You and several of your colleagues have an idea that client anxiety is decreased in direct proportion to the amount of teaching that they receive preoperatively. Describe how you might use computer applications to look at this issue and prepare a proposal for funding consideration.

• • •

You and your classmates are expected to conduct a health teaching project in a public high school as one of the requirements for your Community Health Nursing course. Identify and discuss resources that you might use to gather material for this project.

• • •

You are working the night shift at your local community hospital. One of your clients was newly diagnosed today with a rare disorder that is unknown to you and your peers. Mrs. Prado is unable to sleep and is asking for more information about her diagnosis. None of the reference books on your unit provide information about her diagnosis. Your unit does, however, have an Internet connection. How might you use resources on hand to meet Mrs. Prado's needs?

SUMMARY

- Research provides data that allows better allocation of scarce resources and supports the development of knowledge.
- Computer applications can aid every facet of nursing research.
- Electronic literature searches, on-line discussion groups, and research reports all assist the potential researcher to identify topics for further study.
- Both CD-ROM and on-line literature searches quickly locate articles and provide abstracts. Full text retrieval is available with some on-line searches.
- Data collection instruments may be located, developed, and even administered on-line.
- Data analysis is facilitated via the use of software for both qualitative and quantitative analyses.
- Nurmetrics is a branch of nursing science that uses mathematical form and statistics to test solutions to problems. One branch of nurmetrics known as computational nursing uses models and simulations to test solutions and proposed models for care.

- Several organizations maintain databases that contain information useful to nurses conducting research, including CRISP, the National Library of Medicine, the *American Journal of Nursing*, and Sigma Theta Tau.
- The implementation of the CPR will provide information required to deliver health care more effectively and at lower costs.
- The lack of a common language to facilitate data collection is a problem in health care. Several projects are underway to address this issue, including the Unified Medical Language System and the Unified Nursing Language System.
- Automation and the implementation of the CPR are expected to increase multi-institutional research efforts as well as research in real time and collaborative research.
- Students in the health care professions may reap the benefits of research tools without formally conducting research.

REFERENCES

Amatayakul, M. (1995). CPR definition becoming clearer. *Health Management Technology, 16*(8), 66(2).

ANA revises criteria for evaluating nursing vocabularies, classification systems. (November/December 1996). *The American Nurse,* 9.

Bair, A. H., Brown, L. P., Pugh, L. C., Borucki, L. C., and Spatz, D. L. (1996). Taking a bite out of CRISP. *Computers in Nursing, 14*(4), 218–224.

Burns, N., and Grove, S. K. (1997). *The practice of nursing research*, 3rd ed. Philadelphia: W. B. Saunders.

Chang, B. L. (1993). CARIN system: Database for Bayers' theorem applications. *Western Journal of Nursing Research, 15*(5), 644–648.

Community of Science Web Server. (1997). On the Web at: *http://cos.gdb.org/.*

Daly, J. M., Button, P., Prophet, C. M., Clarke, M., and Androwich, I. (1997). Nursing interventions classification implementation issues in five test sites. *Computers in Nursing, 15*(1), 23–29.

DeGruy, K. B. (2000). Healthcare applications of knowledge discovery in databases. *Journal of Healthcare Information Management, 14*(2), 59–69.

Delaney, C., Gardner-Huber, D., Mehmert, M., Crossley, J., and Ellerbe, S. (1994). A nursing management minimum data set. In S. J. Grobe and E. S. P. Pluyter-Wenting (Eds.). *Nursing informatics: An international overview for nursing in a technological era, Proceedings of the Fifth IMIA International Conference on Nursing Use of Computers and Information Science* (pp. 155–157). New York: Elsevier.

DePalma, J. A. (1994). Computers and nursing research in acute care settings. In S. J. Grobe and E. S. P. Pluyter-Wenting (Eds.). *Nursing informatics: An international overview for nursing in a technological era,*

Proceedings of the Fifth IMIA International Conference on Nursing Use of Computers and Information Science (pp. 495–499). New York: Elsevier.

Frawley, K. (April 1995). Achieving the CPR while keeping an ancient oath. *Healthcare Informatics, 12*(4), 28–30.

Hirsch, M., Chang, B. L., and Gilbert, S. (1989). A computer program to support patient assessment and clinical decision-making in nursing education. *Computers in Nursing, 7*(4), 157–160.

Houston J. D., and Fiore, D. C. (1998). Online medical surveys: Using the Internet as a research tool. *M.D. Computing, 15*(2), 116–120.

Jones, R., and Jedrasik, E. (2000). Using audio computer-assisted self-interview in AIDS risk research. *Connect: Information Technology at NYU, 10*(2), 29–31.

Kouzes, R. (1997). Can we work together apart? *Scientific Computing and Automation, 14*(2), 52–54.

Martin, K. S. (1994). The Omaha system: A model for nursing care information systems. In S. J. Grobe and E. S. P. Pluyter-Wenting (Eds.). *Nursing informatics: An international overview for nursing in a technological era, Proceedings of the Fifth IMIA International Conference on Nursing Use of Computers and Information Science* (pp. 398–401). New York: Elsevier.

McCloskey, J., and Bulechek, G. (1993). The NIC taxonomy structure. *Image: Journal of Nursing Scholarship, 25*(3), 187–192.

Meintz, S. L. (1994). High performance computing for nursing research. In S. J. Grobe and E. S. P. Pluyter-Wenting (Eds.). *Nursing informatics: An international overview for nursing in a technological era, Proceedings of the Fifth IMIA International Conference on Nursing Use of Computers and Information Science* (pp. 448–451). New York: Elsevier.

Murphy, J. (1994). CPR development tunnel longer than expected. *Health Management Technology, 15*(11), 45(3).

Murray, P. J. (1996). Nurses' computer-mediated communications on NURSENET. *Computers in Nursing, 14*(4), 227–234.

Paul, S. M. (1994). Computer support for power analysis in nursing research. In S. J. Grobe and E. S. P. Pluyter-Wenting (Eds.). *Nursing informatics: An international overview for nursing in a technological era, Proceedings of the Fifth IMIA International Conference on Nursing Use of Computers and Information Science* (pp. 491–494). New York: Elsevier.

Pilkington, F. B. (1996). The use of computers in qualitative research. *Nursing Science Quarterly, 9*(1), 5–6.

Prohaska, J. L., and Chang, B. L. (1996). Computer use and nursing research. *Western Journal of Nursing Research, 18*(3), 365–370.

Ryan, P., Coenen, A., Devine, E. C., Werley, H. H., Sutton, J., and Kelber, S. (1994). Prevalence and relationships among elements of the Nursing Minimum Data Set. In S. J. Grobe and E. S. P. Pluyter-Wenting (Eds.). *Nursing informatics: An international overview for nursing in a technological era, Proceedings of the Fifth IMIA International Conference on*

Nursing Use of Computers and Information Science (pp. 174–178). New York: Elsevier.

Ryan, S. A., and Nagle, L. M. (1994). Nursing informatics: The unfolding of a new science. In S. J. Grobe and E. S. P. Pluyter-Wenting (Eds.). *Nursing informatics: An international overview for nursing in a technological era, Proceedings of the Fifth IMIA International Conference on Nursing Use of Computers and Information Science* (pp. 443–447). New York: Elsevier.

Sheil, E. P., and Wierenga, M. E. (1994). The use of the Nursing Minimum Data Set in several clinical populations. In S. J. Grobe and E. S. P. Pluyter-Wenting (Eds.). *Nursing informatics: An international overview for nursing in a technological era, Proceedings of the Fifth IMIA International Conference on Nursing Use of Computers and Information Science* (pp. 129–143). New York: Elsevier.

SIByl Program information. (1995). On the Web at: *http://www.gamma.rug.nl/files/p531.html and p534.html.*

Wegman, E. J., Carr, D. B., King, R. D., Miller, J. J., Poston, W. L., Solka, J. L., and Wallin, J. (1996). Statistical software, siftware and astronomy. On the Web at: *http://www.galaxy.gmu.edu/papers/ast.html.*

Appendix A:
Internet Primer

This primer is a supplemental reference guide designed to get you up and running on the Internet. The Internet, generally referred to as the "Net," encompasses many different methods of manipulating information and communicating, including the World Wide Web, electronic mail, newsgroups, and file transfer.

TOOLS TO GET ON-LINE

If you are not already on-line through your school or place of work, there are a few things you need in order to hook up to the Net:

- A computer
- A modem
- A telephone line (if you use your regular telephone line, callers will hear a busy signal when you are on-line; you can also get a dedicated line) or cable or wireless connection
- An Internet service provider (ISP)

Modems

A modem is a piece of equipment that changes computer information to the kind of information that can be passed over telephone or cable lines. It can be an external box or an internal card.

Modems come in different speeds. The speed of a modem determines how quickly you can download or access information from the Internet. Modem speeds keep getting faster but as of this writing 56K is the most common speed available over telephone wire.

Some older computers cannot provide the same level of Internet access as newer, faster computers, and might not be able to handle this rate of transfer. Check with your local computer hardware store to see what modem might be right for you.

INTERNET SERVICE PROVIDERS

To access the Internet, most users go through an Internet service provider (ISP). ISPs are companies that run the computers that enable you to get onto the Net; these computers are called servers. When you connect to the Net, your modem lights up and dials the number of your ISP. Your modem actually connects to the server's modem. Some cable and telephone companies also provide Internet access.

When choosing an ISP, you should consider:

- *Price.* There are a variety of fee structures for Internet service. It is possible to obtain Internet access at no cost, but these providers generally bombard users with advertisements and may offer little or no technical support. Some ISPs allow unlimited usage for a flat fee, some offer a certain amount of time per month before they begin charging extra, and some charge by the amount of time you are on-line from the moment you go on-line.

- *Traffic.* Find out the "dial up" number (the number your modem calls to link up) of an ISP and call it at different times during the day. Some ISPs get a lot of traffic and it can be difficult to get on-line (particularly the larger, national companies).

ELECTRONIC MAIL (E-MAIL)

E-mail is a way of transmitting messages across a phone line, network, or cable connection to other computers through your ISP. It works like this: You have a program called a mail browser (such as Eudora or Microsoft Mail) that enables you to send and read e-mail messages. To send e-mail, first type in the e-mail address. E-mail addresses look like this: username@servername.domainname. For example, ClaraBarton@nursingnet.com.

Make sure to put what the message is about in the "subject" line. After writing your text in the "body" of the message, you can send it. The message is transmitted across phone, cable, or network lines to the server, which sorts the mail and sends it to the correct e-mail address.

Whether you use e-mail for work or play, it is generally somewhat informal and not very lengthy. E-mail can be used for sending out memos, writing a note to a friend, and exchanging documents and files. You can even send someone your resume over e-mail (see Appendix B).

Some things to remember when using e-mail:

- Try to check your mail every day, especially if you belong to a mailing list (see section on listservs). It's amazing how quickly your mailbox can fill up with messages.

- Don't send lengthy material via e-mail.
- Know your netiquette (see page 328 of this Appendix).
- Don't send anything too confidential or sensitive over e-mail; e-mail is easily accessed by others.
- Try to proofread your e-mail before you send it; it is all too common to see typos in e-mail messages, many of which could be eliminated if the messages were read over just once.
- Most of all, have fun with it. E-mail is a good way to keep in touch, get messages out to a lot of people, and make new friends!

THE WORLD WIDE WEB (WWW)

The World Wide Web provides a way to access Internet resources by content instead of file names. Since it was launched in 1992, the Web has virtually exploded into mainstream culture.

Browsers

To get to the Web, you must to have a computer program called a Web browser. Some of the more popular Web browsers include Netscape and Microsoft Explorer. Once you are on-line with your server, you simply open the browser and you are ready to "surf" the Net.

Web Addresses

The Web is made up of millions of Web sites (or Web pages). Each Web site has an address, which is known as the URL (uniform resource locator). A typical URL looks like this: *http://www.prenticehall.com/health.* This is the address for the Prentice Hall Web site for the health professions. To get to any Web site, all you have to do is type in the URL in the browser's "go to" box (or something similar, depending on which browser you are using).

You can dissect Web site addresses and figure out who and what they stand for:

- "http," or HyperText Transport Protocol, appears in every Web site address (with a few exceptions). You will *always* see "://" after "http."
- Generally you will see "www," which tells the server to get the information from the World Wide Web.
- The last two parts of the address are the domain name; in this case, prenticehall.com is the domain name. The domain indicates what kind of site it is. In our case it is ".com" (pronounced "dot-com"), which stands for "commercial." Other domains you will probably come across include: ".edu" = education, ".org" = organization, and ".gov" = government. You get the idea.

Note: Don't get http and HTML confused. HTML stands for HyperText Markup Language, the programming language that enables you to develop a Web site. Also, when you read the address for a Web site out loud, remember that every "." is pronounced "dot."

Web Sites

Web sites are generally developed around a particular topic, such as nursing or health care. The amount of information available on the Web today is staggering and continues to grow. You can use the Web for general research, as an educational tool, as a shopping mall, to find a long lost friend, to get a new job (see Appendix B), or to answer practically any question you might have.

The first page you come to is called the *home page*, or sometimes the *splash page*. This page should convey the main ideas behind the entire web site. It generally contains a menu for the entire site.

The home page contains *links* to other pages. They send you into further detail by a click of the mouse. Links are generally marked by keywords or images. It's like an outline: the home page is your thesis, and each link is a breakdown of main ideas to be covered on that topic. To "follow a link" from the home page, look for highlighted text, buttons, or images and click on them with your mouse. For example, go to *http://www.prenticehall.com/health* and click on the word "nursing." This is a link to resources for nurses that includes the Prentice Hall book catalog as well as other sites of interest.

Search Engines

Now that you have a basic idea of the workings of the Web, how do you go about finding Web sites that may interest you? There are a number of popular directories on the Web called search engines. Search engines are Web sites that contain Web site information (i.e., the URL and a short description) on virtually every topic imaginable.

Some of the larger and more popular search engines are

- Yahoo! at *http://www.yahoo.com*
- Alta Vista at *http://altavista.digital.com*
- Excite at *http://www.excite.com*
- Hot Bot at *http://www.hotbot.com*
- Lycos at *http://www.lycos.com*
- Go at *http://www.go.com*
- WebCrawler at *http://webcrawler.com*

To use a search engine, type in one of the addresses listed above. When the home page for that site comes up, you will notice a search box in which you can type in a keyword or phrase. The site will then bring up all the information that it has available on that topic as a list of sites. Sometimes you will need to narrow your search; for example, if you type in "nursing," hundreds of site listings will return. On the other hand, if you are too specific, you may not have any sites returned. You may have to try a few different word combinations to find the sites you are looking for.

Bookmarks

One very useful component of your Web browser is the bookmark tool. Whenever you come to a site that you may want to return to, you can bookmark it. To bookmark a site, go to that site. After it has loaded, choose "bookmark" or a similar command, depending on your browser. Your browser will record the address of that site in your bookmark folder. Anytime you want to return to that site, you simply open the bookmark folder and click on the title of that Web site.

Patience

Have patience when using the World Wide Web. Accessing Web sites can take time, depending on how elaborate the site is (how large it is, how many pictures are on it, and so on), how fast your modem can download the information, and what time of day you are surfing. You can speed things up a bit by turning off the autoload image option in your browser.

Also, because information is generally sent via phone lines, all sorts of hiccups can occur in the transfer process. Sometimes the server of the Web site you are trying to reach may be down, there may be a lot of activity on that site, or there may be line noise. Just try a couple of more times to load the site.

Finally, because the Web is so dynamic, sites and links change every day. You might find numerous links on Web pages that go nowhere. There are many reasons for this: people move their pages to new servers, get new Web site addresses, or take the pages down. Don't get discouraged; chances are there is another site right around the corner that contains all the information that you need. You can search for a particular site by enclosing the name in quotation marks.

MAILING LISTS AND LISTSERVS

Mailing lists are electronic discussion groups that take place through e-mail. They are groups of people who "get together" on-line to discuss a specific topic. There are numerous mailing lists on nearly every topic imaginable.

A listserv is the software program that is used to run the mailing list. Here's how it works:

- You find out about a mailing list dealing with a subject you are interested in discussing with others (such as culture and nursing).

- To get involved in this discussion group, you have to subscribe to it. To subscribe, send an e-mail message to that mailing list's listserv.

- Most often, the listserv automatically will subscribe you to the list and send you instructions on how to post to the group. *Posting* means that you send out a comment to the entire mailing list that you have subscribed to.

- Once you have subscribed, you will begin to receive e-mail messages from the mailing list. Be careful: some discussion groups have a large following and you may find your mailbox filling up rather quickly.

To find out about mailing lists that might interest you, see Appendix C.

Newsgroups/Usenet

Newsgroups, like mailing lists, are another popular way of discussing specific topics over the Internet with other people who share the same interest. Unlike a mailing list, however, newsgroups take place on an entirely different network called Usenet.

Usenet is composed of thousands of newsgroups. Individual comments that people make to one another on a newsgroup are called articles. You *post an article* when you want to make a comment. The lines of discussion within a newsgroup are called *threads*. To read the discussions on any newsgroup, you must have a software program called a newsreader.

Generally, your ISP will provide you with a newsreader program as part of the software package. When you open the newsreader it should download any new newsgroups that have been added. You can look through the entire list and choose which newsgroups interest you. When you find one of interest, just open it up and begin reading the articles.

Newsgroup addresses are called hierarchies. Listed below are some of the standard hierarchies with examples of each. There are many other categories, some of which are from foreign countries.

alt—groups generally alternative in nature (e.g., alt.education.distance, alt.alien.visitors)

bionet—groups discussing biology and biological sciences (e.g., bionet.general, bionet.immunology)

comp—groups discussing computer or computer science issues (e.g., comp.infosystems)

misc—groups that don't fit into other categories (e.g., misc.fitness, misc.jobs)

news—groups about Usenet itself (e.g., news.groups)

rec—groups discussing hobbies, sports, music, and art (e.g., rec.food, rec.humor) *sci*—groups discussing subjects related to the science and scientific research (e.g., sci.med.nursing, sci.psychology)

soc—groups discussing social issues, including politics, social programs, etc. (e.g., soc.culture, soc.college)

talk—public debating forums on controversial issues (e.g., talk.abortion, talk.religion)

One word of caution: People take newsgroups very seriously. If you want to post an article, be sure you understand the threads (lines of discussions) that have been taking place on the newsgroup. Read a number of articles and understand the threads before putting up your own opinion.

Remember that these discussion groups are frequented by people from all over the world; because of this, newsgroups can offer a wealth of information. Many field experts frequent newsgroups. There may even be groups out there that you can monitor and to which you can provide expert advice.

To find out about newsgroups that might interest you, see Appendix C.

PORTALS AND VIRTUAL COMMUNITIES

Portals are Web sites that offer a personalized view for you based on information provided when you register. Portals organize data into a single, easy-to-use menu providing services such as e-mail, search capability and on-line shopping. America On-Line (AOL) and Yahoo represent general portal sites. There are also special-interest or niche portals. Some examples of nursing and health care portals include Nursing Net, WebMD, HealthGate, OnHealth, and HealthCentral. Portals continue to evolve.

The term virtual community refers to a group of people who share common interests, ideas, and feelings on-line. This may occur through bulletin boards, chat rooms, or user groups. Special interest portals may serve as a tool to create a virtual community that models the features of a neighborhood, complete with shopping and other services.

FTP

FTP stands for *file transfer protocol*. FTP is a means by which you can send and receive (upload and download) documents and software over the Internet. FTP sites house these documents and software. Not all sites permit two-way traffic. Look for help with the FTP process under your brower's Help button.

NETIQUETTE

Netiquette is just like it sounds: etiquette on the Internet. It's just basic, common courtesy to others. Because no single person owns or controls the Internet, it is left to the individual user to be facilitative and kind when participating in discussion groups, authoring Web pages, or sending e-mail messages.

The following list contains general netiquette standards that most people on the Net attempt to abide by:

- Don't make assumptions
- Don't be judgmental
- Don't use all capital letters; this is interpreted as SHOUTING
- Do proofread your messages carefully
- Do be facilitative
- Do be honest
- Do be timely in your replies
- Do try to make postings brief and to the point

CONCLUSION

All of this information can be overwhelming at first, but, with time, you can learn to use the many invaluable resources the Internet has to offer. Understanding the many components that make up the Internet and using this knowledge to be discriminatory in the information that you find on-line will enable you to use the Internet as a research tool, an educational source, a meeting place, and a library. Now that you have this knowledge, you are ready to start surfing the Net.

Appendix B: Career Resources on the Internet

JOB HUNTING IN THE TWENTY-FIRST CENTURY

The advent of computers and the Internet has revolutionized the job search process. If you want to maximize your chances of finding a great job, using the Internet can help. Whether you are a recent nursing school graduate or an experienced nurse, sending out a traditional resume may no longer be enough to land an interview. The Internet and other computer technologies can help you get the attention of employers, network with colleagues, and research potential new jobs.

JOB SEARCHING ON THE INTERNET

The Internet can help you with your job search in several ways. The first that may come to mind is on-line job listings. Literally hundreds of sites on the World Wide Web contain help wanted listings. Most have search engines, so you can enter keywords describing the job you are seeking to see whether there are any matches in that database. Looking through all the job listings on the Web can be very time-consuming, so you may want to narrow your search to health care–related sites (see Appendix C). At this point in time, the majority of job listings on the Web are for computer professionals. However, listings in the health care professions will likely continue to grow.

Another way to use the Internet in your job search is to post your resume to a database. Again, it is probably best to choose a database that is specific to health care or nursing. For guidelines on writing and posting an electronic resume, see the Creating and Posting an Electronic Resume section of this Appendix.

Some of the most powerful ways to use the Internet to help find a job may be less obvious. The Internet can be a great way to make contacts all over the country. Interested in getting into home health care in Florida? There is bound to be someone out there, in a chat room or newsgroup, who knows all about it. She or he may even know of a place that is hiring. Many people who spend time on-line are friendly and willing to help, so post your inquiry anywhere you think you may get a response. As always, be careful about divulging personal information. You can also use e-mail to network with contacts and stay in touch with former classmates, co-workers, and others who may be able to help you find a job.

The World Wide Web can be a great tool for researching careers and potential employers. Many hospitals and other employers have Web sites you can peruse. There are also sites for professional organizations, educational institutions, and other groups that may post useful information (see Appendix C). Be inquisitive and creative.

HOW RESUME DATABASES WORK

More and more employers are turning to automated applicant-tracking systems to sort and track resumes. These systems are actually databases that allow prospective employers to use keywords to search for applicants who meet certain criteria. For example, say a health maintenance organization is looking for a pediatric acute care nurse. The employer enters words describing her ideal candidate into the automated applicant-tracking system. In this case she may type in "pediatric," "acute care," and "registered nurse" as required keywords that resumes must include to come up in her search results. She may add other keywords if she likes, such as criteria that would be helpful for the job but are not mandatory. The tracking system then searches all the resumes in its system and retrieves those with the keywords the employer specified. Some tracking systems may display a list of resume "titles" or header lines for each resume retrieved, such as "LVN/home health care/Massachusetts." The employer can then select which resumes she wants to see in full.

How do you find these resume databases? Some employers have their own in-house automated tracking systems. Employers scan resumes received by mail into the system, and when a position opens up they log onto the database to search for a candidate. Some employers are able to receive electronic applications via e-mail; these are also stored in the database.

Employers who don't have their own database may use other generic applicant-tracking systems on the Internet (see the Resources at the end of this appendix for a listing of on-line applicant-tracking systems). Some of these encompass all job seekers in any field; others are geared to specific areas such as health care. With these systems it is up to the job seeker to enter a resume into the database. There are several ways to do this, and the available techniques vary among systems. One common way to post your resume on-line is to type it directly into the database once you've logged on to the site. Many systems allow you to paste your resume from your word processor onto the database. You can often send it via e-mail. Employers search these databases according to keywords, which may include information about your skills, education, or geographic area.

CREATING AND POSTING AN ELECTRONIC RESUME

The electronic resume has many things in common with the traditional resume. Both prominently display your name, address, and phone number, and list your work experience, education, and special skills. However, there are several differences. An electronic resume will be seen by prospective employers only if it contains the keywords the employers are searching for. Many electronic resumes contain a keyword summary section toward the top, listing the standard phrases that describe the applicant's skills, areas of expertise, job titles, and credentials (see Figure B–1). It's a good idea to put the keywords in ascending order of importance. Also use common abbreviations, synonyms, or acronyms for words used in the body of the resume to increase your odds of matching the employer's keyword specifications. For example, if you list "registered nurse" in the body of your resume, use "RN" in the keyword summary. To determine what keywords to use, look at the words used in the job listings and use those that describe you. If you have access to electronic resumes, either on your computer or at your library, you can see what keywords others have used as well.

Since your electronic resume may either be scanned into a computer or sent to a database via e-mail, you'll need to ensure that the formatting you use will be readable to any system. Some kinds of formatting and typefaces will turn to gibberish or become unreadable in some circumstances. To make sure this doesn't happen, follow these rules of thumb:

- Choose a common typeface, such as Times Roman, Helvetica, or Palatino. Avoid fancy scripts, which are likely to degrade when scanned. Use 12- or 14-point type. Do not use graphics, shading, italics, or underlining; for emphasis, use boldface or capital letters.

- If you are sending your resume electronically over the Internet, check whether there are formatting specifications you must meet. Some databases require that you meet certain margins or not use tabs. And many require that resumes be sent in plain text or ASCII format.

- If you're sending a hard copy of your resume, use a printer that produces clean easy-to-read copy. Be sure to send an original print, not a photocopy. If you must fax it, use the fine setting.

- Use plain white 8½ × 11-inch paper with no folds or staples.

Mary Lou Johnson
1234 Elm Street
Springfield, MO 12345
Home: (222) 345-6789
Work: (222) 456-7890

Keyword Summary: Nursing. Health Care. RN. BSN. Manager. Home Health Care. Geriatric Extended Care. Geriatric Preventive Care. Infection Control. Psychosocial Care. Teaching. Spanish. Relocation.

Current Position

1994–present   Nursing Supervisor, Large Nursing Home, Springfield, MO. Coordinated and supervised a nursing team responsible for 24-hour care of geriatric clients at an extended care home. Expanded program of preventive care and reduced hospitalization rate by 20%. Taught in-service programs for floor staff on geriatric care issues. Co-chaired committee on infection control and product evaluation. Effectively represented the unique interests and priorities of the nursing home staff; turnover dropped by 25%.

Previous Positions

1989–1994   Teaching Assistant, School of Nursing, Private School of Nursing, Kansas City, MO.

1983–1989   Staff Registered Nurse, Large Medical Center, Kansas City, MO.

Education

1983   Bachelor of Science, Nursing, University of Missouri.

Continuing Education Sampling

1997   Seminar: "New Perspectives on Aging"

1997   Workshop, "Care of People with Alzheimer's Disease"

1996   Evening course, "The Changing Face of Aging in America"

1995   In-service: "New Studies on Diabetes"

Professional Memberships

1984–present   American Nurses Association

FIGURE B–1 • Sample Electronic Résumé

ISSUES TO CONSIDER WITH AUTOMATED APPLICANT TRACKING SYSTEMS

The advantage of getting your resume into an automated applicant-tracking system is that you will maximize your exposure to employers. There are, however, some disadvantages to consider. It may be difficult for a recent graduate with little experience to shine in a database system, since qualities like independence, perseverance, and reliability aren't usually entered as keywords in a search. If you are looking for your first job as a health care professional you may not want to rely solely on an electronic resume.

There are also confidentiality issues with database resume systems. While some systems restrict access to subscribers only, others do not. Either way, anyone, including your current boss (who could be a subscriber to the database you're using), can see your resume posted there. Some services will provide users with a list of subscribers, but this is no guarantee that the information won't get back to your current employer. One way to help protect your privacy is to leave out identifying information about your current employer in your resume. For example, you could write that you work at "a university medical center" instead of "The University of Texas Medical Center."

Before you post your resume on any on-line system, be sure you understand the user guidelines. They will let you know any details about formatting to use or avoid, how long your resume will remain in the system, how to update it, and whether any fees are charged.

Appendix C: Internet Resources for Nurses and Health Care Professionals

Due to the dynamic nature of the Internet, the Web sites, listservs, and newsgroups listed below may change, move to another URL, or cease to exist. With this appendix we hope to provide an introduction to the diversity and wealth of information available on the Internet.

WEB SITES

Career Resources

American Mobile Healthcare
http://www.americanmobile.com/
Agency that offers temporary nursing and allied health care positions all over the United States.

CareerPath.com
http://www.careerpath.com
Database of help wanted ads from across the United States; includes job search and employer profiles.

MediStaff
http://www2.portal.ca/~wwide/Nurses.html
Job search service; a division of Worldwide Staffing Inc.

Monster Healthcare
http://www.medsearch.com/
National medical employment Web site with resume entry form and job listings.

NursesPortal.Com
http://www.healthcareerweb.com/
Provides resources for health care professionals looking for new opportunities.

Nurseweek Career Planning and Development Guide
http://www.nurseweek.webnexus.com/features/career/one.html
Resources for new, experienced, and veteran nurses.

Nursing Job Search Handbook
http://www.upenn.edu/careerservices/nursing/jobhandbookindex.html
Provides useful information on writing a cover letter, writing a resume, job search and interview skills, sample interview questions, and suggested follow-up after an interview.

Nursing Spectrum
http://www.nursingspectrum.com/
This site provides the capability to search for jobs or employers as well as career management information, continuing education, and discussions.

PRN Med Search
http://www.halcyon.com/prnmed
National medical employment Web site lets you search its database for job listings and contact prospective employers.

SpringNet
http://www.springnet.com/
This portal by Lippincott, Williams and Wilkins provides numerous links of interest to nurses, including job listings, information useful for career planning, and links to conferences, continuing education, and their on-line bookstore.

General Nursing Resources

Cybernurse
http://www.cybernurse.com/
A portal run by nurses for nurses to enhance nursing as a profession. It contains links to newsletters, CEUs, job opportunities, on-line shopping for books, as well as chats and search capability.

The NursesPortal
http://virtualnurse.com/
A portal developed by the innovators of Virtual Nurse. Features include moderated specialty nursing chats, message boards, free e-mail, search capability, information on education and employment, guestbooks, and conferencing.

Nurseweek/Healthweek
http://www.nurseweek.com/
Health care, nursing, and allied health hot links by category.

Nursing Net
http://www.nursingnet.org/
This popular site features links, chat rooms, and message boards and provides a forum in which nurses can communicate with each other.

Resources for Nurses and Families
http://pegasus.cc.ucf.edu/~wink/home.html
A comprehensive list of links maintained by Dr. Diane Wink from the University of Central Florida School of Nursing.

The Virtual Nursing Center
http://www.sci.lib.uci.edu/HSG/Nursing.html
Thousands of articles and links to a virtual plethora of information.

Whole Nurse
http://www.wholenurse.com/
Articles, chats, book reviews, education information, and a variety of other resources for nurses, students, and other health care professionals.

Organizations and Associations

American Academy of Ambulatory Care Nursing
http://aaacn.inurse.com/
Provides information about membership, certification, and links relevant to practice in the ambulatory care setting.

American Academy of Pediatrics
http://www.aap.org/
Professional organization "committed to the attainment of optimal physical, mental, and social health for all infants, children, adolescents, and young adults."

American Association of Colleges of Nursing
http://www.aacn.nche.edu/
Resources include an interactive issues forum, institutional data and research, and career resources for nurses.

American Association of Critical Care Nursing
http://www.aacn.org/
Web site of the professional organization for critical care nurses.

American Association of Nurse Anesthetists
http://www.aana.com/
Home page of the AANA includes client, professional, and member resources. Highlights include an Internet hotline and a CRNA Internet discussion list.

American College of Nurse-Midwives
http://www.acnm.org/
This organization's Web site serves as a resource to nurse-midwives through education, certification, and professional information.

American Holistic Nurses' Association
http://www.ahna.org/home/home.html
The AHNA Web site contains conference listings, chat rooms, and message boards for those interested in holistic nursing.

American Hospital Association
http://www.aha.org
This site contains conference and press announcements, information related to services for members and links related to the health care industry with an emphasis on issues related to legislation and reimbursement.

American Medical Association
http://www.ama-assn.org
The official AMA Web site contains information on medical science and education, advocacy and communication, and membership, as well as the AMA catalog and links to other medical sites.

American Nurses Association/*Nursing World*
http://www.ana.org/
Nursing World is the American Nurses Association's on-line magazine. Highlights include Capital Watch, Market Place, News Kiosk, and the Credentialing Center.

American Psychiatric Nurses Association
http://www.apna.org/
This organization provides links to job opportunities, conferences, and legislation pertinent to the practice of psychiatric nursing.

Association of Pediatric Oncology Nurses
http://www.apon.org/
The Association of Pediatric Oncology Nurses (APON) is the leading professional organization for registered nurses caring for children and adolescents with cancer and their families.

Association of Perioperative Registered Nurses
http://www.aorn.org/
The official site of the Association of Perioperative Registered Nurses provides links to education, standards, services, and legislation of interest to nurses working with patients in the perioperative, operative, and postoperative phases of surgery.

American Society of Perianesthesia Nurses
http://www.aspan.org/
This organization serves the interest of nurses working in ambulatory surgery, preanesthesia, and postanesthesia care. Information is provided about the organization and membership with relevant links to areas of interest for this area of practice.

AMIA WWW Home Page
http://www.amia.org/
The Web site for the American Medical Informatics Association includes

member information and the *Journal of AMIA*. See also the AMIA Nursing Informatics Working Group at *http://amia-niwg.org/*

Canadian Nurses Association (CNA)
http://www.cna-nurses.ca/
The Canadian Nurses Association Web site includes a calendar of events, links, publications, and more. In English and French.

CPRI-HOST
http://www.CPRI.org/
This organization and site focus on the development and use of electronic health information systems as a means to improve health and the delivery of care. Resources include documents on the evolution of the electronic record, security guidelines, and conferences.

Data Interchange Standards Association
http://www.disa.org/
The Data Interchange Standards Association (DISA) contains information on electronic data interchange, links to conferences and other standards organizations.

Electronic Transactions Criteria for the Health Care Industry
http://www.ehnac.org/
This nonprofit group establishes standards for the electronic exchange of health care information. The home page includes links to related information sources.

Emergency Nurses Association
http://www.ena.org/
ENA is the world's largest emergency nursing organization devoted entirely to the advancement of emergency nursing practice. Founded in 1970, the Association has more than 24,500 members in more than 20 countries.

Health Care Financing Administration
http://www.hcfa.gov/
This federal agency provides information on the Medicare, Medicaid, and Children's Health Insurance programs that it administers, as well as its initiatives, quality-focused activities, and legislation that impacts the health care delivery system. Links to other government agencies are also included.

Healthcare Information and Management Systems Society
http://www.himss.org/
The HIMSS site provides information about the organization, educational programs, health industry news, job search capability, a forum for discussion, and links to its journal and an on-line bookstore.

HomeCare On-Line
http://www.nahc.org/
The Web site for the National Association for Home Care, this site lists

membership information along with other resources for those interested in the specialty.

Institutes of Medicine
http://www.iom.edu/
The IOM address a wide range of health care issues, including recommendations for patient records. Specific information on IOM activities, reports, and links to other sites are found here.

Joint Commission on Accreditation of Healthcare Organizations
http://www.jcaho.org/
JCAHO Web site. The Joint Commission is the nation's oldest and largest standards-setting and accrediting body in health care. It evaluates and accredits more than 15,000 health care organizations in the United States.

Midwest Nursing Research Society
http://www.mnrs.org/
This site provides information about the organization and provides links to other sites relevant for researchers.

National Association of Neonatal Nurses
http://www.nann.org/
The National Association of Neonatal Nurses' Web site features member information, conference schedules, and neonatology links.

National Council of State Boards of Nursing, Inc. (NCSBN)
http://www.ncsbn.org/
The official Web site for the NCSBN, developers of the NCLEX Examination. Includes a database on acts and regulations, licensure requirements and maintenance, educational issues, multistate regulation information, and much more.

National Institute of Nursing Research
http://www.nih.gov/ninr/
The nursing arm of the National Institutes of Health, the National Institute of Nursing Research features research and clinical information for nurses.

National League for Nursing (NLN)
http://www.nln.org/
Resource center for nursing practice, education, and research; includes the latest information about NLN membership, Constituent Leagues, accreditation, testing services and tests, and meetings and workshops.

National Student Nurses Association (NSNA)
http://www.nsna.org/
A national nonprofit organization open to all nursing students; includes links to state chapters.

Sigma Theta Tau International Honor Society of Nursing
http://www.nursingsociety.org/
Web site of Sigma Theta Tau, the Honor Society of Nursing. Offers access to research materials, links, and information about the organization.

Southern Nursing Research Society
http://www.snrs.org/
Provides links to other research organizations and opportunities, information about the organization on-line access for members to a newsletter and journal.

Telemedicine Information Exchange
http://tie.telemed.org/
This page is maintained by the Telemedicine Research Center with support from the National Library of Medicine. It has numerous links to telehealth funding, programs, vendors, related organizations, publications, news, and conferences.

Tri-State Nursing Computer Network
http://homepage.third-wave.com/tncn/index.htm
TNCN is a resource organization for health care professionals seeking to expand their knowledge and use of computers. This site contains membership information, job opportunities, and links to other informatics sites.

General Health Care Resources

CenterWatch, Clinical Trials Listing Service
http://www.CenterWatch.com/
International listing of clinical research trials. Also features information about newly approved drugs.

Department of Health and Human Services, GrantsNet
http://www.os.dhhs.gov:80/progorg/grantsnet/index.html
An on-line tool for finding and exchanging information about federal grant programs.

E-Health and Telemedicine
http://www.arentfox.com/quickGuide/businessLines/e-health/
e-health_telemed/e-health_telemed.html
The focus here is on legal issues surrounding e-health with links to news, legislation, and guidelines from professional organizations.

Healthweb Nursing
http://www.lib.umich.edu/hw/nursing.html
University of Michigan/Taubman Medical Library collaboration that features career information and links to a variety of on-line health science resources.

Internet Grateful Med U.S. National Library of Medicine
http://igm.nlm.nih.gov/
This site offers assisted searching in Medline and other on-line databases of the U.S. National Library of Medicine.

MedConnect: Information Services for the Medical Community
http://www.medconnect.com/
Features interactive education, an interactive jobs line, updates on meetings and educational programs, and health: A Search Engine for Health and Medicine.

The Merck Manual
http://www.merck.com/pubs/manual/
The entire *Merck Manual* on-line is free for registered users.

National Institutes of Health
http://www.nih.gov/
NIH Web site contains extensive health information, grants and contracts opportunities, and scientific resources.

Pharmaceutical Information Network
http://pharminfo.com/
A wealth of pharmaceutical resources, including drug updates, discussion groups, and disease center information.

The Rehabilitation Accreditation Commission (CARF)
http://www.carf.org/
The Web site for the Rehabilitation Accreditation Commission. Information is provided about the organization and its services to ensure the delivery of quality rehabilitation services.

RxList The Internet Drug List
http://www.rxlist.com/
An on-line database of drugs, interactions, and uses.

World Health Organization
http://www.who.ch/
Features include the world health report, the weekly epidemiological report, and newsletter.

Current Health Care News

CNN Interactive, Health Main Page
http://cnn.com/HEALTH/
CNN's magazine-style site has a wide range of health care–related articles.

Journal of the American Medical Association (JAMA)
http://www.ama-assn.org/public/journals/jama/jamahome.htm
"Peer-reviewed, primary source, highly selected clinical science, disease prevention, and health policy information for physicians and other health professionals."

New England Journal of Medicine
http://www.nejm.org/current.htm
New England Journal of Medicine on-line.

Reuters Health Information Services
http://www.reutershealth.com/
Reuters, the international news organization, has gathered health-related information from a variety of sources. Excellent resource.

LISTSERVS

Nursing

CASEMGR
To subscribe, send an e-mail message to: prnmed@halcyon.com
In the body of the message, write only:
subscribe yourfirstname yourlastname

Clinical Alerts (CLINALRT)
To subscribe, send an e-mail message to: listproc@list.umaryland.edu
In the body of the message, write only:
subscribe clinalrt yourfirstname yourlastname

Culture and Nursing (GLOBALRN)
To subscribe, send an e-mail message to: listserv@itssrv1@ucsf.edu
In the body of the message, write only:
subscribe globalrn yourfirstname yourlastname

International Telenurses Association (ITNA)
To subscribe, send an e-mail message to: listserv@listserv.bcm.tmc.edu
In the body of the message, write only:
subscribe ITNA yourfirstname yourlastname

Intravenous Therapy Nurses (IVTHERAPY-L)
To subscribe, send an e-mail message to: majordomo@ohsu.edu
In the body of the message, write only:
SUBSCRIBE VENOUS

Midwife
To subscribe, send an e-mail message to: midwife-request@fensende.com
In the body of the message, write only:
Subscribe

Nurse Practitioners (NPINFO)
To subscribe, send an e-mail message to: Majordomo@npl.com
In the body of the message, write only:
SUBSCRIBE NPINFO Youremailaddress

Nurse Practitioners (NPCHAT)
To subscribe, send an e-mail message to: listproc@listproc.listproc.net
In the body of the message, write only:
subscribe yourfirstname yourlastname

Nursing Care Plans List (CAREPL-L)
To subscribe, send an e-mail message to:
listserv@listserv.acsu.buffalo.edu
In the body of the message, write only:
subscribe yourfirstname yourlastname

Nursing Education (NRSINGED)
To subscribe, send an e-mail message to:
LISTSERV@ULKYVM.LOUISVILLE.EDU
In the body of the message, write only:
SUBSCRIBE NRSINGED Yourfirstname Yourlastname

Nursing Informatics (NRSING-L)
To subscribe, send an e-mail message to: listserv@library.ummed.edu
In the body of the message, write only:
SUBSCRIBE NRSING-L Yourfirstname Yourlastname

Nursing Issues (NURSENET)
To subscribe, send an e-mail message to:
LISTSERV@LISTSERV.UTORONTO.CA
In the body of the message, write only:
SUBSCRIBE NURSENET yourfirstname yourlastname

Nursing Learning Resource Center (NurseLRC)
To subscribe, send an e-mail message to:
MAJORDOMO@DOUGLAS.BC.CA
In the body of the message, write only:
Subscribe NurseLRC

Nursing Research (NURSERES)
To subscribe, send an e-mail message to:
LISTSERV@LISTSERV.KENT.ED
In the body of the message, write only:
SUBSCRIBE NurseRes Yourfirstname Yourlastname

Perinatal Nursing (PNATALRN)
To subscribe, send an e-mail message to:
LISTSERV@UBVM.CC.BUFFALO.EDU
In the body of the message, write only:
subscribe pnatalrn yourfirstname yourlastname

Psychiatric Nurses (PSYCHIATRIC-NURSING)
To subscribe, send an e-mail message to:
MAILBASE@MAILBASE.AC.UK
In the body of the message, write only:
JOIN PSYCHIATRIC-NURSING Yourfirstname Yourlastname

School Nurse (SCHLRN-L)
To subscribe, send an e-mail message to:
LISTSERV@UBVM.CC.BUFFALO.EDU

In the body of the message, write only:
SUBSCRIBE SCHLRN-L Yourfirstname Yourlastname

Student Nurse (SNURSE-L)
To subscribe, send an e-mail message to:
listserv@listserv.acsu.buffalo.edu
In the body of the message, write only:
Sub SNURSE-L [Your name]

Telenursing (ITNA)
To subscribe, send an e-mail message to:
listserv@listserv.bcm.tmc.edu
In the body of the message, write only:
Subscribe itna [Your name]

Health Care

Alternative Medicine Research (ALTMED-RES)
To subscribe, send an e-mail message to: majordomo@virginia.edu
In the body of the message, write only:
subscribe ALTMED-RES [Your name]

Aromatherapy
To subscribe, send an e-mail message to: Majordomo@metron.com
In the body of the message, write only:
Subscribe aromatherapy

Biomedical Ethics (BIOMED-L)
To subscribe, send an e-mail message to: listserv@vm1.nodak.edu
In the body of the message, write only:
subscribe BIOMED-L [Your first and last names]

Health and Wellness Issues (WELLNESSLIST)
To subscribe, send an e-mail message to: majordomo@wellnessmart.com
In the body of the message, write only:
subscribe Wellnesslist [Your name]

Health Economics (HEALTHECON)
To subscribe, send an e-mail message to: mailbase@mailbase.ac.uk
In the body of the message, write only:
join healthecon-discuss [Your name]

Health Info-Com Network Medical Newsletter (MEDNEWS)
To subscribe, send an e-mail message to: listserv@asuvm.inre.asu.edu
In the body of the message, write only:
sub MEDNEWS yourfirstname yourlastname

Health Informatics (MEDNFORM)
To subscribe, send an e-mail message to:
LISTSERV@SJUVM.stjohns.edu
In the body of the message, write only: subscribe

HEALTH-L
To subscribe, send an e-mail message to: listserv@listserv.hea.ie
In the body of the message, write only:
subscribe HEALTH-L [Your name]

Health Management (HEALTHMGMT)
To subscribe, send an e-mail message to: listserv@ursus.jun.alaska.edu
In the body of the message, write only:
Subscribe HEALTHMGMT [Your name]

Health Professionals (HEALTH-PRO)
To subscribe, send an e-mail message to: Listserv@NETCOM.COM
In the body of the message, write only:
Subscribe health-pro [Your e-mail address]

Health Promotion (CLICK4HP)
To subscribe, send an e-mail message to: listserv@yorku.ca
In the body of the message, write only:
Subscribe click4hp [Your name]

Holistic Health Care (HOLISTIC)
To subscribe, send an e-mail message to: listserv@suivmb.bitnet
In the body of the message, write only:
Subscribe holistic [Your name]

Home Health Care (HOMEHEALTH)
To subscribe, send an e-mail message to: listserv@usa.net
In the body of the message, write only:
SUBSCRIBE HOMEHEALTH [Your name]

Hospice Care (HOSPICE)
To subscribe, send an e-mail message to: majordomo@po.cwru.edu
In the body of the message, write only:
subscribe hospice [Your e-mail address]

Medical Libraries (MEDLIB-L)
To subscribe, send an e-mail message to:
LISTSERV@LISTERV.ACSU.BUFFALO.EDU
In the body of the message, write only:
Subscribe Medlib-L [Your name]

Midwife
To subscribe, send an e-mail message to:
midwife-request@csv.warwick.ac.uk
In the body of the message, write only:
Subscribe midwife

PUBLIC-HEALTH
To subscribe, send an e-mail message to: mailbase@mailbase.ac.uk
In the body of the message, write only:
subscribe PUBLIC-HEALTH [Your name]

Quality in Health Care Issues (QP-HEALTH)
To subscribe, send an e-mail message to: majordomo@quality.org
In the body of the message, write only:
Subscribe qp-health [Your e-mail address]

NEWSGROUPS

alt.abuse.recovery
alt.education.disabled
alt.health.ayurveda
   (Indian medicine)
alt.health.oxygen-therapy
alt.infertility
alt.med.allergy
alt.med.behavioral
alt.med.ems
   (emergency medical services)
alt.med.equipment
alt.med.fibromyalgia
alt.med.outpat.clinic
alt.npractitioners
   (nurse practitioners)
alt.psychology.help
alt.recovery
alt.society.mental-health
alt.support.abortion
alt.support.abuse-partners
alt.support.anxiety-panic
alt.support.arthritis
alt.support.asthma
alt.support.attn-deficit
alt.support.breast-implant
alt.support.cancer
alt.support.cerebral-palsy
alt.support.chronic-pain
alt.support.crohns-colitis
alt.support.depression
alt.support.diabetes.kids
alt.support.eating-disord
alt.support.epilepsy
alt.support.food-allergies
alt.support.glaucoma
alt.support.grief
alt.support.headaches.migraine
alt.support.hearing-loss
alt.support.hemophilia

alt.support.herpes
alt.support.inter-cystitis
alt.support.kidney-failure
alt.support.menopause
alt.support.mult-sclerosis
alt.support.obesity
alt.support.ostomy
alt.support.prostate.prostatitis
alt.support.sinusitis
alt.support.skin-diseases.psoriasis
alt.support.spina-bifida
alt.support.stop-smoking
alt.support.stuttering
alt.support.thyroid
alt.support.tinnitus
alt.support.tourette
alt.support.trauma-ptsd
bionet.audiology
bionet.biology.cardiovascular
bit.listserv.aidsnews
bit.listserv.autism
bit.listserv.blindnws
bit.listserv.c+health
   (computers and health)
bit.listserv.deaf-l
bit.listserv.down-syn
bit.listserv.easi
   (computer access for people
   with disabilities)
bit.listserv.l-hcap
bit.listserv.medforum
bit.listserv.medlib-l
bit.listserv.mednews
bit.listserv.snurse-l
bit.listserv.tbi-sprt
   (traumatic brain injuries)
bit.listserv.transplant
bit.med.resp-care.world
misc.emerg-services

misc.handicap
misc.health.aids
misc.health.alternative
misc.health.arthritis
misc.health.diabetes
misc.health.infertility
misc.health.therapy.occupational
misc.kids.health
misc.kids.pregnancy
sci.bio
sci.bio.microbiology
sci.bio.technology
sci.chem
sci.cognitive
sci.med
sci.med.aids
sci.med.diseases.cancer
sci.med.diseases.mental
sci.med.dentistry

sci.med.immunology
sci.med.informatics
sci.med.laboratory
sci.med.nursing
sci.med.nutrition
sci.med.pharmacy
sci.med.prostate.cancer
sci.med.psychobiology
sci.med.telemedicine
sci.med.vision
sci.psychology
sci.psychology.research
soc.support.depression.crisis
soc.support.depression.family
soc.support.depression.treatment
soc.support.pregnancy.loss
soc.support.transgendered
talk.politics.medicine
    (politics and health care)

Appendix D: Case Study Exercises—Suggested Responses

CHAPTER 1

A client arrives in the emergency department short of breath and complaining of chest pain. Describe how informatics can help nurses as well as other health care providers to more efficiently and effectively care for this client.

- *Old records (including prior medical history and medications) are available quickly through the use of information systems to all parties involved in the patient's care, no matter what their location.*
- *High-quality care is readily available through telemedicine (electronically submit EKG and chest x-ray to on-call specialists off site).*
- *The latest research on the patient's drugs and presenting symptoms is available via the Internet.*
- *Expert systems and care maps guide the treatment plan.*

CHAPTER 2

You are appointed to the hospital's information technology committee as the representative for your nursing unit. The charges of the committee include the following:

Identify PC software that is needed to accomplish unit work, such as word processing, spreadsheets, and databases.

- *Word processing aids the following efforts: committee minutes, writing and revising unit policies and procedures, authoring and revising patient instructions, developing care maps.*

- *A database can be used to maintain and display personnel information.*
- *The availability of a statistical package fosters unit-based research.*
- *Browser software provides access to materials housed on the intranet such as announcements, policies and procedures, institutional phone numbers, patient education materials, and programs mandated for regulatory bodies. Internet access provides the means to retrieve reference material such as literature search results, drug information, continuing education, and professional groups.*
- *E-mail provides the capability to share information with professional colleagues within the institution and in other facilities.*

Determine criteria for the selection and placement of hardware on the units. Discuss these issues and how they affect patient care and work flow.

- *Avoid high traffic zones—they are subject to multiple interruptions.*
- *Have enough devices for all users.*
- *Provide good lighting and place monitors to avoid screen glare.*
- *Consider ergonomics.*
- *Avoid placing computers in areas subject to liquid or food spills.*
- *Ensure that work surfaces are free from clutter.*

· · ·

Your committee is charged with setting up a computer system that will automate transcription of physician orders and reporting of results. Identify the support personnel that you need at this point and write job descriptions for each identified position.

- *Have staff who do the everyday work identify the current work flow.*
- *Have staff and administrators identify information needed by each level of worker.*
- *Meet with staff and information services staff to discuss screen design, information that needs to be exchanged among systems, and desired output.*
- *Get physician and medical record approval for the information displayed in on-line reports.*
- *Consider whether results will be reported in pending and/or final forms.*
- *Evaluate whether charges for procedures or medications will occur at the time of order, completion, or documentation (or remain a separate process).*
- *Identify a plan for training and implementing the new system.*

CHAPTER 3

Agnes Gibbons was admitted through the hospital's emergency department in congestive heart failure. During her admission she was asked to verbally acknowledge whether her demographic data were correct. Ms. Gibbons did so. Extensive diagnostic tests were done, including radiology studies. It was later discovered that all of Ms. Gibbons' information had been entered into another client's file. How would you correct this situation? What departments or other agencies would need to be informed of this situation?

- *Contact all clinical parties involved in Ms. Gibbons' care to look at whether she was treated appropriately and review her records in respective ancillary systems. Look at what drugs or blood products she may have been given and potential consequences.*
- *Involve information services, registration, medical records, and the billing department to correct the records.*
- *What was the length of time to discover the error and how was it discovered?*
- *Contact legal counsel regarding the situation.*
- *Educate all staff to seek more than one means of validation of patient identity upon admission (health insurance and photo identification in addition to verbal affirmation). Have client view information to validate that it is correct.*
- *Next time have Ms. Gibbons review the printout of her information and sign it to verify that it is correct. Be prepared to read the information to her.*
- *Delete Ms. Gibbons' information from the other patient's record and/or create a new medical record number for the second patient.*

• • •

A non–English-speaking Vietnamese male was admitted through the emergency department with suspected TB. The system carried information under his name. Mr. Nguyen nodded his head when the admitting clerk pointed to the demographic screen. Mr. Nguyen was tested and treated for TB. When the public health nurse went to Mr. Nguyen's address for follow-up, the man there was not the Mr. Nguyen who had been treated for TB. How would you address this problem? Explain your rationale.

This situation is similar to the one above. A response of "yes" or nodding the head does not ensure that the patient has heard or understood what was said. Validate identity through photo identification plus name and social security number. Obtain a translator as necessary. Notify all departments involved in the care of this patient. Review patient treatment relative to chart information for potentially harmful treatments.

. . .

You volunteered to serve on a committee to identify information from prior admissions that would be helpful to staff caring for current inpatients. What information, if any, would you select for ready access, and how long would you recommend that it remain active in the system? Remember that your system has limited capacity so that items must be carefully selected and prioritized. Identify the priority assigned to each item and provide your rationale for this priority.

Useful information: demographics, medical history, present medications, allergy information, over-the-counter products and herbal or other nontraditional treatments, and advanced directives, in that respective order. Availability of information eliminates repetitious questions and improves care.

CHAPTER 4

As the representative for your medical center's Better Care Initiative, a project with the purpose of identifying ways that services can be delivered in a more efficient manner, you have suggested that the Internet be made available to clinicians at the point of care. You must develop a report listing the potential uses of the Internet, as well as potential problems that might occur.

Potential uses

- *Intranet: to access policies and procedures, telephone numbers, human resources information, institution-specific references without worry about different versions*
- *Internet: to access to on-line databases and research, continuing education and degree programs, full text retrieval of articles, increased access to experts in the field due to the ease of use of e-mail.*

Potential problems

- *Internet: Staff may spend more time on the Web than expected, taking them from their other responsibilities.*
- *Some staff may surf non–work-related sites.*
- *Personnel may accept information found at face value without evaluating information for quality.*

. . .

One of your clients has a rare genetic defect. The client is requesting additional information about this from you, but no reference books on the unit describe this condition. Discuss strategies for how you might obtain this information using the Internet and electronic communication.

Try a Web search looking for support groups for the client. Medline or one of the other literature databases should have information, possibly in full-text form. Use e-mail to write to specialists to request information.

CHAPTER 5

You are a nurse participating in the customization and implementation of a medication documentation system. Define the data that must be included in the medication order entry process and the medication administration record documentation process.

- *Identify the drug by generic name (and trade name if desired), route, dose, administration times.*
- *Define times associated with daily, twice daily, three times daily, four times daily, bedtime, and before and after meals medication administration times.*
- *Develop a mechanism to display medications administered as well as medications not given.*
- *Provide a means to indicate why a medication was not given as well as that it was given by another person.*

. . .

You are participating in the customization and implementation of the radiology system. Define the data that must be included in the order entry process. Define the information that the nursing staff would like to view or print from the radiology system.

- *Must include the name of the exam, any modifiers that specify the exact body part to be filmed, date for the exam, and reason for the exam during order entry for treatment and reimbursement purposes.*
- *Output should include the test preparation instructions for staff and the patient, notification that the exam has been done, and on-line results (preliminary and/or final).*

CHAPTER 6

You are a nurse manager in a hospital that has recently merged with two other hospitals, forming a large health care enterprise. Each of the three hospitals currently uses a different nursing information system. You are a member of the strategic planning committee, which is charged with the task of selecting which of the three systems will be used throughout the enterprise. Describe the process you would use to scan the internal and external environments, as well as the types of data you would collect.

- *Consider the strategic plan for the combined and separate institutions.*
- *Determine current staff satisfaction with each nursing information system.*
- *Look at whether the system is due for major upgrades as well as associated costs. Which one would be easier to expand? Which one has the most capability for the future? What technology is used?*

. . .

Develop a tool to evaluate each of the three nursing information systems for the scenario described above.

Develop a weighted tool that considers ease of use, expandability, compatibility with other systems, ability to customize, ability to generate reports, time needed for training, time frame for implementation, and overall costs.

•   •   •

Your facility belongs to one of three health care delivery systems in the city. Competition is fierce. You have been asked to serve on a committee to study and recommend the retention or deletion of certain clinical services. Develop a plan for how you would do that and for how information services might facilitate that task via the use of benchmarking.

Compare services delivered to those provided by competitors for total number of cases served, quality of services inclusive of patient satisfaction, length of stay as appropriate, cost per case, and profits or loss per cost center. Commercial packages may aid this task.

CHAPTER 7

You are a member of a committee that will select a clinical documentation system for nurses. Prepare a time line for the needs assessment and system selection phases. These processes should be accomplished over a 6-month period.

- *Set the target implementation date, then work backward to set other key dates.*
- *Start with a "kickoff" meeting to provide an overview of the process.*
- *Establish an ongoing meeting schedule and develop a project plan.*
- *Anticipate change.*
- *Collect information about work flow processes from end users and administrators.*
- *Identify problems with the current process.*
- *Review the Request for Proposal requirements and compare available products.*
- *Schedule vendor demonstrations and site visits.*
- *Narrow the selection.*
- *Develop a list of "musts" and "wants" and assign a weight to each item. Define what your weighting scale will be.*
- *Choose a model for the system such as care mapping.*
- *Discuss how the new system will impact other systems.*
- *Develop a numeric scale, say 1–10, with 10 as the most desirable.*
- *Evaluate each of the systems using this scale.*
- *Create a list of questions related to this system selection process that you will ask at site visits: Is it easy to use? What reports and printouts are produced or may be produced? How long is needed for implemen-*

tation? training? What roadblocks were encountered? What would you do differently? Can it be adapted easily?

CHAPTER 8

You are the project director responsible for creating an implementation time line that addresses the training and go-live activities for a nursing documentation system that will be implemented on 20 units and involve 350 users. Determine whether the implementation will be staggered or occur simultaneously on all units, and provide your rationale.

This decision may be influenced by the following:

- *Whether a system is in place now*
- *Administrative support*
- *Staffing and training resource availability*
- *Ability to pull staff from other areas to the pilot unit(s)*
- *Weighing the advantages and disadvantages of doing one or all units at a time*

• • •

Create the time line for the training and go-live schedule for this implementation.

- *Start at least 1 year in advance, then work backward to get all activities in.*
- *Plan for 24-hour IS coverage for at least 1 week (from IS).*
- *Obtain administrative support and a budget.*
- *Plan for the unexpected.*
- *Choose a training system (core trainers, educators versus outside parties).*
- *Determine the number of training hours per staff.*
- *Determine training costs for equipment, trainers, replacement staffing.*
- *Provide flexibility in the scheduling. Build in extra time before implementation.*
- *Do not start training too early, because folks forget.*

• • •

Your present manual medication administration record is being replaced by an automated information system. Discuss the specifications that you would recommend for reports that the system will generate to notify the nurses when medications are due. Determine how often the reports should print and what information they should contain.

Medication administration records need to identify drug name, dose, scheduled time, route, and special instructions. The format for reminders should be one determined to be most useful for the staff nurse (i.e., shift overview or list by a particular time, patient or group of patients, items not charted or charged). Staff need to determine the most useful frequency for these reports (every 1 or 2 hours or prior to the end of the shift?).

· · ·

You have been selected to develop test scripts for interface testing for a new patient care system. Develop a test script with multiple interfaces. Define the output that you should see for each system.

A nursing documentation system would have demographic information, lab results from an outside system, radiology results plus any other diagnostic results, and a monitor interface and possibly a charge interface. Output differs for each interface and function. It must be accurate, and where it should be when it is needed. For example, demographic information passes from the registration system and is displayed in the nursing system. Diagnostic results need to pass from other systems into the documentation system. In the case of a charge interface a message is sent to accounting when a service, supply, or medication is administered.

CHAPTER 9

Kevin Gallagher, RN, has access to all client records on his medical–surgical unit. Consider each of the following situations:

- Kevin's mother is admitted to the unit. Is it appropriate for him to peruse his mother's electronic medical record? Why or why not? *No, not unless he is doing so directly on her behalf; otherwise, it is a violation of her privacy.*
- Kevin's unit clerk also has access to Mrs. Gallagher's record. Is it appropriate for her to view Mrs. Gallagher's record? *Only on a need-to-know basis.*
- Kevin's co-worker Kaneesha is a client on the unit assigned to another staff nurse's care. Is it appropriate for Kevin to review her chart or lab results? *Only on a need-to-know basis if he is involved in her care.*

· · ·

Nancy Whitehorse, RN, routinely accesses client records on her medical unit. Does she violate her confidentiality statement if she performs the following actions?

- She reviews the information and doesn't discuss it with anyone else. *This is a violation.*
- She discusses information obtained from client records with other health care workers on the unit. *This is a violation.*
- She discusses clinical cases, omitting names, in social situations. *This is a violation.*

· · ·

Grace Elizaga has been given the charge of training the RNs and unit clerks from the first three client care units slated to start automated order entry at Potter's Medical Center (PMC). The target implementation date is in 2 months. A total of 93 RNs and 11 unit clerks must receive training prior to that time. Based on information from other agencies that have the same information system as PMC, 8 hours of training time is projected for each individual. As the nurse manager responsible for those units, you have been asked to work with Grace to develop a detailed plan to accomplish this task and submit this plan to your vice-president of Client Care Services. Include the following in your plan and provide your rationale:

- Staffing—*Replacement staffing is needed while others train.*
- Costs for your personnel—*Replacement staffing is needed while others train. People also need practice time and time to apply newly learned skills.*
- Training start and completion dates—*Training must start early and be completed 1–2 weeks before GL to take care of last-minute stragglers and new hires and to allow practice time.*
- Length and number of training sessions—*Consider the ability of personnel and trainers to get away from the unit, the appropriateness of the training location, and the ability of personnel to learn over a longer session.*

CHAPTER 10

In the course of conversation, your nurse manager tells you that she loaded a copy of the spreadsheet program she uses on her home office PC onto one of the unit PCs so that she can work on projects at both locations. Your institution has a well-publicized policy against the use of unauthorized, unlicensed software copies. As a staff nurse, what should you do? Explain your response.

Talk with your nurse manager, telling her that this is a violation of copyright law and can result in large fines and is probably a violation of institutional policy.

• • •

You notice several of the new residents playing computer games on the nursing unit. You had not been aware of these games previously. What, if any, action should you take? Explain your rationale.

Remove them. Ask the IS department to "lock" down the machines so that additional software cannot be added without authorization. Approach the residents if necessary and ask them to restrict use on this machine to clinical uses.

• • •

To remember her computer system password, university nursing instructor Pat Pawakawicz taped her password to the back of her name pin. When Ms. Pawakawicz lost her name pin recently, it was turned into hospital security and subsequently the IS department with her password still attached. When Ms. Pawakawicz picked up her name pin, she expressed intent to use the same password. Is this an appropriate way to treat a password? Should she use the same password again? Provide your rationale. What, if any, legal ramifications might there be for Ms. Pawakawicz regarding use of her password by unauthorized users?

Passwords need to be kept private. When there is any question as to whether they have been compromised they should be changed immediately. This instructor's behavior may compromise someone's confidentiality. Unless she was clear when her badge was lost, she may face civil or other disciplinary action.

• • •

The administration at St. John's Hospital takes pride in their strong policies and procedures for the protection of confidential client information. In fact, St. John's serves as a model for other institutions in this area. However, printouts discarded in the restricted-access IS department are not shredded. On numerous occasions, personnel working late observed the cleaning staff reading discarded printouts. What action, if any, should these personnel take relative to the actions of the cleaning staff? What action, if any, should be taken by IS administration? Provide your rationale. If current practices are maintained, are there any additional potential risks for unauthorized disclosure of client information? If you answer yes, identify what these risks might be.

The IS department needs to practice what it preaches. Printouts should be shredded at the time that they are discarded or at the very least the housekeeping personnel should receive an inservice and sign a confidentiality statement.

• • •

The secretary on 7 Tower Oncology receives a fax transmission about a client consult. The fax was intended for a physician's office in the adjacent building. She places the fax in the out bin of her desk to be delivered later by volunteers. No in-house mailer was used. Is this action appropriate? Explain why or why not.

This action is not appropriate. All faxes should have cover sheets and be placed in a confidential mailer. Staff need an inservice and reprimand in this case.

CHAPTER 11

You have been selected as a member of the Integration Project Team, which is charged with identifying ways that system integration could improve information flow. You work on an inpatient unit that uses a stand-alone nursing documentation system that is not interfaced or integrated with any other hospital information system. Identify the implications of this situation, and suggest integration options that could improve information flow.

This situation creates extra work and can compromise data integrity, leading to several different versions of information for every patient. Data entry should occur once whenever possible at a point closest to the source. Substantial cost savings may result for the entire organization by eliminating redundant data entry.

. . .

You are working to identify elements in your health care enterprise that could be used for a master patient index (MPI). List five basic elements and describe how each could be used for an MPI.

Obvious elements for an MPI include the patient's name, medical record, social security number, and date of birth. Name and insurance may change. Eventually, the universal patient identifier will be a crucial element. Used in combination, these elements help to ensure access to the correct record.

CHAPTER 12

You are a member of the committee charged with designing the computer-based patient records (CPRs) at your facility. Identify which components of nursing documentation should be retained in the clinical data repository. For example, would you want to include all client vital signs from the current hospital admission? Explain why you would include or exclude the various components.

History and assessment, operative notes, allergies and drug reactions, medications, specific lab data, such as blood type, and some diagnostic tests need to be retained. Items such as all patient temperatures would clutter the record.

. . .

Identify several external sources of information that would be useful as part of the CPR for access by a home health nurse.

Ancillary test results, social history, history and assessment, operative notes, allergies and drug reactions, and medications are useful in every care setting.

. . .

Discuss the implications of providing nurses in a hospital setting with access to all electronic client information. Identify which types of information are appropriate for access by nurses.

Nurses need clinical information but generally do not require billing and payment information. In some cases, it is not necessary for a nurse to know about every aspect of the patient's history. One example might be that the emergency department patient who has a laceration from an automobile accident doesn't need to relate his history of abuse as a child.

CHAPTER 13

You are teaching an undergraduate course titled "Nursing Informatics." One class session is scheduled for a discussion on the protection of client record information. How would you summarize the current status of legislative safeguards in the United States? What, if anything, would you suggest that students might personally consider to improve this situation?

Traditionally, protection of patient information has been patchy from state to state. HIPAA provides protection at a federal level, although many issues remain unclear. Students can uphold standards and serve as advocates for patient privacy and write their legislators and senators to view their opinions on the need for additional safeguards or changes to legislation.

•   •   •

You have been appointed to the Clinical Information Systems Committee, which is charged with looking at ways that automation can facilitate data collection for the next JCAHO accreditation visit. List examples of how your community hospital demonstrates adherence to JCAHO information standards, and state your rationale for why you feel these examples display compliance.

Examples include

- *The existence and use of confidentiality and privacy safeguards, such as individual log-ons, different levels of access based on a need-to-know basis, and user sign-on statements.*
- *Improved access from different locations and by different types of providers at one time for more efficient patient care.*
- *24-hour access with protection against loss via file backup.*
- *Documentation of patient education is more legible and complete than traditional records.*
- *Improved turnaround time for documentation.*
- *Collection of aggregate data to support clinical research and patient care is improved.*

•   •   •

You are the general information systems liaison at Wilson Rehabilitation Institution. CARF accreditation is coming up. What would you do to ensure that your automated documentation is in compliance with CARF standards? Explain your rationale.

This preparation should be similar to preparation done with a manual system, although automation can be used to facilitate the process. Reports can be run to show the extent to which required data is collected and in some cases system prompts added to guarantee that data is provided. Automation also makes it easier to review treatment plans for completeness of documentation and to determine if they are up-to-date. These practices can be used prior to accreditation as a means to pinpoint and correct problem areas.

CHAPTER 14

You are the administrator of a home health care agency in a community that has recently developed a CHIN. Explain how access to this network will improve the ability of your staff to provide appropriate client care.

Network access to patient information will eliminate redundant data entry and improved data integrity. The time saved can be used for direct patient care. Agency staff should have a more comprehensive view of the patient since information spans treatment episodes.

• • •

Describe the types of information that your staff will be accessing from the CHIN, as well as the data that will be added to the CHIN from your agency.

The types of information accessed from the CHIN may include prior referrals for home health care, social service notes, history and assessment information, medications, treatment records, and diagnostic results. Home health staff may add the following information to the CHIN: assessment of living conditions and ability to live independently, response to home health care interventions, evidence that teaching was understood, changes that have been made in the lifestyle, and additional referrals.

CHAPTER 15

As the clinical representative for your unit on the Disaster Planning Committee, you are charged with identifying all forms in your area that require completion of a physical vital records inventory sheet. What forms would you list and why?

Look at forms that are frequently consulted, such as staff telephone and pager numbers. Consider whether unavailability to the information creates difficulties. If the answer is yes, then add these forms to the vital records inventory sheet.

• • •

Work crews at Wilmington Hospital inadvertently cut the cable connecting all terminals at the hospital with the computer center. As the on-duty nursing supervisor, what should you tell your employees, and why? Who would you contact for further information? How do you determine whether to initiate manual alternatives?

Tell employees the truth rather than giving the appearance that someone is hiding something. Next try to get an estimate for the expected time frame that the system will be unavailable. If the downtime is expected to be more than 2 hours, the institution needs to implement manual alternatives; otherwise, nonemergency procedures may be entered into the system once it is restored, rather than manually.

• • •

An early-morning train wreck near St. Luke's Hospital derailed seven freight cars carrying chemicals that can emit toxic fumes. The accident took out power lines for the neighborhood and for St. Luke's. Emergency crews evacuated a seven-block area, stopping just outside of the hospital's main entrance. Power has already been out for 12 hours and restoration is not expected for at least another 12–24 hours. You are on an executive administrative committee charged with determining what information will be brought on-line first and what will remain in paper form. What would you restore first? What records, if any, would you not restore? Explain your rationale. How would you document, for record-management purposes, that part of the record is automated and part is manual?

Demographics and registration information would be restored first because the patient must be in the system in order to perform any action. One of the next features would be the medication administration records (MARs). Not only do MARs have the capability to minimize med errors but in many settings charges occur when the medication is charted as given. Beyond these areas consideration must be given to treatments and system features that are considered as essential for care. There should be notation in record of what is in manual form. It may be far too expensive to backload data into the system when a paper record also exists.

• • •

As IS project manager you are responsible for helping the renal department select a new database. One of the top vendors must cancel its Web-based demonstration because its server was stolen. What questions should this raise for disaster planning with the use of vendor-supported applications?

Security of patient information, because information resides on the vendor's equipment.

CHAPTER 16

You are on the education committee at your small community hospital. Your staff development department was eliminated several years ago. You and your colleagues are charged with developing strategies to meet the educational needs of agency RNs and LPNs. Limited capital and the isolated location of your community make this a difficult assignment. Your institution does have Internet and Web access in the medical library, as well as teleconferencing capability. Develop a proposal to meet your charge using available resources. Be prepared to defend your proposal to an administration loathe to part with monies beyond those already budgeted.

Internet access to continuing education eliminates hours of travel and expenses associated with travel

• • •

You are the client educator at a medical center in the Pacific Northwest. Your clientele are drawn from a 150-mile radius and beyond. For this reason it is difficult to have clients complete diabetic education or other classes. You have been told to improve client completion of classes or face elimination of your department. The medical center has both teleconferencing capability presently used for consults and an established Web page that provides basic information about the institution. How might you use these resources to develop alternative strategies for client education? Address budget considerations, necessary resources, target populations that might be better served, and how you propose to link distant clients with instructional offerings.

Submit a proposal to administration to provide education via the Web as well as in the traditional classroom setting. The proposal should address provisions for access for all clients that might include use of computers in local libraries, schools, and senior citizen centers as well as the possibility of submitting a grant to obtain PCs for clients who do not otherwise have access. Work with the Webmaster for assistance in placing the material on the Web. Consider low-tech options, such as videotapes and the use of the telephone, as well.

• • •

You recently joined the faculty at a small, private rural college. Because you express an interest in computers and are slightly more knowledgeable about computers than your faculty colleagues, you have been asked to establish a computer lab for the nursing department and incorporate computer use in all of the nursing courses. Current resources are quite limited. Provide a detailed plan of how you would accomplish this charge from start to finish. Identify potential stumbling blocks and ways that you would address them.

This type of effort needs to be in concert with the overall strategic plan for computing within the institution, school, and department. Find out what is happening. Determine your goals. Do a project plan and establish a target time line. Conduct a needs assessment. Investigate funding, including the possibility of writing a grant. Use institutional standards when looking at equipment. Be advised that the remainder of the institution may see this as taking resources away from them, so salesmanship is important.

CHAPTER 17

You are the nurse practitioner in St. Theresa's emergency department. A client is brought in with obvious psychiatric problems. You have no psychiatrist available and the nearest psychiatric facility is a 1-hour drive away. St. Theresa is a Tri-State Health Care Alliance Member. Tri-State has telehealth links with the regional hospital, where a psychiatrist is in the emergency department. What steps would you take to initiate a productive teleconference? Justify your response.

Be prepared to introduce the situation to the psychiatrist as well as to the patient. The patient may or may not be receptive, although the same can be true without a telemedicine link. Ensure that technical support as well as emotional support is available.

• • •

Erin O'Shell, home health nurse, just set up teleconference equipment for Dr. Bobby to evaluate Mr. Richard Goldstein for possible hospitalization for congestive heart failure. Dr. Bobby and the hospital are a 1-hour drive away. Just as the teleconference started, but before Dr. Bobby could listen to Mr. Goldstein's lungs or complete other key portions of the exam, a power outage severed the teleconference link. How should Ms. O'Shell handle this situation? Provide your rationale.

The backup situation is that the nurse uses the telephone and communicates her findings to the physician. The patient is probably experiencing distress already, which will probably increase without some action. The physician and nurse must work together to determine if this patient needs to go to the hospital or may receive further treatment in the home.

CHAPTER 18

You are the staff nurse in a busy medical–surgical department at your community hospital. You and several of your colleagues have an idea that client anxiety is decreased in direct proportion to the amount of teaching that they receive preoperatively. Describe how you might use computer applications to look at this issue and prepare a proposal for funding consideration.

This issue could be addressed in a patient satisfaction survey done during or after the hospitalization. This survey might be completed via telephone or possibly on-line. An argument for funding this project might be twofold. First, it provides a way to improve patient satisfaction and return visits and is therefore good for business. Second, patient stay may be decreased with cost savings to the institution. The organization may fund the survey or funding may be obtained from a number of different sites that might include professional organizations or various foundations, particularly for a specific population.

• • •

You and your classmates are expected to conduct a health teaching project in a public high school as one of the requirements for your Community Health Nursing course. Identify and discuss resources that you might use to gather material for this project.

There are a huge number of resources that can be tapped for this project. These may include the government, sites such as the National Library of Medicine, as well as information available through other agencies and professional groups, such as the American Academy of Pediatrics. Information from all sites should be evaluated for accuracy, authenticity, and currency before it is shared with others.

. . .

You are working the night shift at your local community hospital. One of your clients was newly diagnosed today with a rare disorder that is unknown to you and your peers. Mrs. Prado is unable to sleep and is asking for more information about her diagnosis. None of the reference books on your unit provide information about her diagnosis. Your unit does, however, have an Internet connection. How might you use resources on hand to meet Mrs. Prado's needs?

Either access your library through your intranet connection to conduct a search and full text retrieval or access one of the on-line databases such as Medline through the National Library of Medicine site to do a search and retrieve literature. Consider a Web search as well, although the quality of information obtained will vary greatly and should be reviewed prior to your giving it to Mrs. Prado.

GLOSSARY

Access code A unique identifier generally provided by a name and password for the specific purpose of restricting computer or information system use to persons who have legitimate authority to view or use information found in the computer or information system.

Administrative information systems Systems that support patient care by managing financial and demographic information and providing reporting capabilities.

Aggregate data Data that is derived from large population groups.

Ambulatory Payment Classification (APC) Describes new reimbursement criteria for ambulatory procedures.

Antivirus software A set of computer programs capable of finding and eliminating viruses and other malicious programs from scanned diskettes, computers, and networks.

Application security Measures designed to protect a specific set of computer programs and the information that they create or store from harm. A common example of application security in health care information systems is timed or automatic sign-off, which prevents unauthorized access by others when users forget to sign off the system.

Architecture The structure of the central processing unit and its interrelated elements within an information system.

Arden Syntax A standard language used in the health care industry for writing rules.

Arithmetic logic unit (ALU) The component of the central processing unit that executes arithmetic instructions.

Asynchronous Transfer Mode (ATM) A high-speed data transmission method suitable for voice, data, image, text, and video information. It can use fiber or twisted pair. It is faster than ISDN, but less frequently used for reasons of cost, availability, and a lack of standards.

Audit trail An electronic tool used by information system administrators that is capable of showing system access by individual user, user class, or all persons who viewed a specific client record.

Authentication An action that verifies the authority of users to receive specified data.

Authoring tools Software programs that allow persons with little or no programming expertise to create instructional computer programs.

Automatic sign-off A mechanism that logs a user off the system after a specific period of inactivity on the terminal or computer.

Backup procedure May refer to the creation of a second copy of files and information found on a computer, or information system, for the intent of restoring information when the primary copy is lost or damaged; or an alternative means to accomplish tasks normally done with an information system when that system is not available to authorized users for some reason.

Batch processing The manipulation of large amounts of data into meaningful applications at times when computer demands are lowest as a means to maintain system performance during peak utilization hours. Batch processed information is not available prior to processing and is little used today except to run reports.

Benchmarking The continual process of measuring services and practices against the toughest competitors in the industry.

Bennett Bill Although not passed into law, the Medical Records Confidentiality Act of 1995 was a significant piece of legislation because it attempted to establish the role of health care providers in the protection of client information; fix conditions for the inspection, copying, and disclosure of protected information; and institute legal protection for health-related information.

Biometrics A unique, measurable characteristic or trait of a human being for automatically recognizing or verifying identity.

Browser A retrieval program that allows the user to search and access hypertext and hypermedia documents on the Web by using HTTP.

Bulletin Board Systems (BBS) An on-line service that offers a computerized dial-in meeting and announcement system, allowing users to make announcements, share files, and conduct limited discussions.

Central processing unit (CPU) The electronic circuitry that actually executes computer instructions. The CPU reads stored programs one instruction at a time, keeps track of the execution, and directs other computer parts and input and output devices to perform required tasks.

Client–server A distributed approach to computing where different computers work together to carry out a task. The computer that makes requests is known as the client, while the high-performance computer that contains requested files is known as the server.

Clinical data repository A database where information from many different information systems is stored and managed, allowing retrieval of elements without regard to their point of origin.

Clinical information systems (CIS) Large computerized database management systems utilized by clinicians to access patient data that is used to plan, implement, and evaluate care. Clinical information systems may also be referred to as patient care information systems.

Clinical pathway A suggested blueprint for the care of a client by diagnosis that includes specific interventions by health care professionals, desired outcomes, and even the projected length of stay of inpatient treatment.

Cold site A company that maintains electronic records and backup media in secure, climate-controlled storage so that stored information can be used to restore information system capability in the event that information and/or system functionality have been lost.

Commission on Accreditation of Rehabilitation Facilities (CARF) A health care accrediting body. Its focus is the improvement of rehabilitative services to people with disabilities and others in need of rehabilitation.

Community Health Information Network (CHIN) An organization that electronically links providers, payers, and purchasers of care for the exchange of financial, clinical, and administrative information via a wide-area network in a particular geographic area.

Computational nursing A branch of nurmetrics that uses models and simulation for the application of existing theory and numerical methods to new solutions for nursing problems.

Computer An electronic device that collects, processes, stores, retrieves, and provides information output under the direction of stored sequences of instructions known as computer programs.

Computer-assisted instruction (CAI) The use of a computer to organize and present instruction primarily for use by an individual learner.

Computer-based patient record (CPR) An automated patient record designed to enhance and support patient care through the availability of complete and accurate data as well as bodies of knowledge and other aids to care providers.

Computer-based patient record system (CPRS) The components that provide the mechanism by which patient records are created, used, stored, and retrieved. These components include people, data, rules and procedures, as well as computer and communications equipment and support facilities.

Confidentiality The tacit understanding that private information shared in a situation in which a relationship has been established for the purpose of treatment or delivery of services will remain protected.

Connectivity The process that allows individual users to communicate and share hardware, software, and information using technology such as modems and the Internet.

Data A collection of numbers, characters, or facts that are gathered according to some perceived need for analysis and possibly action at a later point in time.

Database A file structure that supports the storage of data in an organized fashion and allows data retrieval as meaningful information.

Database administrator A person who is responsible for overseeing all activities related to maintaining a database and optimizing its use.

Data dictionary A tool that defines terms used in a system to ensure consistent understanding and application among all users in the institution. This process may be also achieved through the use of an interface engine.

Data exchange standards A set of agreed-upon rules that permit the uniform capture and exchange of data between information systems from different vendors and between different health care providers.

Data integrity The ability to collect, store, and retrieve correct, complete, and current data so that it is available to authorized users when it is needed.

Data management The process of controlling the storage, retrieval, and use of data to optimize accuracy and utility while safeguarding integrity.

Data retrieval The process that allows the user to access previously collected and stored data.

Decision-support software Computer programs that organize information to aid decision making related to patient care or administrative issues.

Desktop videoconferencing (DTV) A real-time encounter that uses a specially equipped personal computer with a telephone line hookup to allow persons to meet face-to-face or view the same images simultaneously.

Digital Image Communication in Medicine (DICOM) A standard that promotes the communication, storage, and integration of digital image information with other hospital information systems.

Disaster planning An organized approach that anticipates potential system problems, maintains security of client information under adverse conditions, and provides an alternative means to support the retrieval and processing of information in the event that the information system fails.

Distance learning The use of print, audio, video, computer, or teleconference capability to connect faculty and students who are located at a minimum of two different sites.

Distributed processing The use of a group of independent processors that contain the same information but may be at different sites as a means to maintain information services in the event of a power outage or other disaster.

Document imaging Scanning paper records to convert them to files on computer disks or other media, in order to facilitate electronic storage and handling.

Downtime The period of time when an information system is not operational and available for use.

Electronic communication The ability to exchange information through the use of computer equipment and software.

Electronic data interchange (EDI) The communication of data in binary code from one computer to another.

Electronic mail (e-mail) The use of computers to transmit messages to one or more persons. Delivery is almost instant, and attachment files may accompany text messages.

Electronic mail software A computer program that assists the user to send, receive, and manage e-mail messages.

Electronic medical record An electronic version of the patient data found in the traditional paper record.

Electronic signature A means to authenticate a computer-generated document through a code or digital signature that is unique to each authorized system user.

Encryption A process that uses mathematical formulas to code messages when content needs to be kept secure and confidential.

Ergonomics The scientific study of work and space, including details that affect workers productivity and worker health.

Error message Computer-generated text message that warns the user when entries are missing or improperly constructed for proper processing. May appear on the monitor screen as data are entered or later via a paper printout.

Expert systems The use of computer artificial intelligence to arrive at a decision that experts in the field would make.

Extranet A network that sits outside the protected internal network of an organization, and uses Internet software and communication protocols for electronic commerce and use by outside suppliers or customers.

File Transfer Protocol (FTP) A set of instructions that controls both the physical transfer of data across a network and its appearance on the receiving end.

Firewall A type of gateway that is designed to protect private network resources from outside hackers, network damage, and theft or misuse of information.

Frames per second (FPS) The number of still images that are captured, transmitted, and displayed in one second of time in a video transmission. The higher the FPS, the smoother the picture. Also referred to as frame rate.

Freezing A situation in which a computer will not accept further input and does not process what has already been entered.

Frequently asked questions (FAQ) A document or file, used by many World Wide Web sites, that serves to introduce the group or topic, update new users on recent discussions, and eliminate repetition of questions.

Gateway A combination of hardware and software used to connect local area networks with larger networks. A firewall is a type of gateway that is designed to protect private network resources from outside hackers, network damage, and theft or misuse of information.

Goal An open-ended statement that describes what is to be accomplished in general terms, and is often used in the strategic planning process.

Go-live The date when an information system is first used, or the process of starting to use an information system.

Grand rounds A traditional teaching tool for health care professionals in training that involves reviewing a client's case history and present condition inclusive of examination findings prior to a mutual determination of the best treatment options.

Graphical user interface (GUI) Provides a set of menus, windows, and other standard screen devices that are intended to make using a computer as intuitive as possible.

Hardware The physical components of a computer.

Header The section at the top of an electronic mail message that tells who sent the message, when, to whom and at what location, and the address to which a reply should be directed if different from the senders' address.

Health Insurance Portability and Accountability Act (HIPAA) Also known as Kennedy–Kassebaum Bill, represents the first federal legislation to protect automatic client records.

Health Level 7 (HL7) A standard for the exchange of clinical data between information systems by means of an extensive set of rules that apply to all data sent.

Help desk A support service, rather than a specific location, for computer users. In health care institutions it is usually available 24 hours a day by calling a special telephone number. Help desk staff generally have an information system or computer backgrounds and are familiar with all of the software applications and hardware in use.

Helper program A computer application that supports a browser by providing added functionality and performs specific tasks.

Help screens Computer messages that are displayed on the monitor screen in response to a request by the user for assistance by pressing an identified key, or in response to an inappropriate entry by the user. Help screens provide specific directions that the user may follow to reach a desired outcome.

Hospital information system (HIS) A group of information systems used within a hospital or enterprise that support and enhance patient care. The HIS consists of two major types of information systems: clinical and administrative.

Hot site A facility located at a separate location than the health care provider that replicates the provider's information systems for the purpose of quickly restoring information system function in the event of a disaster or disruption to services.

HyperText Markup Language (HTML) A language or set of instructions that is frequently used to write home pages for the Internet, and includes text as well as special instructions known as tags for the display of text and other media. HTML also includes highlighted references to other documents that the user may choose if additional information about that topic is desired.

Hypertext Transfer Protocol (HTTP) A transfer protocol used on Internet pages that establishes a TCP/IP connection between the client and server that sends a request in the form of a command when a link or hypertext is clicked with the mouse.

Information A collection of data that has been interpreted and examined for patterns and structure.

Information privacy The right to choose the conditions and the extent to which information and beliefs are shared with others. Informed consent for the release of medical records represents the application of information privacy.

Information security The protection of confidential information against threats to its integrity or inadvertent disclosure.

Information system A computer system that uses hardware and software to process data into information in order to solve a problem.

Information system security The protection of information systems and the information housed on them from unauthorized use or threats to integrity.

Input devices Hardware that allows the user to put data into the computer. Basic input devices include the keyboard, mouse, track ball, touch screens, light pens, microphones, bar code readers, fax/modem cards, joysticks, and scanners.

Integrated services digital network (ISDN) A high-speed data transmission technology that allows simultaneous, digital transfer of voice, video, and data over telephone lines but at higher speeds than available via modem.

Integrated video disk (IVD) A technology that uses the interactivity, information management, and decision-making capability of computers with audiovisual capabilities of videodisk or tape to enhance CAI. IVD has largely been replaced by CD-ROM.

Interface engine A software application designed to allow users of different computer systems to access and exchange information without any special effort on their part or the need to customize equipment or write specific instructions to allow several different systems to communicate.

International standard H.320 A standard for passing audio and video data streams across networks, allowing videoconferencing systems from different manufacturers to communicate.

Internet A worldwide network that connects millions of computers and serves to link government, university, commercial institutions, and individual users.

Internet service provider (ISP) A company that furnishes Internet access for a fee.

Intranet A private computer network that uses Internet protocols and technologies, including Web browsers, servers, and languages, to facilitate collaborative data sharing.

JAVA A programming language that enables the display of moving text, animation, and musical excerpts on Web pages.

Jobs aids Written instructions that are designed to be used for reference in both training and work settings.

Joint Photographic Experts Group Compression (JPEG) A standard for the compression of digital images for transmission and storage. Although not developed for use with diagnostic images, JPEG is used for that purpose.

Keyboards Input devices with keys that represent those of a typewriter.

Knowledge The synthesis of information derived from several sources to produce a single concept or idea.

Learning aids Materials intended to supplement or reinforce lecture or computer-based training. Examples may consist of outlines, diagrams, charts, and maps.

Legacy systems Mainframe vendor-based information systems.

Life cycle A well-defined process that describes the recurring process of developing and maintaining an information system.

Links Also known as hypertext, links are words or phrases used on Internet pages that are distinguished from the remainder of the document through the use of highlighting or a different screen color. Links allow users to skip from point to point within or among documents, escaping conventional linear format.

Listserv An e-mail subscription list program that copies and distributes all e-mail messages to everyone who is a subscriber.

Live data Actual patient and health care system data as opposed to fictitious data used for training purposes.

Main Memory The component of memory that is permanent and remains when power is off. Also known as read only memory (ROM).

Mapping A process by which the definition of terms used in one information system are associated with comparable terms in another information system, thereby facilitating the exchange of information from one system to another.

Master patient index (MPI) A database that lists all identifiers used in connection with one particular client in a health care alliance. Identifiers may include items such as social security number, birth dates, and name.

Memory The computer storage device in which programs reside during execution. It comprises main memory and random access memory.

Menu A list of related commands that can be selected from a computer screen to accomplish a task.

Microprocessor chip The electronic circuits of the CPU etched onto a silicon chip.

Mission The purpose or reason for an organization's existence, representing the fundamental and unique aspirations that differentiate it from others.

Modem A communication device that transmits data over telephone lines from one computer to another.

Monitor A screen that displays text and graphic images.

Monitoring systems Devices that automatically monitor biometrics measurements in critical care and specialty areas.

Multimedia Presentations that combine text, voice or sound, and still or video images, as well as hardware and software that support the same.

Network A combination of hardware and software that allows communication and electronic transfer of information between computers.

Nurmetrics A branch of nursing science that uses mathematics and statistics to test, estimate, and quantify nursing theories and solutions to problems.

Nursing informatics The use of computer technology to support nursing.

Nursing informatics specialist A nurse with formal education and practical experience using computers, who supports the automation needs of all facets of nursing practice.

Nursing information system An information system that supports the use and documentation of nursing processes and provides tools for managing the delivery of nursing care.

Nursing Minimum Data Set (NMDS) A consistent collection of data comprising nursing diagnosis, interventions, and outcomes that attempts to collect data that is comparable across different health care settings, to project trends, and to stimulate research.

Objective A statement that describes how a goal will be accomplished and the time frame for this activity.

Off-line storage A form of data storage that utilizes secondary storage devices for data that is needed less frequently, or for long-term data storage.

On-line A term indicating a connection to various computer resources, including information systems, the Internet, and the World Wide Web.

On-line storage A form of data storage that provides access to current data. An example is a high-speed, hard disk drive.

On-line tutorials Detailed instructions available to a user while he or she is using a computer, software application, or information system that show or tell how a particular software application or feature can be implemented.

Open architecture An information system architecture that uses protocols and technology that follow publicly accepted conventions and are employed by multiple vendors, so that various system components can work together.

Open system See *open architecture.*

Output devices Hardware that allows the user to see processed data. Terminals or video monitor screens, printers, speakers, and fax/modem boards are types of output devices.

Outsourcing The process in which an organization contracts with outside agencies for services.

Password An alphanumeric code required for access and use of some computers or information systems as a security measure against unauthorized use. The password does not appear on the monitor display when it is keyed in.

Personal digital assistants (PDAs) Specialized handheld devices used primarily to keep appointments, calendars, addresses, and phone numbers.

Picture archiving communications systems (PACS) Storage systems that permit remote access to diagnostic images at times convenient to the physician.

Plug-in programs Computer applications that have been designed to support browsers by performing specific tasks. Plug-in programs require the browser to be running.

Point-of-care devices Computer or terminal located at the actual work site, which is at the patient's bedside with the delivery of health care.

Portal Term that refers to some Web sites. Portal sites require registration and collect information from the user that can be used to personalize features for individual users.

Privacy Freedom from intrusion or control over the exposure of self or personal information.

Production environment The point at which a planned information system is actually used to process and retrieve information and support the delivery of services.

Public key infrastructure (PKI) Provides a unique code for each user that is embedded into a storage device.

Radiology information system (RIS) Provides scheduling of diagnostic tests, communication of patient information, generation of patient instructions and preparation procedures, and file room management.

Random access memory (RAM) The component of memory that can be accessed, used, changed, and rewritten repeatedly while the computer is turned on.

Read-only memory (ROM) The component of memory that contains startup instructions for each time the computer is turned on. ROM is permanent and remains when power is off.

Real-time processing Entry and access to information occurs almost as soon as it is provided.

Remote access The ability to use the resources contained on a network, or an information system, from a location outside of the facility where it is physically located.

Remote backup service (RBS) A company that provides backup services for customers from an off-site location to an off-site location.

Request for Information (RFI) An RFI is a letter or brief document sent to vendors that explains the institution's plans for purchasing and installing an information system. The purpose of the RFI is to obtain essential information about the vendor and the system capabilities in order to eliminate those vendors that cannot meet the organization's basic requirements.

Request for Proposal (RFP) A document sent to vendors that describes the requirements of a potential information system. The purpose of this document is to solicit proposals from many vendors that describe their capabilities to meet these requirements.

Resolution A term used to refer to the sharpness, or clarity, of an image on a computer monitor. Resolution itself is determined by the number of pixels, or tiny dots or squares, displayed per inch on a monitor screen.

Response time The amount of time between a user action and the response from the information system.

Sabotage The intentional destruction of computer equipment or records to disrupt services.

Scope The statement in an organization's mission that defines the type of activities and services that it will perform.

Search engines A tool to help users find information on the World Wide Web. Each search engine maintains its own index or list of information on the Web and uses its own method of organizing topics.

Search engine unifier Programs that search servers and databases, such as the World Wide Web, and can shorten search time by looking at several search engines at one time, often yielding more comprehensive data in less time.

Secondary storage A format of computer memory that retains data even when the computer is turned off. Any one of the following devices can provide secondary storage: hard drives, CD-ROM disks, redundant array of inexpensive disks (RAID), optical disks, magnetic disks, magnetic tape, and floppy disks.

Serial Line Internet Protocol (SLIP) A protocol that allows passage of data through communication lines and is used to access the Internet and World Wide Web.

Site license An agreement between the computer lab and the software publisher on the terms of use.

Smart card A storage device for patient information that resembles a plastic credit card. The card is kept by the client and presented to health care providers when services are rendered, eliminating redundant data entry and the need to store this information on a network.

Software Computer programs, or stored sequences of instructions to the computer.

Software shredder A set of computer programs that prevents recovery of deleted, or discarded, computer files by writing meaningless information over them.

Strategic planning The development of a comprehensive long-range plan for guiding the activities and operations of an organization.

Strategy A comprehensive plan used by an organization that states how its mission, goals, and objectives will be achieved.

Structured data Data that follows a prescribed format, often presented as discrete data elements.

Superuser A staff person who has become proficient in the use of the system and mentors others.

Switched multimegabit data service (SMDS) A high-speed data transmission service that uses telephone lines, also known as a T1 line. SMDS is faster than ISDN but slower than ATM.

System check A mechanism provided by a computer system to assist users by prompting them to complete a task, verify information, or prevent entry of inappropriate information.

Technical criteria The hardware and software requirements needed to attain a desired level of overall computer or information system performance.

Teleconferencing The use of computers, audio and video equipment, and communication links to provide interaction between two or more persons at two or more sites.

Telehealth The provision of information to health care providers and consumers as well as the delivery of services to clients at a site separate from the health care professional through the use of telecommunication and computer technology.

Telemedicine The use of telecommunication technologies and computers to provide medical information and services to clients at another site.

Telenursing The use of telecommunications and computer technology for the delivery of nursing care to clients at another location.

Test environment A separate software program like that used for the actual application or information system, which permits trial of programming changes prior to their implementation in the actual system, thereby protecting the "real" system from unwanted alterations.

Thin client technology A computing model that allows PCs to connect to a server using a highly efficient network connection.

Training environment A separate software application that mirrors the actual information system but permits learners to practice skills without fear of harming the system or data contained in it. In the case of health care information systems, the training environment consists of fictitious clients and scenarios that can be used for instruction and practice.

Training hospital A collection of simulated, or fictitious, client data assembled and stored in a database separate from the actual information system for the purposes of instruction and practice. Most, if not all, features available on the actual information system are available for use with the fabricated database.

Training plan An organized approach for the delivery of instruction that should include a philosophy; identification of instructional needs, approaches, and persons responsible for instructional design and delivery; a target date for completion; a budget; and methods for evaluation.

Unified Medical Language System An attempt to standardize terms used in health care delivery.

Unified Nursing Language System An attempt to standardize and link nursing databases as a means to extend nursing knowledge.

Uniform Hospital Data Set (UHDS) The most commonly used data set in the United States, even though it does not include data on nursing care and outcomes.

Uniform resource locator (URL) A string of characters that provides an address that identifies a document's World Wide Web location and the type of server it resides on.

Unique patient identifier A single, universal identifier for client health information that ensures availability of all data associated with a particular client. A critical element in the development of CHINs, given that no universal identifier has yet been agreed upon.

Unstructured data Data that does not follow a prescribed format such as may be seen in narrative charting.

Usenet news groups A popular Internet feature similar to listservs in content and diversity, with each newsgroup dedicated to a different topic. These groups provide a forum where any user can post messages for discussion and reply.

User class A group of individuals who perform similar functions, and for the purpose of information system training and use, require instruction in how to access and use the same set of system features.

Vendor Company or corporation that designs, develops, sells, and/or supports a product, which in the context of this book is generally a computer, peripheral device, and, more often, an entire information system.

Videoconferencing The face-to-face meeting of persons at separate locations through the use of telecommunications and computer technology.

Virus A malicious program that can disrupt or destroy data.

Web-based instruction (WBI) Uses the attributes and resources of the World Wide Web, such as hypertext links and multimedia, for educational purposes.

Webmaster The person responsible for creating and maintaining a World Wide Web site.

World Wide Web (WWW) An information service for access to Internet resources by content instead of file names. The World Wide Web uses a graphical user interface (GUI) and supports text, images, and sound, as well as links to other documents.

Index

AANurses, 66
Access:
  code, 149
  levels, 173–74
  remote, 169
Accreditation:
  Commission on Accreditation of Rehabilita-
    tion Facilities (CARF), 217, 219
  Joint Commission on Accreditation of
    Healthcare Organizations (JCAHO),
    164, 193, 217–19
  role of, 216–17
Active portals, 57
ActiveX, 59
Administrative information systems, 83,
  94–95
Administrative issues, security and, 172–77
Admission/discharge/transfer (ADT) systems,
  95
Agency for Health Care Policy and Research
  (AHCPR), 281
Aggregate data, 5
Alphanumeric characters, 22
AltaVista, 60
Ambulatory Payment Classifications (APCs),
  217, 220–21
American Cancer Society, 63
American Civil Liberties Union (ACLU),
  212–13, 214
American Heart Association, 63

American Journal of Nursing Career Guide,
  The, 66
American Nurses Association (ANA), 3, 10,
  11, 191, 289, 296, 314, 315
American Nurses Credentialing Center, 11
American Society for Testing and Materials,
  192
America On-Line (AOL), 50
AmericasDoctor.com, 63
Analyst, 29
Antivirus software, 172
Application security, 171
Application service providers (ASPs), 69
Applications software, 25, 27, 28
AQUAD, 311
Architecture, 120
Arden syntax, 90
Arithmetic logic unit (ALU), 15
Artificial intelligence, 27
Asynchronous Transfer Mode (ATM), 292–93
Audit trails, 176, 177
Authentication, user, 174
Authoring tools, 268
Automatic sign-off, 168–69

Backloaded, 138
Backup:
  planning, 243–44
  procedures, 150–51
  system, 19

Batch processing, 187–88
Benchmarking, 110–11
Bennett, Bill, 212–13
Binary code, 22
BIOS (basic input/output system), 23
Bit, 20, 22
Bits per second (bps), 20
BMDP, 310
Bookmarks, 326
Browsers, 59, 324
Bulletin Board Systems (BBSs), 62
Byte, 22

Capacity, disk, 19
Career resources, Web sites, 335–36
Carpal tunnel syndrome, 24
CD-ROM drive, 19, 40
Center for Democracy and Technology, 214
Central processing unit (CPU), 15
Charting:
  by exception, 87
  flowsheet, 87
  narrative, 87
Chief Information Officer (CIO), 30–31
Client, 21
Client/consumer education, 265–66
Client/server, 21
Clinical data repository, 188, 192, 202, 228
Clinical information systems (CISs):
  clinician information system, 88
  defined, 83
  goal of, 84
  laboratory information systems, 89–90
  monitoring systems, 88–89
  nursing information systems, 85–88
  order entry systems, 89
  other systems, 93–94
  pharmacy systems, 92–93
  radiology information systems, 90–91
Clinical liaisons, 29–30
Clinician information system, 88
Cold sites, 243–44
Commission on Accreditation of Rehabilitation Facilities (CARF), 217, 219
Committee to Study National Cryptography Policy, 291
Community Health Information Networks (CHINs):
  benefits of, 231–32
  components of, 227–28
  confidentiality issues, 232
  connectivity, 229–30
  costs of, 232–33
  current status of, 233
  data elements, 230

data repository, centralized, 230–31
  defined, 227
  development of, 229–31
  limiting factors, 232–33
  ownership of, 232
  patient identifier, 230
  services provided by, 229
Compact discs, 16
CompuServe, 50
Computer-aided research in nursing (CARIN), 312–13
Computer-assisted instruction (CAI), 6, 260, 266–67
Computer-assisted self-interview software (CASI), 307–8
Computer-based patient record (CPR), 228
  benefits of, 203–4
  characteristics of, 199–203
  concerns associated with, 206–8
  current status of, 204–6
  data integrity, 207
  defined, 198–99
  future issues, 208–9
  impediments to, 205–6, 313–14
  ownership of, 207
  privacy and confidentiality issues, 207
  smart cards, 208
Computer-Based Patient Record Institute, 192
Computer-based patient record system (CPRS), 199
Computer-based training (CBT), 155
Computer Emergency Response Team (CERT), 70
Computer printouts, monitoring, 178
Computer Retrieval of Information on Scientific Projects (CRISP), 313
Computers: (*See also* Education, computer applications; Research, computer applications)
  defined, 14
  how they work, 22–23
  networks, 20–22
  related injuries, 24–25
  selecting, 23–25
  types of, 16–17
  viruses, 53, 72, 167–68
Confidential information, handling and disposal of information, 177–80
Confidentiality:
  Community Health Information Networks and, 232
  computer-based patient records and, 207
  defined, 164
  legislation regarding, 212–16
  telehealth and, 290–91

Connectivity, 49
Consultants, use of, 118
Consumers, information for, 63
Continuing education, 265, 287
Control unit, 15
Critical pathway/protocols approach, 88, 285
Cumulative Index of Nursing and Allied Health
  Literature (CINAHL), 85, 305, 307

Data:
  analysis, 106, 309–11
  defined, 34
  dictionary, 190
  examples of, 35
  exchange, 42–43
  exchange standards, 191–92, 202–3
  graphic presentation, 311–12
  integrity, 35–37, 207
  live, 152
  mining, 310
  retrieval, 41–42
  storage, 38–41
  structured, 199
  unstructured, 198–99
  warehouse, 38
Database, 38
  on-line access to, 313
Database administrator (DBA), 38
Data collection and entry:
  ensuring correct, 36–37
  tools, 306–9
  verification techniques, 37
DataDesk, 310
Data management:
  defined, 38
  exchange of data, 42–43
  outsourcing, 39–41
  retrieval of data, 41–42
  storage of data, 38–39
Decision-support software, 8
Decision support systems, 95–96
Delphi, 50
Desktop videoconferencing (DTV), 282, 294
Digital credentialing, 53
Digital Image Communication in Medicine
  (DICOM) standard, 295
Digital subscriber lines (DSL), 293
Disaster planning:
  advantages of, 237–40
  backup and storage, 243–44
  defined, 236–37
  environmental disaster versus system fail-
    ure, 238–40
  essential information, identifying, 240–41
  feedback to improve, 252

manual versus automated alternatives,
    244–46
  steps, 240–46
Disaster recovery:
  costs, 249–50
  focus of, 247–48
  insurance coverage, recommended, 250
  restarting the system, 250–52
  salvaging damaged records, 248
  techniques, 249
Discs/diskettes, 16
Disk drives, 19
Distance learning, 269, 270
Distributed processing, 247–48
Document imaging, 38
Dogpile, 60
Downtime, 121
DrPaula.com, 63
DVD-ROM disks, 41

E-business, 68
E-care, 68
E-commerce, 68
Education:
  continuing, 265, 287
  telehealth applications, 286–87
Education, computer applications:
  for client education, 265–66
  computer-assisted instruction (CAI), 6,
    260, 266–67
  for continuing education, 265
  distance learning, 269, 270
  e-learning, 260–61, 265
  for formal nursing education, 262–64
  labs, 271–74
  learner resistance, 261
  multimedia, 267–68
  teleconferencing, 268–69
  Web-based instruction (WBI), 259–60,
    269–71, 272
E-health, 67–69, 281
E-learning, 260–61, 265
Electronic communication: (*See also* E-mail;
    Internet; On-line information)
  access to health care information and ser-
    vices, 62–65
  browsers, 59
  Bulletin Board Systems (BBSs), 62
  defined, 49–50
  listservs, 60–61
  marketing services, 66–67
  news groups, 61–62
  search tools, 60
  World Wide Web (Web or WWW), 50,
    54–59

Electronic data interchange (EDI), 42–43, 65

Electronic medical record (EMR), 7–8, 198–99

Electronic Privacy Information Center, 214

Electronic signature, 208

E-mail:
 advantages and disadvantages of, 52
 description of, 50–53, 323–24
 informal rules for using, 54
 monitoring, 180
 package, 52
 privacy, 71
 as a training method, 155

Encryption, 53, 71

Enterprise portals, 57

Environment:
 production, 138
 test, 135
 training, 137–38

Environmental scanning, 105–6

Ergonomics, 24, 26

Error messages, 150

Ethics, 174–76

Expert systems, 95–96

External environment, 105

Extranets, 22, 74

Fair Health Information Practices Act (1995), 212, 213

Faxes, monitoring, 178–79

Fax modem, 20

Federal Communications Commission (FCC), Advisory Committee on Telecommunications and Health Care, 296–97

Federation of State Medical Boards, 290

File, 19

File transfer, 51, 53

File Transfer Protocol (FTP), 53, 328

Firewalls, 69–70, 171

Floppy disk drive, 19

Floppy diskettes, 16

Frame rate, 295

Frames per second (FPS), 295

Freezing, 150

Frequently asked questions (FAQ), 61

Gateway, 70

Geriatric and long-term facilities, 222–23

Gigabytes, 19

Goals and objectives, 101–2, 105

Go-live planning, 138–39

Grand rounds, 286

Graphical presentation, 311–12

Graphical user interface (GUI), 27

Handheld computers, 16, 17

Hard disk drives, 16, 19, 41

Hardware:
 central processing unit, 15
 defined, 14
 input devices, 14
 output devices, 16
 peripheral items, 18–20
 requirements for information systems, 136
 secondary storage, 15–16
 training, 152

Harvard Graphics, 312

Header, 51

Health care, listservs, 345–47

Health care delivery, current status of, 6

Health Care Financing Administration (HCFA), 292

Healthcare information system (HIS), 28–29

Health care news, Web sites for current, 342–43

Health Care Personal Information Nondisclosure Act (1998), 214–15

Health care resources, Web sites for general, 341–42

Health Insurance Portability and Accountability Act (HIPAA) (1996), 164, 212, 287:
 compliance, 216
 objectives, 215
 standards, 215–16

Health Internet Ethics (Hi-Ethics) Alliance, 64

Health Level 7 (HL7), 43, 191–92, 229–30

Health on the Net Foundation (HON), 64

Help desk, 140

Help desk technician, 29

Helper programs, 59

Help screens, 150

Homegrown software, 96

Home health care, 287

Home page, 55, 58

Hospital information system (HIS), 83, 263–64

Hot sites, 247

H.320, 295

HyperText Markup Language (HTML), 55–56

HyperText Transfer Protocol (HTTP), 57, 59

Implementation (*See* Information systems, implementation of)

Individual Privacy Act (1991), 212, 213

Information: (*See also* On-line information)
 characteristics of quality, 43–45
 defined, 34
 examples of, 35
 minimizing fraudulent, 37

privacy, 164–65
security, 165
threats to, 44
Information handling, role of nurses, 8–9
Information systems (IS):
administrative, 83, 94–95
clinical, 83–94
decision support and expert, 95–96
defined, 83
hospital, 83
strategic planning for, 103–4
Information systems, implementation of:
committee for, 133, 134
development of procedures and documentation, 136–37
go-live planning, 138–39
hardware requirements, 136
installing, 133–35
pitfalls, common, 139–40
testing, 137
timeline for, 135
training, providing, 137–38
Information systems, life cycle of:
definition of life cycle, 115
needs assessment, 115–24
system implementation, 133–40
system maintenance, 140–42
system selection, 124–30
Information systems, maintenance of:
system maintenance, 141
technical maintenance, 141–42
user feedback and support, 140–41
Information systems, selecting, 124
contract negotiations, 130
request for information, 125–26
request for proposal, 126–30
sources of information, 125
Input devices, 14
Institutes of Medicine, 192, 199
Integrated delivery systems (IDS), 191
Integrated services digital network (ISDN),
230, 293
Integration:
benefits of, 187, 192–93
defined, 186
factors that slow, 189
implications of, for nursing, 193–94
standards, need for, 190–92
Web-based solutions, 194
Interface, defined, 186
Interface engines, 229
benefits of, 188
defined, 187
role of, 188–89
Internal environment, 105

International Medical Informatics Association,
Nursing Informatics Special Interest
Group of, 3
International Nursing Library (INL), 313
International Standard, H.320, 295
International TeleNurses Association (ITNA),
296
Internet:
concerns, 69–72, 180
defined, 22, 49
description of, 50–69
job searching on, 330–34
monitoring, 180
overload, 72
Internet-based training (IBT), 260
Internet Explorer, 59
Internet Relay Chat (IRC), 51
Internet service providers (ISPs), 50, 323
Intranets, 22, 72–74

Java, 59
JMP, 310
Job aids, 157
Job searching, Internet, 330–34
Joint Commission on Accreditation of Health-
care Organizations (JCAHO), 164, 193,
217–19
Joint Photographic Experts Group (JPEG)
compression standard, 295
Journal of the National Cancer Institute, 281
Joystick, 18

**Kennedy–Kassebaum Bill [*See* Health In-
surance Portability and Accountabil-
ity Act (HIPAA) (1996)]**
Keyboards, 18
Kilobits (kbps), 20
Knowledge, 34
Knowledge discovery in databases (KDD),
309–10

**Laboratory information systems (LIS),
89–90, 202**
Language, uniform, 191
Laptops, 16, 17
Learning aids, 154, 157
Legacy systems, 107
Legal issues, telehealth and, 287–91
Legislation regarding privacy and confiden-
tiality, 212–16
Liability, telehealth and, 289
Licensure issues, telehealth and, 290
Licensure preparation software, 263
Life cycle, defined, 115 (*See also* Information
systems, life cycle of)
Links, 57

Listservs, 60–61, 303, 305, 326–28
  health care, 345–47
  nursing, 343–45
Literature searches, 305–6
Live data, 152
Local area networks (LANs), 20–21
LookSmart, 60

Macintosh computers (Macs), 27
Magnetic resonance imaging (MRI), 91
Magnetic tape, 40
Magneto-optical media, 40
Mailing lists, 326–28
Mainframes, 16, 17
Maintenance (*See* Information systems, main-
  tenance of)
Mapping, 188
Marketing services, 66–67
Master patient index (MPI), 190–91
Medical Records Confidentiality Act (1995),
  212–13
Medical Records Privacy Act (1997), 214
Medical World Search, 60
Medication administration, documentation of,
  87–88
Medication administration record (MAR), 87
Medication dispensing, automatic, 92–93
Medication errors, 93
MEDIX International Standards Organization,
  192
MedLine, 85, 305
Megahertz, 23
Memory, 15
Menu, 85
MetaCrawler, 60
Microcomputers, 16, 17
Microcomputer specialist, 29
Microprocessor chip, 22–23
Microsoft Corp.:
  ActiveX, 59
  Internet Explorer, 59
  Network, 50
Minicomputers, 16, 17
MINITAB, 310
Mission statement, 100–1
Modems, 20, 49, 322
Monitoring systems, 88–89
Monitors, 18
Mosaic, 59
Motherboard, 23
Mouse, 18
Multimedia, 267–68

NASA, 282
National Center for Supercomputing Applications (NCSA), 59

National Coalition of Patient Rights, 214
National Council Licensure Examination
  (NCLEX), 262
  for Registered Nurses (NCLEX-RN), 263,
  264
National Council of Nurses, 290
National Information Infrastructure Testbed
  (NIIT), 292
National Institutes of Health (NIH), 313
National Library of Medicine, 283, 286, 313
National Nursing Informatics Project of
  Canada, 3–4
Needs assessment, 115–16
  consultants, 118
  determining requirements, 119–24
  developing a common vision, 118–19
  steering committee, 117–18
  understanding current system, 119
Net (*See* Internet)
Netiquette, 328–29
Netscape Navigator, 59
Network administrator, 30
Network interface card, 23
Networks, 20–22, 136 [*See also* Community
  Health Information Networks (CHINs)]
Newsgroups, 61–62, 327–28
  lists of, 347–48
News reader software, 61
North American Nursing Diagnosis Associa-
  tion (NANDA), 314–15, 316
Notebooks, 16, 17
Nurmetrics, 311
NURSERES, 303
Nurses and Nursing, 56
Nursing, listservs, 343–45
NursingCenter.com, 313
Nursing informatics:
  applications of, 4–6
  benefits of, 6–8
  defined, 3–4
  educational opportunities, 274
  model, 4
Nursing informatics specialist:
  certification/education for, 11
  role of, 10
Nursing information systems, 85–88
Nursing Interventions Classification (NIC),
  314, 316
Nursing Minimum Data Set (NMDS), 315
Nursing Net, 56

Objectives, goals and, 101–2
Office of Rural Health Policy, 292
Off-line storage, 38–39
Off-the-shelf software, 96

OMAHA, 316
On-line, 49
On-line information:
  access to, 62–65, 313
  citation of, 71
  evaluation of, 63–65
  literature searches, 305–6
  publications and journals, 65–66
On-line storage, 38
On-line tutorials, 150, 155
On-the-job training, 156
Open system, 120
  technology, 187
Operating systems, 26–27
Optical disk drives, 19
Optical media, 40
Order entry systems, 89
Organizational policy, for Internet use,
  71–72
Organizations and associations, Web sites for,
  337–41
Output devices, 16
Outsourcing, 39, 41
Outsourcing companies, 41

Passwords, 169–71
Patient identifier, unique, 230
PC specialist, 29
Peer training, 156
Peripheral device interface cards, 23
Peripheral hardware, 18–20
Personal Computer Memory Card Interna-
  tional Association (PCMCIA), 23
Personal computers (PCs), 16, 17
Personal digital assistants (PDAs), 16, 17
Personnel issues, security and, 172–77
Pharmacy systems, 92–93
Picture archiving communications systems
  (PACS), 91, 295
Pixels, 18
Plug-in programs, 59
Point-of-care devices, 136
Point-to-Point (PPP) protocol, 50
Portals, 56–57, 328
PowerPoint, 312
Prescriptions, electronic, 68
Printers, 20, 136
Privacy:
  computer-based patient records and, 207
  defined, 164
  information, 164–65
  legislation regarding, 212–16
  telehealth and, 287–91
Privacy Act (1974), 213–14
Prodigy, 50

Production environment, 138
Programmers, 30
Programming languages, 25–26
Programs, 25
Psychiatric facilities, 223
Public key infrastructure (PKI), 53, 174
Public Law 104–91 [*See also* Health Insur-
  ance Portability and Accountability Act
  (HIPAA) (1996)]

Qualitative analysis, 311
Quantitative analysis, 310–11

Radiology information systems (RIS),
  90–91, 202
Random access memory (RAM), 15
Read-only memory (ROM), 15
Real-time processing, 187
Recovery (*See* Disaster recovery)
Redundant array of inexpensive/independent
  disks (RAIDs), 19, 41
Refresh rate, 18
Registration systems, 95
Reimbursement issues, 219
  Ambulatory Payment Classifications
    (APCs), 217, 220–21
  telehealth and, 287–88
Relational database, 38
Remote access, 169
Remote backup services (RBSs), 244
Repetitive motion injuries, 24
Repetitive stress injuries (RSIs), 24
Request for information (RFI), 125–26
Request for proposal (RFP), 126–30
Research:
  collaborative, 317
  funding sources for, 314
  impediments to, 313–17
  multi-institutional, 315–16
  need for unified language, 314–15
  real time, 316–17
Research, computer applications:
  computer-aided research in nursing
    (CARIN), 312–13
  data analysis, 309–11
  data collection tools, 306–9
  graphical presentation, 311–12
  literature searches, 305–6
  on-line access to databases, 313
  topics, identifying, 303, 305
Resolution, 18, 294–95
Response time, 121
Resumes, electronic, 331–34
Retrieval, data, 41–42
Rule, 90

Sabotage, 166–67
SAS (System for Statistical Analysis), 310
Savvysearch, 60
Scanners, 20
Scanning, environmental, 105–6
Scheduling systems, 95
Scope, mission statement, 100–1
Search engines, 60, 325–26
Search engine unifiers, 60
Search indexes, 60
Search tools, 60
Secondary storage, 15–16
Security:
    access levels, 173–74
    administrative and personnel issues, 172–77
    antivirus software, 172
    application, 171
    automatic sign-off, 168–69
    defined, 165
    disasters/errors, 167
    firewalls, 69–70, 171
    information, 165
    Internet, 69–72, 180
    mechanisms, 168–72
    monitoring, 176–77
    passwords, 169–71
    physical, 169
    sabotage, 166–67
    system penetration, 165–66
    unauthorized users, 166
    user authentication, 174
    viruses/malicious programs, 53, 72,
        167–68, 169
Security officer, 30
Selecting information systems (*See* Information systems, selecting)
Serial Line Internet Protocol (SLIP), 50
Server, 21
Site licenses, 274
Site visits, 129–30
Smart cards, 208
Snowe–Rockefeller Amendment, 283
Software:
    antivirus, 172
    applications, 27, 28
    defined, 14, 25
    homegrown, 96
    instructional, evaluation criteria for, 263
    licensure preparation, 263
    off-the-shelf, 96
    operating systems, 26–27
    shredder, 180
    training, 152
    types of, 25–26
    utility programs, 27–28

S-Plus, 310
Springhouse Publishing, 66
SPSS, 310
Standards, need for integration, 190–92
Steering committee, 117–18
Storage, data, 38–41, 180, 243–44
Strategic planning:
    data analysis, 106
    defined, 100
    developing strategies, 102–3
    environmental scanning, 105–6
    goals and objectives, 101–2, 105
    implementation, 109
    for information systems, 103–4
    mission, 100–1
    ongoing evaluation and feedback, 110–11
    selecting a course of action, 107
    solutions identified, 107
    steps for, 104–11
Strategy, defined, 102
Structured data, 199
Supercomputers, 16, 17
Superuser, 29, 156, 158
Support personnel, roles of, 28–31
Switched multimegabit data service (SMDS),
    293
SYSTAT, 310
System check, 36–37

Tape drives, 19
TCP/IP (Transmission Control Protocol/Internet Protocol), 57
Telecommunications Act (1995), 283
Teleconferencing, 268–69, 281–82
Telehealth:
    applications, 284–87
    barriers to, 290
    benefits of, 283–84
    costs, 294
    defined, 280
    establishing, 291–95
    future for, 296–97
    historical background, 282–83
    legal and privacy issues, 287–91
    terms related to, 280–82
Telemedicine, 280
Telenursing, 281, 295–97
Telephone Nursing Telezine, 296
Terminals, 18
Test environment, 135
Testing, proficiency, 157–58
Textbase Alpha, 311
Thin Client Technology, 21–22
Thornbury Nursing Portal, 56
T1, 293

Touchpads, 18–19
Trackballs, 19
Trainers, 30
  selecting, 157–58
Training:
  center/site, 152–53
  class content, 149–51
  costs, 152
  environment, 137–38
  hardware and software requirements, 152
  hospital, 154
  methods, 153–57
  needs, identifying, 147–49
  plan, 146–47
  proficiency testing, 157–58
  reevaluating, 159
  schedules, 151

Unified Medical Language System, 314
Unified Nursing Language System, 314–15
Uniform Hospital Data Set (UHDS), 315
Uniform language, 191, 314–15
Uniform resource locator (URL), 57, 324
Unique patient identifier, 230
U.S. Department of Commerce, 292
U.S. Department of Defense, 292
University of Missouri, neurosurgery Web site, 63
UNIX, 27, 52
Unstructured data, 198–99
Usenet news groups, 61–62, 327–28
User authentication, 174
User class, 147–48, 174
User interface, 27
Utility programs, 27–28

Vanilla system, 139
Vectors, 167–68
Vendors, 125–26
Videoconferencing, 282

Videos, for training, 156
Virtual Doctor, 63
Viruses, computer, 53, 72, 167–68
  antivirus software, 172

Web (World Wide Web/WWW):
  addresses, 324–25
  advantages and disadvantages of, 55
  defined, 50
  description of, 54–59, 324–26
  integration and, 194
  security, 70–71, 180
Web-assisted instruction (WAI), 260
Web-based instruction (WBI), 259–60, 269–71, 272
Web-based learning (WBL), 260
Web-based training (WBT), 260
Web interactive training (WIT), 260
Webmaster, 31
Web sites, 325
  career resources, 335–36
  consumer, 63
  health care news, current, 342–43
  health care resources, general, 341–42
  nursing resources, general, 336–37
  organizations and associations, 337–41
Wide area networks (WANs), 21
Wireless computers, 16, 17
Wisconsin Health Information Network, 233
Workstations, 136
World Wide Web [*See* Web (World Wide Web/WWW)]

Your Family Doctor, 63